# ANNALS OF
# THE NEW YORK ACADEMY
# OF SCIENCES

*Volume 432*

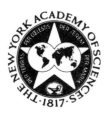

EDITORIAL STAFF
*Executive Editor*
**BILL BOLAND**
*Managing Editor*
**JOYCE HITCHCOCK**
*Associate Editor*
**JUSTINE CULLINAN**

*The New York Academy of Sciences*
*2 East 63rd Street*
*New York, New York 10021*

# CLINICAL PHARMACOLOGY OF CARDIAC ANTIARRHYTHMIC AGENTS: CLASSICAL AND CURRENT CONCEPTS REEVALUATED

ANNALS OF THE NEW YORK ACADEMY OF SCIENCES
Volume 432

# CLINICAL PHARMACOLOGY OF CARDIAC ANTIARRHYTHMIC AGENTS: CLASSICAL AND CURRENT CONCEPTS REEVALUATED

*Edited by Oscar B. Garfein*

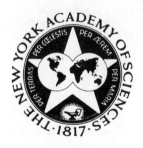

*The New York Academy of Sciences*
*New York, New York*
*1984*

**Library of Congress Cataloging in Publication Data**

Main entry under title:

Clinical pharmacology of cardiac antiarrhythmic agents.

(Annals of the New York Academy of Sciences; v. 432)
Result of a conference held Oct. 3–5, 1983 by the
New York Academy of Sciences.
Includes bibliographies and index.
1. Arrhythmia—Chemotherapy—Congresses.   2. Myocardial
depressants—Congresses.   I. Garfein, Oscar B.   II. New
York Academy of Sciences.   III. Series. [DNLM: 1. Anti-
Arrhythmia Agents—pharmacodynamics—congresses.
2. Arrhythmia—drug therapy—congresses.
W1 AN626YL v. 432   /   QV 150 C6417 1983]
Q11.N5 vol. 432        500s        84-27165
[RC685.A65]          [616.1′28061]
ISBN 0-89766-258-X
ISBN 0-89766-259-3 (pbk.)

BiC/PC
*Printed in the United States of America*
**ISBN 0-89766-258-X (cloth)**
**ISBN 0-89766-259-8 (paper)**

ANNALS OF THE NEW YORK ACADEMY OF SCIENCES

Volume 432

December 21, 1984

# CLINICAL PHARMACOLOGY OF CARDIAC ANTIARRHYTHMIC AGENTS: CLASSICAL AND CURRENT CONCEPTS REEVALUATED*

*Editor*

OSCAR B. GARFEIN

## CONTENTS

* This volume is the result of a conference entitled Clinical Pharmacology of Cardiac Antiarrhythmic Agents: Classical and Current Concepts Reevaluated, held on October 3–5, 1983 by the New York Academy of Sciences.

**Financial assistance was received from:**

ABBOTT LABORATORIES,
  DIAGNOSTICS DIVISION
  PHARMACEUTICAL PRODUCTS DIVISION
ASTRA PHARMACEUTICAL PRODUCTS, INC.
AYERST LABORATORIES
BAYER AG/MILES
BOEHRINGER INGELHEIM, LTD.
BRISTOL-MYERS COMPANY
BURROUGHS WELLCOME CO.
CIBA-GEIGY CORPORATION, PHARMACEUTICALS
  DIVISION
E.I. DuPONT de NEMOURS & COMPANY, BIOCHEMICALS DEPT.
HOFFMANN-La ROCHE INC.
KNOLL PHARMACEUTICAL COMPANY
LILLY RESEARCH LABORATORIES
McNEIL PHARMACEUTICAL
MERCK SHARP & DOHME RESEARCH LABORATORIES
OFFICE OF NAVAL RESEARCH
PARKE-DAVIS
RIKER LABORATORIES, INC.
A.H. ROBINS COMPANY
SCHERING-PLOUGH CORP.
G.D. SEARLE & CO.
STUART PHARMACEUTICALS, DIVISION OF ICI
  AMERICAS, INC.
SYNTEX LABORATORIES
SYVA COMPANY
WYETH LABORATORIES

# Preface

OSCAR B. GARFEIN

*Department of Medicine*
*College of Physicians & Surgeons of*
*Columbia University*
*New York, New York 10032*

The clinical pharmacology of cardiac antiarrhythmic drugs has developed at an extraordinary rate in the past two decades. Advances in clinical research techniques, such as computer-assisted arrhythmia recognition programs, long-term electrocardiographic recording, intracardiac electrocardiography, and clinical electrophysiological techniques, as well as an increased understanding of the complexities of experimental design, have led to a more rational use of potent and valuable cardiac antiarrhythmic drugs. Qualitatively similar progress in the understanding of the basic physiology of arrhythmias, the basis of action of drugs on a cellular level and in the intact organism, the physical chemistry of antiarrhythmic drugs (especially as it pertains to protein binding and mode of metabolism), and new and ingenious techniques of measuring the concentrations of these agents in biological fluids have all aided in converting what historically was an empirically based medical discipline to a field endowed with a strong scientific base.

Some of these developments may properly be called revolutionary since they have mandated revisions of long-held and deeply cherished notions of drug action and effectiveness. To determine an antiarrhythmic drug's efficacy, for example, it is obvious that one must know the intrinsic variability of the arrhythmia to be treated so as to be able to separate drug-induced responses from those that might be expected as a result of a random decrease. Yet Morganroth *et al.* first accurately quantitated, indeed recognized, the natural variability of chronic ventricular premature contraction (PVC) frequency in 1978.[1] Using 8 hours of control electrocardiographic monitoring and 8 hours of monitoring following drug administration, they calculated that a greater than 90% reduction in mean hourly PVC frequency was required to demonstrate an antiarrhythmic drug effect. This observation requires that most of the drug studies showing an effect against chronic PVCs be redone or reconsidered, since therapeutic response was often determined somewhat arbitrarily by a clinician, or on the basis of a 50% reduction in arrhythmia frequency.

Routledge *et al.* first demonstrated the clinical importance of determining free plasma drug levels of cardiac antiarrhythmic agents in 1980.[2] These investigators showed that lidocaine undergoes progressive binding by acute-phase proteins in the plasma of patients with acute myocardial infarction. Thus, if total plasma lidocaine levels remain unchanged, a progressive decline of free, active drug ensues in this critical setting. This study, while pertaining only to lidocaine, points out the need for similar studies with other antiarrhythmic agents under circumstances that might alter protein binding characteristics.

From the field of clinical chemistry have come dramatic advances in technology, that, when most fully applied, offer the promise of accurate, inexpensive, rapidly performable assays of drug concentrations, including measurement of free drug concentration. These techniques include high-performance liquid chromatography, enzyme-mediated immunoassays, and radioimmunoassays.

Reports from the University of Pennsylvania, Stanford University, and Harvard have firmly established the role of acute drug testing and electrophysiological studies in identifying those patients with serious arrhythmias who require antiarrhythmic prophylaxis. These reports have all been widely disseminated within the past 3 to 4 years.

These are but a few examples of major advances in this field that have affected and will continue to affect and remold thinking about clinical pharmacology both in its current form as well as in its historical entirety.

In the light of these striking and far-ranging developments, this volume evaluates this field in a critical fashion, appraising its current strengths and identifying its weaknesses. We view classical data with an eye to discerning which may have to be discarded as flawed and inaccurate, and which can still be viewed as correct and can be used as building blocks for further growth and development in the field. It is hoped that the papers presented here will let us know what we are entitled to know, and will provide us with guidance to find the answers to what is not known.

This symposium is constructed on three levels: The theoretical, technological and technical fields that support clinical pharmacology are reviewed with the intent of providing the reader with an up-to-date vision and understanding of the infrastructure upon which it is based. Then, the current status of the several areas that properly lie within the purview of classical clinical pharmacology are reviewed. This includes a review of classical as well as experimental antiarrhythmic agents and an evaluation of the arrhythmias against which they may be effective. And finally we discuss several different aspects of drug research and action that might be incorporated most easily under the term the ecology of clinical pharmacology. In this we explore the interactions of patients, the pharmaceutical industry, and human psyches as determinants of drug use, availability, and effect.

I am deeply indebted to the investigators who have participated in this conference and shared their knowledge, expertise, and experience with us. The many members of the New York Academy of Sciences, ranging from the program subcommittee, which offered wonderful guidance in the early days of this conference's development, to Mrs. Ellen Marks and her tireless and remarkably efficient aides, who have made this entire conference not only a reality but a perfectly packaged one at that, receive my most sincere thanks. I am also grateful for the painstaking editorial work done by Justine Cullinan and the Academy's Editorial Department, who have seen that the papers presented at the Conference reach book form. And finally I wish to acknowledge my appreciation to all the sponsors who have provided generous support to this conference.

## REFERENCES

1. MORGANROTH, J. et al. 1978. Limitations of routine long-term electrocardiographic monitoring to assess ventricular ectopic frequency. Circulation **207:** 976–82.
2. ROUTLEDGE, P. A. et al. 1980. Alpha-1 acid glycoprotein and the disposition of lidocaine in health and myocardial infarction (abstract). Clin. Pharmacol. Ther. **27:** 282.

# Cellular Electrophysiologic Mechanisms of Cardiac Arrhythmias

ANDREW L. WIT[a]

*Department of Pharmacology*
*College of Physicians & Surgeons*
*Columbia University*
*New York, New York 10032*

Arrhythmias result from abnormalities of impulse generation or impulse conduction or a combination of both.[1] In the 20 years since this classification of arrhythmia mechanisms was first proposed by Hoffman and Cranefield, the basic classification has been continuously modified to the point where we now believe that there are a variety of mechanisms that can cause abnormal impulse initiation or abnormal conduction. TABLE 1 outlines these mechanisms.[2]

## ARRHYTHMIAS CAUSED BY ABNORMAL IMPULSE GENERATION

Abnormal impulse generation occurs because of localized changes in ionic currents which flow across the membranes of single cells or groups of cells. Such impulse generation may be expressed as automaticity or triggered activity.

### *Automaticity*

Automaticity, the ability to initiate spontaneous action potentials, is a normal property of cardiac cells in the sinus node, in some parts of the atria, in the atrioventricular (AV) junctional region and in the His-Purkinje system. Automaticity can also be caused by cardiac disease in cells in which it is not a normal property.

#### *Normal Automatic Mechanism*

The basis for normal automaticity is a slow fall in membrane potential during the diastolic interval. This is referred to as phase 4 or diastolic or pacemaker depolarization. When the membrane reaches its threshold potential, an impulse is initiated and the pacemaker conductance is then reactivated (FIG. 1). The decrease in membrane potential during phase 4 reflects a gradual shift in the balance between inward and outward current components in the direction of net inward (depolarizing) current. For many years the pacemaker potential in Purkinje fibers, and perhaps in other cardiac fibers as well, was considered to result from an outward pacemaker current carried by $K^+$, which gradually declines, thereby

[a] Address for correspondence: Dr. Andrew L. Wit, Department of Pharmacology, College of Physicians & Surgeons, 630 West 168th Street, New York, New York 10032.

TABLE 1. Mechanisms for Arrhythmias[a]

| Abnormal Impulse Generation | Abnormal Impulse Conduction | Simultaneous Abnormalities of Impulse Generation and Conduction |
|---|---|---|
| A. Automatic impulse initiation <br> 1. Normal automatic mechanism <br> 2. Abnormal automatic mechanism | A. Slowing and block (SA block, AV block, etc.) | A. Parasystole (see Refs. 32 and 33) |
| B. Triggered activity <br> 1. Early afterdepolarization <br> 2. Delayed afterdepolarization | B. Unidirectional block and reentry <br> 1. Random reentry <br> 2. Ordered reentry <br> 3. Summation and inhibition (see Ref. 59) | B. Slow conduction because of phase 4 depolarization (see Ref. 2) |
| | C. Conduction block, electrotonic transmission and reflection (see Refs. 62 and 63) | |

[a] Modified from Hoffman and Rosen.[2]

allowing the background inward $Na^+$ current to depolarize the cell membrane.[3,4] Now, however, recent studies on pacemaker mechanisms have questioned the results of earlier experiments that led to this concept.[5-8] The recently proposed alternative is that an inward $Na^+$ pacemaker current (called $I_f$) increases with time, thereby depolarizing the membrane, while the outward $K^+$ current is constant. The exact cause of diastolic depolarization is still far from settled.

In the normal heart, the rate of impulse initiation due to automaticity of cells in the sinus node is sufficiently rapid that potentially automatic cells (latent pacemakers) elsewhere in the heart are excited by propagated impulses before they can depolarize spontaneously to threshold potential. Not only are ectopic pacemakers prevented from initiating an impulse because they are depolarized before they have a chance to fire, but also the diastolic depolarization of the latent pacemaker cells is actually inhibited by the impulses from the sinus node. This inhibition is called overdrive suppression.[9,10] Overdrive suppression results from driving a pacemaker cell faster than its intrinsic spontaneous rate and is mediated by enhanced activity of the $Na^+/K^+$ exchange pump.[9] When subsidiary pace-

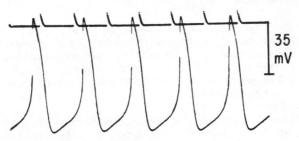

35 mV

**FIGURE 1.** Automaticity in an AV nodal fiber. The transmembrane potentials shown were recorded from an isolated 2 × 2-mm preparation dissected from the rabbit AV node and superfused with Tyrode's solution. Automaticity is commonly found when the connections between the AV node and surrounding tissue are severed. Time marks are at 250-msec intervals.

maker cells are driven faster than their intrinsic rate, the enhanced outward current generated by this pump[11] suppresses spontaneous impulse initiation in these cells. When the dominant (overdrive) pacemaker is stopped, this suppression is responsible for a period of quiescence which lasts until the intracellular $Na^+$ concentration, and hence the pump current, becomes small enough to allow subsidiary pacemaker cells to depolarize spontaneously to threshold.[9] A shift in the site of impulse initiation to a region other than the sinus node would be expected to occur when the sinus rate falls considerably below the intrinsic rate of the subsidiary pacemakers having the capabilities for normal automaticity. Impulse initiation by the sinus node may be slowed or inhibited altogether either by the parasympathetic nervous system or as a result of sinus node disease. Alternatively, there may be block of impulse conduction from the sinus node to the atrium.

Another mechanism that may suppress subsidiary pacemakers is the electrotonic interactions between the pacemaker cells and nonpacemaker cells.[12,13] For example, it has been proposed that the electrotonic interactions between atrium and AV node suppress automaticity of nodal cells through the atrionodal connections.[12] The atrial cells have more negative resting potentials than do the nodal cells and are not latent pacemakers. Because of the more negative potentials of the atrial cells, current flow between them and the nodal cells should be in a direction that prevents spontaneous diastolic depolarization of the nodal cells. Any intervention, then, that decreases intercellular coupling might increase automaticity (FIG. 1).[14] This could result from physical separation of the node from the atrium, as might occur during fibrosis of the junctional region, which causes heart block. Uncoupling might also be caused by factors that increase the intracellular concentration of $Ca^{++}$,[15] such as digitalis.[16]

Subsidiary pacemaker activity can also be enhanced, causing impulse initiation to shift to ectopic sites even when sinus node function and impulse conduction through the heart are normal. Norepinephrine released locally from sympathetic nerves enhances pacemaker activity by steepening the slope of diastolic depolarization of most ectopic pacemaker cells.[17] Norepinephrine also diminishes the inhibitory effects of overdrive.[18]

*Abnormal Automatic Mechanism*

Working atrial and ventricular myocardial cells do not normally show spontaneous diastolic depolarization. However, when the resting potential of these cells is experimentally reduced to less than about $-60$ mV, spontaneous diastolic depolarization may occur and cause repetitive impulse initiation.[19-22] This is called abnormal automaticity. Likewise, cells such as Purkinje fibers, which have the property of normal automaticity at normal levels of membrane potential, also show abnormal automaticity when membrane potential is reduced.[22] However, if a low level of membrane potential is employed as the only criterion for abnormal automaticity, the automaticity of the sinoatrial (SA) node would have to be considered abnormal. Therefore, an important distinction for abnormal automaticity is that the membrane potentials of fibers showing this type of activity are markedly reduced from the normal level.[2]

At the low level of membrane potential at which abnormal automaticity occurs, it is likely that at least some of the ionic currents causing the automatic activity are not the same as those causing normal automatic activity.[2,23] Since the ionic currents may not be the same, the two kinds of automaticity may not respond to antiarrhythmic drugs in the same way. In addition, because of the low level of membrane potential, the spontaneously occurring action potentials may be slow responses (action potentials with upstrokes dependent on slow inward current).[22] The decrease in membrane potential of cardiac cells required for abnormal automaticity to occur may be caused by a variety of factors related to cardiac disease which have been described in detail in other papers.[24-28]

An abnormal automatic focus should manifest itself and cause an arrhythmia when the sinus rate decreases below the intrinsic rate of the focus, as was discussed for latent pacemakers with normal automaticity. However, there may be an important distinction between the effects of the dominant sinus pacemaker on the two kinds of foci. Unlike normal automaticity, abnormal automaticity may not be "overdrive-suppressed."[29,30] Therefore, even transient sinus pauses or occasional long sinus cycle lengths may permit the ectopic focus to capture the heart for one or more impulses. On the other hand, an ectopic pacemaker with normal automaticity would probably be quiescent during relatively short transient sinus pauses because they are overdrive-suppressed.

It is also possible that the depolarized level of membrane potential at which abnormal automaticity occurs might cause entrance block into the focus and prevent it from being overdriven by the sinus node.[31] This would lead to parasystole, an example of an arrhythmia caused by a combination of an abnormality of impulse conduction and initiation as outlined in TABLE 1. Entrance block may also occur into regions of normal automaticity if they are surrounded by depolarized or inexcitable fibers.[32,33]

## Triggered Activity

Triggered activity is impulse generation caused by afterdepolarizations. An afterdepolarization is a second subthreshold depolarization that occurs either during repolarization (referred to as an early afterdepolarization) or after repolarization is complete or nearly complete (referred to as a delayed afterdepolarization.[34,35]

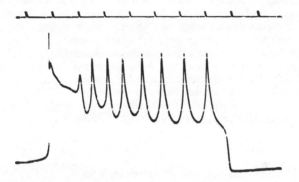

**FIGURE 2.** Early afterdepolarization and repetitive activity in canine cardiac Purkinje fiber. The maximum diastolic potential was −87 mV. A "burst" of rhythmic activity arising from a low level of membrane potential occurred during repolarization of the action potential. The slow responses during this burst peaked near 0 mV. Time marks occur at 1-sec intervals. (From Wit et al.[35] Reproduced by permission.)

### Early Afterdepolarizations and Triggered Activity

Early afterdepolarizations usually occur during repolarization of an action potential which has been initiated from a high level of membrane potential, usually between −75 and −90 mV (FIG. 2). Early afterdepolarizations appear as a change in membrane potential in a positive direction, relative to the expected membrane potential during normal repolarization. Under certain conditions early afterdepolarizations can lead to second upstrokes[34]; membrane potential during the early afterdepolarization reaches threshold potential for activation of the slow inward current and a second action potential occurs prior to complete repolarization of the first. The second upstroke is triggered in the sense that it is evoked by an early afterdepolarization which follows and is caused by the preceding action potential. The second action potential may also be followed by other action potentials, all occurring at the low level of membrane potential characteristic of the plateau or phase 3. These action potentials presumably are slow responses (FIG. 2).[22,34,35] The sustained rhythmic activity may continue for a variable number of impulses and terminates when the increase in membrane potential associated with repolarization of the initiating action potential returns membrane potential to a high level (FIG. 2).

There are some conceptual difficulties associated with triggered activity caused by early afterdepolarizations.[34] According to the definition of triggered activity there is no problem in characterizing the second upstroke that follows an action potential arising from a high level of membrane potential as being triggered. But if a series of action potentials arise before the cell repolarizes to a high resting potential, are these action potentials triggered or do they occur only because the membrane potential has been shifted into a region where automatic activity occurs? (We have discussed in the previous section how abnormal automaticity occurs at reduced membrane potentials.) Perhaps only the first action potential is triggered and the remaining are automatic.[34]

Early afterdepolarizations leading to triggered activity in isolated cardiac preparations may be caused by factors that are present in the heart *in situ* under some pathologic conditions. Among these factors are hypoxia,[36] high $pCO_2$,[37] and high concentrations of catecholamines.[38] Since catecholamines, hypoxia and elevated $pCO_2$ may be present in an ischemic or infarcted region of the ventricles, it is possible that early afterdepolarizations may cause some of the arrhythmias that occur soon after myocardial ischemia. Some drugs which are used clinically and which markedly prolong the time course for repolarization, such as the beta-receptor blocking drug sotolol and the antiarrhythmic drug *N*-acetyl procainamide,[39,40] cause early afterdepolarizations and triggered activity. These drugs may cause cardiac arrhythmias which may be a result of this triggered activity.

### Delayed Afterdepolarizations and Triggered Activity

A delayed afterdepolarization is a transient or oscillatory depolarization that occurs after the terminal repolarization of an action potential and that is induced by that action potential. Delayed afterdepolarizations may be subthreshold, as shown in FIGURE 3, but when they are large enough to bring the membrane potential to threshold, a nondriven (triggered) impulse arises that also is followed by an afterdepolarization. The impulse is said to be triggered since it would not have occurred without the preceding action potential.[22,34,35]

Delayed afterdepolarizations occur under a number of conditions in which there is a large increase in the intracellular Ca.[41–45] One of the most widely recognized causes is toxic amounts of cardiac glycosides.[45] Catecholamines can also cause delayed afterdepolarizations, possibly because they enhance $Ca^{++}$ entry into cardiac fibers by increasing the slow inward current.[46–48] Delayed afterdepolarizations may sometimes occur in the absence of drugs or catecholamines but may still be related to an increase in intracellular $Ca^{++}$ or abnormal handling of $Ca^{++}$ by the sarcoplasmic reticulum.[49–53] The possible mechanisms by which an increase in $Ca_i$ may cause afterdepolarizations are discussed in the publications of Tsien and his coworkers.[41–43]

Delayed afterdepolarizations may not reach threshold, in which case triggered activity does not occur. In fibers showing subthreshold delayed afterdepolarizations, triggering may result if the rate at which the fiber is driven is increased (FIG. 3). The amplitude of the afterdepolarizations increases as the drive rate increases. Beyond a certain drive rate the afterdepolarizations reach threshold and triggering occurs. A decrease in the length of even a single drive cycle, that is, a premature impulse, may increase the amplitude of the afterdepolarization of the action potential that follows the short cycle. The afterdepolarization may reach threshold and initiate triggered activity.

There are some differences in the characteristics of triggered activity, depending upon the cause. In particular, triggered activity caused by digitalis toxicity may sometimes have different properties than triggered activity caused by catecholamines. The initial period of triggered activity in coronary sinus atrial fibers

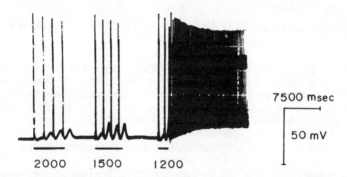

**FIGURE 3.** Afterdepolarizations and triggering in canine coronary sinus fiber in the presence of norepinephrine, 0.5 μg/ml. The record shows the effects of decreasing stimulus cycle length on afterdepolarization amplitude and triggering. At the *left*, the fiber was stimulated at a cycle length of 2000 msec and four impulses were initiated (underlined by the horizontal bar). The afterdepolarization following the last driven impulse had an amplitude of 10 mV. In the *center*, four impulses were stimulated at a cycle length of 1500 msec (underlined by the horizontal bar). The afterdepolarization following the last driven impulse had an amplitude of 17 mV. At the *right*, after two impulses were stimulated at a cycle length of 1200 msec (underlined by horizontal bar), sustained rhythmic activity was triggered. Maximum diastolic potential immediately decreased by 15 mV and action potential amplitude decreased. (Modified from Wit and Cranefield.[47])

caused by catecholamines is often characterized by a gradual decrease in the cycle length after which a constant cycle length occurs.[47,53] This decrease in cycle length is often accompanied by a decrease in maximum diastolic potential. During triggered activity in Purkinje fibers exposed to toxic amounts of digitalis there is not always a gradual increase in rate.[45,54]

Triggered activity caused by digitalis or by catecholamines often terminates spontaneously, even in the presence of maintained levels of these agents. When catecholamine-induced triggered activity in the coronary sinus terminates, the rate usually slows gradually before termination. This gradual slowing is accompanied by a progressive increase in the maximum diastolic potential. A delayed afterdepolarization usually follows the last triggered impulse. Maximum diastolic potential at the time triggered activity ceases may be more negative than when triggering began.[53] Maximum diastolic potential may continue to increase for some seconds after triggered activity has stopped, but then it returns slowly over the next few minutes to the control level. The spontaneous termination of triggered activity in canine coronary sinus fibers is caused, at least in part, by an increase in the rate of electrogenic sodium extrusion and the outward sodium pump current that is generated.[53] Triggered activity caused by digitalis toxicity probably stops by another mechanism. Termination of a triggered burst is usually not associated with gradual slowing and hyperpolarization, but often by speeding of the rate, a decrease in action potential amplitude and a decrease in membrane potential.[54] Termination is probably not related to activity of the $Na^+$ pump since the pump is inhibited by the digitalis, but may be caused by $Na^+$ or $Ca^{++}$ accumulation in the cell caused by the rapid rate.

## ARRHYTHMIAS CAUSED BY ABNORMAL IMPULSE CONDUCTION AND REENTRY

Under special conditions the propagating impulse may not die out after complete activation of the heart but it may persist to reexcite the atria or ventricles after the end of the refractory period. This is called reentrant excitation (FIG. 4).[55] Hoffman and Rosen have further subdivided this mechanism for arrhythmias into two categories, random reentry and ordered reentry.[2] Random reentry is most often associated with atrial or ventricular fibrillation, whereas ordered reentry can cause most other types of arrhythmias. The main distinction between the two is that during random reentry propagation occurs over reentrant pathways that continuously change their size and location with time, whereas ordered reentry implies a relatively fixed reentrant pathway. However, despite these differences, the basic prerequisite electrophysiologic conditions required for either kind of reentrant excitation are similar. Most mechanisms for reentry require that conduction of the impulse blocks somewhere in part of a reentrant circuit and that the block must either be transient or unidirectional. The block enables an excitable pathway to persist through which the reentering impulse can return to reexcite regions it has already excited. Also, the wave length of the impulse in the reentrant circuit (conduction velocity × refractory period) must be shorter than the length of the circuit so that the tissue into which the impulse is reentering has had time to recover excitability.[56] Because of this requirement, it is clear that the relationship between path length, conduction velocity, and refractory period is crucial (FIG. 4). Reentry can be promoted by slowing conduction velocity, or shortening the refractory period, or a combination of both.

There can be a number of causes for the slowed conduction and block that are necessary in order for reentrant excitation to occur. The speed at which the impulse conducts in cardiac fibers is dependent on certain features of their transmembrane action potentials, their passive electrical properties, and their microanatomy. Different groups of investigators studying mechanisms for reentrant excitation have often focused their attention on one or another of these causes and have at one time attempted to attribute the cause of all or most reentry to one specific mechanism for slow conduction and block; nevertheless, it is most likely that a number of different mechanisms are operative singly or in combination. Several examples of different mechanisms are discussed below, but this discussion is not all inclusive. The cause of slow conduction and block may vary with the type of arrhythmia and the underlying cardiac pathology.

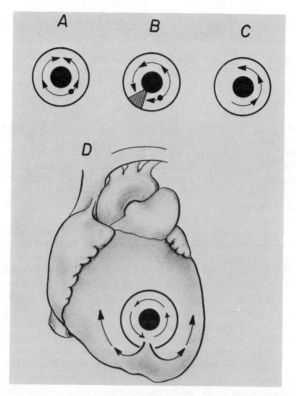

**FIGURE 4.** Schematic representation of reentry in a ring muscle. In **A** the ring was stimulated in the area indicated by the small black dot; impulses propagated away from the point of stimulation in both directions and collided; no reentry occurred. In **B** the cross-hatched area was compressed, while the ring was stimulated again at the black dot. The impulse propagated around the ring in only one direction, having been blocked in the other direction by the area of compression. Then, immediately after stimulation, the compression was relieved, and in **C** the unidirectionally circulating impulse is shown returning to its point of origin and then continuing around the loop. Identical reentry would occur if the cross-hatched area was a region of unidirectional conduction block, with the conduction block in the right to left direction. **D** shows how reentry in a loop of the kind described in **A–C** can cause arrhythmias if located in the heart. In this example, the loop is composed of ventricular muscle that is functionally separated, perhaps because of fibrosis, from the rest of the ventricle along most of its border (*heavy black line*), but is in functional continuity with the ventricle in one place (at its lower end). The *arrows* show how excitation waves could propagate into the ventricles from the continuously circulating impulse to cause ventricular tachycardia. (From Wit.[77] Reproduced by permission.)

### Depressed Resting Membrane Potentials and Premature Action Potentials Cause Slow Conduction, Block, and Reentry

The influence of transmembrane potential characteristics on conduction is very complex and cannot be discussed here in full. Only some basic principles are presented. An important feature of the transmembrane action potentials of working (atrial and ventricular) myocardial and Purkinje fibers which govern the speed of propagation is the magnitude of the inward $Na^+$ current flowing through the fast $Na^+$ channel during the upstroke, and the rapidity with which this current reaches its maximum intensity (the upstroke velocity or $V_{max}$ of phase 0). The intensity of the inward $Na^+$ current depends on the fraction of $Na^+$ channels that open when the cell is excited and the size of the $Na^+$ electrochemical potential gradient (relative concentration of $Na^+$ outside the cells in the extracellular space to $Na^+$ concentration inside the cell).[57,58] The fraction of sodium channels available for opening is determined largely by the level of membrane potential at which an action potential is initiated. Premature activation of the heart can induce reentry because premature impulses conduct slowly in regions of the heart where cells are not completely repolarized (where $Na^+$ channels are to some extent inactivated) and conduction of premature impulses may block in regions where cells have not yet repolarized to about $-60$ mV. Reentry might also occur in cardiac cells with persistently low levels of resting potential (which may be between $-60$ and $-70$ mV) caused by disease. At these resting potentials about 50% of the $Na^+$ channels are inactivated, and therefore are unavailable for activation by a depolarizing stimulus.[24] The magnitude of the net inward current during phase 0 of the action potential is reduced and consequently both the speed and amplitude of the upstroke is diminished, slowing conduction significantly. Such action potentials with upstrokes dependent on inward current flowing via partially inactivated $Na^+$ channels are sometimes referred to as depressed fast responses. Further depolarization and inactivation of the $Na^+$ channel may render cardiac fibers inexcitable so that they may become a site of conduction block. Thus, in a diseased region, there may be some areas of slow conduction and some areas of conduction block, possibly depending on the level of resting potential. The conduction block may be unidirectional.[59] The combination of slow conduction and block may cause reentry.

The slow inward current, under certain conditions, may also underlie the occurrence of reentrant arrhythmias.[22] Although the fast $Na^+$ channels may be largely inactivated at membrane potentials near $-50$ mV, the slow inward channel is not inactivated and still is available for activation.[60] Under certain conditions in cells with resting potentials positive to $-60$ mV (when membrane conductance is very low or when catecholamines are present), this normally weak slow inward current may give rise to the regenerative depolarization characteristic of a propagated action potential. This propagated action potential dependent on slow inward current alone is the slow response.[22] Since this inward current is weak, conduction velocity is slow and both unidirectional and bidirectional conduction block may occur.[59] Slow-response action potentials can occur in diseased cardiac fibers with low resting potentials, but they also occur in some normal regions of the heart, such as in cells of the sinoatrial and atrioventricular nodes where the maximum diastolic potential is normally positive to about $-70$ mV.[22]

Reentrant excitation caused by the slow conduction and block that accompany depression of the action potential upstroke may occur in gross, anatomically distinct circuits (around an anatomic obstacle). This is exemplified by reentry in a loop of cardiac fiber bundles, such as the loops of Purkinje fiber bundles in the distal conducting system. Similar anatomic circuits might be formed by bundles of surviving muscle fibers in healed infarcts or in fibrotic regions of the atria and ventricles. Gross anatomic circuits are also involved in reentry utilizing the bundle branches or accessory AV connecting pathways.[55] The basic principles have been discussed quite extensively in other reviews.[2,22,55,59]

Gross anatomic loops and anatomic obstacles are not a prerequisite for the occurrence of reentry. Reentry caused by slow conduction and unidirectional block can also occur in unbranched bundles or "sheets" of muscle fibers. A kind of reentry called reflection occurs in unbranched bundles of Purkinje fibers in which conduction is slow because the resting and action potentials are depressed.[22,59] Recently Moe and his coinvestigators have described another mechanism that may cause reflection.[62,63] Slow conduction does not occur along the bundles because of depressed transmembrane potentials, as described by Wit *et al.*,[61] but rather there is delayed activation of part of the bundle resulting from electrotonic excitation of a region distal to an inexcitable segment.

### The Leading Circle: A Mechanism for Circus Movement without an Anatomic Obstacle

Repetitive activity can be induced in the atria by appropriately timed single premature stimuli. Such activity may be caused by reentrant excitation occurring in the absence of an anatomic obstacle. This kind of reentry may occur by the leading circle mechanism described by Allessie *et al.*[64,65] The initiation of reentry is made possible by the different refractory periods of atrial fibers in close proximity to each other. The premature impulse that initiates repetitive activity blocks in fibers with long refractory periods and conducts in fibers with shorter refractory periods, eventually returning to the initial point of block after excitability recovers there. The impulse may then continue to circulate. Conduction through the reentrant circuit is slowed because impulses are propagating in partially refractory tissue. The circumference of the pathway may be as small as 6–8 mm.

### Slow Conduction and Reentrant Excitation Caused by the Anisotropic Structure of Cardiac Muscle

Cardiac muscle is anisotropic, that is, its anatomic and biophysical properties vary according to the direction in the cardiac syncytium in which they are measured.[66] Spach and his coworkers have recently published a series of articles on the effects of anisotropy on conduction properties of normal atrial and ventricular muscle and they have shown how anisotropy can cause reentry.[67-69] They have demonstrated that in *uniformly anisotropic* cardiac tissue (in tissue where the cardiac muscle fibers are closely packed together and arranged parallel to each other in a uniform manner) conduction in a direction parallel to the orientation of the myocardial fiber (along the long axis of the myocardial fibers) is much more rapid than in the direction perpendicular to the long axis. Conduction perpendicular to the long axis of the fibers can be very slow in normal atrial or ventricular muscle (0.1 m/sec), even though resting and action potentials of the muscle fibers are normal.[67] The slow conduction is caused by an effective axial resistivity that is higher in the direction perpendicular to fiber orientation than parallel to fiber orientation.[67,68] The higher axial resistivity perpendicular to fiber orientation results in part from fewer and shorter intercalated discs connecting myocardial fibers in a side-to-side direction than in the end-to-end direction. In addition, although it may seem paradoxical, in spite of more rapid conduction down the long axis of the myocardial fibers than that perpendicular to the long axis, premature impulses may block more readily along the long axis because the safety factor for conduction is lower in the direction of the lower axial resistivity.[67] When myocardial fiber bundles are separated by nonmuscular tissue such as connective tissue, the conduction properties will be further altered by the separation and the structural discontinuities. Such separation of myocardial bundles further slows conduction because of a reduction in intercellular connections.[68] The separation of myocardial fibers by connective tissue results in a *nonuniform anisotropic* structure.[68] Spach *et al.* have shown that both uniform and nonuniform anisotropic structural properties can cause reentry in atrial myocardium with normal transmembrane potentials and uniform refractory periods because anisotropy can cause both slow conduction and block.[67,68] It has also been proposed that anisotropy of epicardial muscle surviving over healing canine infarcts may cause reentry.[70]

### Investigating Reentry in the in Situ Heart

The studies on reentry that have just been described were performed on isolated cardiac preparations. This enabled detailed investigations of the cellular electrophysiological mechanisms. In addition to this experimental approach, it is now possible to investigate mechanisms causing reentry in the *in situ* heart by accurate mapping of impulse propagation with techniques that permit extracellular electrograms to be simultaneously recorded from a large number of sites. Isochronal maps of conduction patterns using this approach have shown that reentrant excitation causes experimental atrial flutter[71,72] as well as ventricular tachycardia associated with acute coronary artery occlusion.[73] Reentrant excitation has also been shown in subacute canine infarcts during those ventricular arrhythmias that can be induced by stimulated premature impulses.[74–76]

### REFERENCES

1. HOFFMAN, B. F. & P. F. CRANEFIELD. 1964. The physiological basis of cardiac arrhythmias. Am. J. Med. **37:** 670–684.
2. HOFFMAN, B. F. & M. R. ROSEN. 1981. Cellular mechanisms for cardiac arrhythmias. Circ. Res. **49:** 1–15.
3. VASSALLE, M. 1965. Analysis of cardiac pacemaker potential using a "voltage clamp" technique. Am. J. Physiol. **208:** 770–775.
4. TRAUTWEIN, W. 1973. Membrane current in cardiac muscle fibers. Physiol. Rev. **53:** 793–835.
5. DiFRANCESCO, D. 1981. A new interpretation of the pacemaking current in calf Purkinje fibers. J. Physiol. **314:** 359–376.
6. DiFRANCESCO, D. 1981. A study of the ionic nature of the pacemaker current in calf Purkinje fibers. J. Physiol. **314:** 377–393.
7. YANAGIHARA, K. & H. IRISAWA. 1980. Potassium current during the pacemaker depolarization in rabbit sinoatrial node cell. Pfluegers Arch. **388:** 255–268.
8. NOMA, A., H. IRISAWA, S. KOKUBUN, H. KOTAKE, M. NISHIMURA & Y. WATANABE. 1980. Slow current systems in the A-V node of the rabbit heart. Nature **285:** 228–229.

9. VASSALLE, M. 1970. Electrogenic suppression of automaticity in sheep and dog Purkinje fibers. Circ. Res. **27:** 361–377.
10. VASSALLE, M. 1977. The relationship among cardiac pacemakers: Overdrive suppression. Circ. Res. **41:** 269–277.
11. GADSBY, D. C. & P. F. CRANEFIELD. 1979. Direct measurement of changes in sodium pump current in canine cardiac Purkinje fibers. Proc. Natl. Acad. Sci. USA **76:** 1783–1787.
12. WIT, A. L. & P. F. CRANEFIELD. 1982. Mechanisms of impulse initiation in the atrioventricular junction and the effects of acetylstrophanthidin (abstr.) Am. J. Cardiol. **49:** 921.
13. VAN CAPELLE, F. J. L. & D. DURRER. 1980. Computer simulation of arrhythmias in a network of coupled excitable elements. Circ. Res. **47:** 454–466.
14. KOKUBUN, S., M. NISHIMURA, A. NOMA & A. IRISAWA. 1980. The spontaneous action potential of rabbit atrioventricular node cells. Jpn. J. Physiol. **30:** 529–540.
15. DAHL, G. & G. ISENBERG. 1980. Decoupling of heart muscle cells: Correlation with increased cytoplasmic calcium activity and with changes in nexus ultrastructure. 1980. J. Membr. Biol. **53:** 63–75.
16. WEINGART, R. 1977. The actions of ouabain on intercellular coupling and conduction velocity in mammalian ventricular muscle. J. Physiol. (London) **264:** 341–365.
17. TSIEN, R. W. 1974. Effect of epinephrine on the pacemaker potassium current of cardiac Purkinje fibers. J. Gen. Physiol. **64:** 293–319.
18. VASSALLE, M. & R. CARPENTIER. 1972. Overdrive excitation: Onset of activity following fast drive in cardiac Purkinje fibers exposed to norepinephrine. Pfluegers Arch. **332:** 198–205.
19. KATZUNG, B. O. & J. A. MORGENSTERN. 1977. Effects of extracellular potassium on ventricular automaticity and evidence for a pacemaker current in mammalian ventricular myocardium. Circ. Res. **40:** 105–111.
20. SURAWICZ, B. & S. IMANISHI. 1976. Automatic activity in depolarized guinea pig ventricular myocardium: Characteristics and mechanisms. Circ. Res. **39:** 751–759.
21. BROWN, H. F. & S. J. NOBLE. 1969. Membrane currents underlying delayed rectification and pacemaker activity in frog atrial muscle. J. Physiol. (London) **204:** 717–735.
22. CRANEFIELD, P. F. 1975. The Conduction of the Cardiac Impulse: The Slow Response and Cardiac Arrhythmias. Futura Press. Mt. Kisco, NY.
23. NOBLE D. & R. W. TSIEN. 1968. The kinetics and rectifier properties of the slow potassium current in cardiac Purkinje fibers. J. Physiol. (London) **195:** 185–214.
24. GADSBY, D. C. & A. L. WIT. 1981. Electrophysiologic characteristics of cardiac cells and the genesis of cardiac arrhythmias. In Cardiac Pharmacology. R. G. Wilkersen, Ed.: 229–274. Academic Press. New York, NY.
25. FRIEDMAN, P. L., J. R. STEWART & A. L. WIT. 1973. Spontaneous and induced cardiac arrhythmias in subendocardial Purkinje fibers surviving extensive myocardial infarction in dogs. Circ. Res. **33:** 612–626.
26. LAZZARA, R., N. EL-SHERIF & B. J. SCHERLAG. 1973. Electrophysiological properties of canine Purkinje cells in one-day-old myocardial infarction. Circ. Res. **33:** 722–734.
27. HORDOF, A., R. EDIE, J. MALM, B. F. HOFFMAN & M. R. ROSEN. 1976. Electrophysiological properties and response to pharmacologic agents of fibers from diseased human atria. Circulation **54:** 774–779.
28. SINGER, D. H., C. M. BAUMGARTEN & R. E. TEN ECK. 1981. Cellular electrophysiology of ventricular and other dysrhythmias: Studies on diseased and ischemic heart. Prog. Cardiovasc. Dis. **24:** 97–156.
29. CARMELIET, E. 1980. The slow inward current: Non-voltage-clamp studies. In The Slow Inward Current and Cardiac Arrhythmias. D. P. Zipes, J. C. Bailey & V. Elharrar, Eds.: 97–110. Martinus Nijhoff. The Hague.
30. DANGMAN, K. H. & B. F. HOFFMAN. 1983. Studies on overdrive stimulation of canine cardiac Purkinje fibers: Maximum diastolic potential as a determinant of the response. J. Am. Coll. Cardiol. **2:** 1183–1190.

31. FERRIER, G. R. & J. E. ROSENTHAL. 1980. Automaticity and entrance block induced by focal depolarization of mammalian ventricular tissues. Circ. Res. **47:** 238–248.
32. JALIFE, J. & G. K. MOE. 1976. Effects of electrotonic potentials on pacemaker activity of canine Purkinje fibers in relation to parasystole. Circ. Res. **39:** 801–808.
33. JALIFE, J. & G. K. MOE. 1979. A biologic model of parasystole. Am. J. Cardiol. **43:** 761–772.
34. CRANEFIELD, P. F. 1977. Action potentials, afterpotentials and arrhythmias. Circ. Res. **41:** 415–423.
35. WIT, A. L., P. F. CRANEFIELD & D. C. GADSBY. 1980. Triggered activity. In The Slow Inward Current and Cardiac Arrhythmias. D. P. Zipes, J. C. Bailey & V. Elharrar, Eds.: 437–454. Martinus Nijhoff. The Hague.
36. TRAUTWEIN, W., V. GOTTSTEIN & J. DUDEL. 1954. Der Aktionsstrom der Myokardfaser im Sauerstoffmangel. Pfluegers Arch. Ges. Physiol. **260:** 40–60.
37. CORABOEF, E. & J. BOISTEL. 1953. L'action des taux élevés de gaz carbonique sur le tissu cardiaque étudiée a l'aide de microelectrodes intracellulaires. 1953. C. R. Soc. Biol. (Paris) **147:** 654–668.
38. BROOKS, C. McC., P. F. HOFFMAN, E. E. SUCKLING & O. ORIAS. 1955. Excitability of the Heart. Grune and Stratton. New York, NY.
39. STRAUSS, H. C., J. T. BIGGER, JR. & B. F. HOFFMAN. 1970. Electrophysiological and beta-receptor blocking effects of MJ 1999 on dog and rabbit cardiac tissues. Circ. Res. **26:** 661–678.
40. DANGMAN, K. H. & B. F. HOFFMAN. 1981. In vivo and in vitro antiarrhythmic and arrhythmogenic effects of N-acetyl procainamide. J. Pharmacol. Exp. Ther. **217:** 851–862.
41. KASS, R. S., W. J. LEDERER, R. W. TSIEN & R. WEINGART. 1978. Role of calcium ions in transient inward currents and after contractions induced by strophanthidin in cardiac Purkinje fibers. J. Physiol. **281:** 187–208.
42. KASS, R. S., R. W. TSIEN & R. WEINGART. 1978. Ionic basis of transient inward current induced by strophanthidin in cardiac Purkinje fibers. J. Physiol. (London) **281:** 209–226.
43. KASS, R. S., W. J. LEDERER, R. W. TSIEN & R. WEINGART. 1978. Role of calcium ions in transient inward currents and aftercontractions induced by strophanthidin in cardiac Purkinje fibers. J. Physiol. (London) **281:** 187–208.
44. EISNER, D. A. & W. J. LEDERER. 1979. Inotropic and arrhythmogenic effects of potassium-depleted solutions on mammalian cardiac muscle. J. Physiol. (London) **294:** 255–277.
45. FERRIER, G. R. 1977. Digitalis arrhythmias: Role of oscillatory afterpotentials. Prog. Cardiovasc. Dis. **19:** 459–474.
46. NATHAN, D. & G. W. BEELER. 1975. Electrophysiologic correlates of the inotropic effects of isoproterenol in canine myocardium. J. Mol. Cell Cardiol. **7:** 1–15.
47. WIT, A. L. & P. F. CRANEFIELD. 1977. Triggered and automatic activity in the canine coronary sinus. Circ. Res. **41:** 435–445.
48. WIT, A. L. & P. F. CRANEFIELD. 1976. Triggered activity in cardiac muscle fibers of the simian mitral valve. Circ. Res. **38:** 85–98.
49. SAITO, T., M. OTAGURO & T. MATSUBARA. 1978. Electrophysiological studies on the mechanism of electrically induced sustained rhythmic activity in the rabbit right atrium. Circ. Res. **42:** 199–206.
50. ARONSON, R. S. 1981. Afterpotentials and triggered activity in hypertrophied myocardium from rats with renal hypertension. Circ. Res. **48:** 720–727.
51. MARY-RABINE, L., A. J. HORDOF, P. DANILO, J. R. MALM & M. R. ROSEN. 1980. Mechanisms for impulse initiation in isolated human atrial fibers. Circ. Res. **47:** 267–277.
52. EL-SHERIF, N., R. ZEILER & W. B. GOUGH. 1980. Effects of catecholamines, verapamil and tetrodotoxin on triggered automaticity in canine ischemic Purkinje fibers. (abstr.) 1980. Circulation **62** (Part 2): 281.
53. WIT, A. L., D. C. GADSBY & P. F. CRANEFIELD. 1981. Electrogenic sodium extrusion can stop triggered activity in the canine coronary sinus. Circ. Res. **49:** 1029–1042.

54. ROSEN, M. R. & R. F. REDER. 1981. Does triggered activity have a role in the genesis of cardiac arrhythmias. Ann. Int. Med. **94:** 794–801.
55. WIT, A. L. & P. F. CRANEFIELD. 1978. Reentrant excitation as a cause of cardiac arrhythmias. Am. J. Physiol. **235:** H1–17.
56. MINES, G. R. 1914. On circulating excitations in heart muscle and their possible relations to tachycardia and fibrillations. Trans. R. Soc. Can. Ser 3, Sect IV **8:** 43–52.
57. WEIDMANN, S. 1955. The effect of the cardiac membrane potential on the rapid availability of the sodium carrying system. J. Physiol. (London) **127:** 213–224.
58. REUTER, H. 1979. Properties of two inward membrane currents in heart. Ann. Rev. Physiol. **41:** 413–424.
59. CRANEFIELD, P. F., A. L. WIT & B. F. HOFFMAN. 1973. Genesis of cardiac arrhythmias. Circulation **47:** 190–204.
60. TSIEN, R. W. 1983. Calcium channels in excitable cell membranes. Annu. Rev. Physiol. **45:** 341–358.
61. WIT, A. L., B. F. HOFFMAN & P. F. CRANEFIELD. 1972. Slow conduction and reentry in the ventricular conducting system. I. Return extrasystole in canine Purkinje fibers. Circ. Res. **30:** 1–10.
62. ANTZELEVITCH, C., J. JALIFE & G. K. MOE. 1980. Characteristics of reflection as a mechanism of reentrant arrhythmias and its relationship to parasystole. Circulation **61:** 182–191.
63. JALIFE, J. & G. K. MOE. 1981. Excitation, conduction and reflection of impulses in isolated bovine and canine cardiac Purkinje fibers. Circ. Res. **49:** 233–247.
64. ALLESSIE, M. A., F. I. M. BONKE & F. SCHOPMAN. 1973. Circus movement in rabbit right atrial muscle as a mechanism of tachycardia. Circ. Res. **33:** 54–62.
65. ALLESSIE, M. A., F. I. M. BONKE & F. J. G. SCHOPMAN. 1977. Circus movement in rabbit atrial muscle as a mechanism of tachycardia. III. The "leading circle" concept: A new model of circus movement in cardiac tissue without the involvement of an anatomical obstacle. Circ. Res. **41:** 9–18.
66. CLERC, L. 1976. Directional differences of impulse spread in trabecular muscle from mammalian heart. J. Physiol. (London) **255:** 355–366.
67. SPACH, M., W. T. MILLER, D. B. GESELOWITZ, R. C. BARR, J. M. KOOTSEY & E. A. JOHNSON. 1981. The discontinuous nature of propagation in normal canine cardiac muscle: Evidence for recurrent discontinuities of intracellular resistance that affect the membrane currents. Circ. Res. **48:** 39–54.
68. SPACH, M. S., W. T. MULLER, P. C. DOLBER, J. M. KOOTSEY, J. R. SOMMER & C. E. MOSHER. 1982. The functional role of structural complexities in the propagation of depolarization in the atrium of the dog: Cardiac conduction disturbances due to discontinuities of effective axial resistivity. Circ. Res. **50:** 175–191.
69. SPACH, M. S., J. M. KOOTSEY & J. D. SLOAN. 1982. Active modulation of electrical coupling between cardiac cells of the dog: A mechanism for transient and steady state variations in conduction velocity. Circ. Res. **51:** 347–362.
70. GARDNER, P., P. C. URSELL, T. D. PHAM, J. J. FENOGLIO & A. L. WIT. 1984. Experimental chronic ventricular tachycardia: Anatomic and electrophysiologic substrates. *In* Tachycardias: Mechanisms, Diagnosis and Treatment. M. E. Josephson & H. J. J. Wellens, Eds. Lea and Febiger, Philadelphia, PA.
71. BOINEAU, J. P., R. B. SCHUESSLER, C. R. MOONEY, C. B. MILLER, A. C. WYLDS, R. D. HUDSON, J. M. BORREMANS & C. W. BROCKUS. 1980. Naturally and evoked atrial flutter due to circus movement in dogs: Role of abnormal atrial pathways, slow conduction, non-uniform refractory period distribution and premature beats. Am. J. Cardiol. **45:** 1167–1181.
72. ALLESSIE, M., W. LAMMERS, J. SMEETS, F. BONKE & J. HOLLEN. 1982. Total mapping of atrial excitation during acetylcholine-induced atrial flutter and fibrillation in the isolated canine heart. *In* Atrial Fibrillation. H. E. Kulbertus, S. B. Olsson & M. Schlepper, Eds.: 44–59. AB Hassle. Molndal, Sweden.
73. JANSE, M. J., F. J. L. VAN CAPELLE, H. MORSINK, A. G. KLEBER, F. WILHMS-SCHOPMAN, R. CARDINAL, C. NAUMANN D'ALNONCOURT & D. DURRER. 1980. Flow of "injury" current and patterns of excitation during ventricular arrhythmias in

acute regional myocardial ischemia in isolated porcine and canine hearts: Evidence for two different arrhythmogenic mechanisms. Circ. Res. **47:** 151–165.

74. EL-SHERIF, N., A. SMITH & K. EVANS. 1981. Canine ventricular arrhythmias in the late myocardial infarction period 8: Epicardial mapping of reentrant circuits. Circ. Res. **49:** 255–265.

75. MEHRA, R., R. H. ZEILER, W. B. GOUGH & N. EL-SHERIF. 1983. Reentrant ventricular arrhythmias in the late myocardial infarction period 9. Electrophysiologic-anatomic correlation of reentrant circuits. Circulation **67:** 11–24.

76. WIT, A. L., M. A. ALLESSIE, F. I. M. BONKE, W. LAMMERS, J. SMEETS & J. J. FENOGLIO, JR. 1982. Electrophysiologic mapping to determine the mechanism of experimental ventricular tachycardia initiated by premature impulses: Experimental approach and initial results demonstrating reentrant excitation. Am. J. Cardiol. **49:** 166–185.

77. WIT, A. L. 1979. The genesis of cardiac arrhythmias. *In* Proceedings of the Florence International Meeting on Myocardial Infarction. D. T. Mason, G. G. Neri Seneri & M. S. Oliver, Eds.: 674–695. Excerpta Medica. Amsterdam.

# Demonstration of the Mechanisms for Arrhythmias in Experimental Animals[a]

BRIAN F. HOFFMAN AND KENNETH H. DANGMAN

*Department of Pharmacology*
*College of Physicians & Surgeons*
*Columbia University*
*New York, New York 10032*

Inquiry into the mechanisms responsible for abnormalities of cardiac rhythm can be divided conveniently into two major questions: The first question asks: What abnormalities of electrical activity of cardiac cells and tissues can be responsible for abnormal rhythms? The second question is concerned with demonstrating which of these mechanisms actually do cause arrhythmias of the *in situ* heart of experimental animals and humans. The advent of the intracellular microelectrode permitted systematic investigation of the first question, and there now is reasonable agreement about the general classes of arrhythmogenic mechanisms. According to a scheme that we introduced many years ago, cardiac arrhythmias can result from abnormal impulse generation, abnormal impulse conduction, or simultaneous abnormalities of impulse generation and conduction.[1] Under the heading of abnormal impulse generation, two major classes are apparent. Impulses may arise from automaticity or they may be triggered.[2,3] For the automatic rhythms, the mechanism responsible for impulse generation may be a normal one or an abnormal one. For the triggered rhythms, once again two apparently dissimilar mechanisms may be involved. Triggered rhythms may result from early afterdepolarizations (EAD) or from delayed afterdepolarizations (DAD). For the arrhythmias caused by abnormal impulse conduction, the underlying abnormality may be simple block of propagation or unidirectional block with reentrant excitation. The latter seemingly can result either from circus movement or reflection.[4,5] This general classification is summarized in TABLE 1 and is the subject of Wit's paper in this volume.

There seems little reason to doubt that each of the mechanisms described can, under appropriate conditions, cause some abnormality of cardiac rhythm. Since the response of an arrhythmia to an antiarrhythmic drug or other therapeutic intervention very likely will depend, among other things, on the mechanism responsible for the arrhythmia, it is important to determine (1) which of the possible mechanisms actually operate to cause clinically significant arrhythmias and (2) what means can be employed to identify the specific mechanism responsible for a particular disturbance of rhythm. For some of the postulated mechanisms, such as circus movement, the experimental demonstration of the operation of the mechanism in the *in situ* heart was provided many years ago. For other postulated mechanisms the demonstrations are more recent or, in some cases, not yet quite satisfactory. For the most part, the demonstration of mechanisms for the *in situ* heart has depended on the development of suitable means to record cardiac

[a] Original studies were supported in part by Grants HL-08508, HL-12738, and HL 24354 from the National Heart, Lung and Blood Institute of the National Institutes of Health.

TABLE 1. Mechanisms for Cardiac Arrhythmias

---

I. Abnormal Impulse Generation
   A. Automatic
      1. Normal automaticity
      2. Abnormal automaticity
   B. Triggered
      1. Early afterdepolarizations
      2. Delayed afterdepolarizations

II. Abnormal Impulse Conduction
   A. Block
   B. Unidirectional Block and Reentry
      1. Circus movement
      2. Reflection

III. Simultaneous Abnormalities of Impulse Generation and Conduction

---

electrical activity and on the development of electrophysiologic tests that were appropriate in the sense that they could discriminate among the several mechanisms.

## REENTRANT ARRHYTHMIAS

Reentry as a cause of cardiac arrhythmias has been suspected since the studies of Mines and others,[6,7] and evidence that reentry caused by circus movement of excitation does in fact cause arrhythmias in experimental animals and humans is quite compelling. Lewis[8] provided suggestive evidence that circus movement around the cavae was responsible for induced atrial flutter in the normal dog heart, and Rosenblueth and Garcia-Ramos[9] provided much more convincing data in support of circus movement as the cause of atrial flutter in the dog that had been subjected to an intercaval crush. For the human heart, a number of clinical electrophysiologic studies clearly demonstrated that circus movement was the cause of tachyarrhythmias in patients with anomalous atrioventricular (AV) connections. Studies on the rabbit atrioventricular node with intracellular microelectrodes clearly demonstrated reentrant excitation as a possible cause for junctional tachyarrhythmias,[10] and studies on the human heart provided clear evidence that many atrial tachyarrhythmias resulted from AV nodal reentry.[11] D'Amato provided evidence of macro-reentry in the normal His-Purkinje system of the human heart[12] and subsequent studies that employed implanted electrodes in the dog heart confirmed the possibility of circus movement over the major subdivisions of the specialized ventricular conducting system.[13] Other studies have indicated strongly that the sinus node may be a site of reentrant excitation in both laboratory animals and man. Most recently, interest has focused on ventricular arrhythmias that result from myocardial infarction, and in both experimental animals and humans maps of excitation sequence have provided convincing evidence of reentry resulting from circus movement.[14–16] The demonstration that reentry can and does cause cardiac arrhythmias thus seems reasonably satisfying.

The major questions about reentrant excitation are concerned with the exact mechanism for reentry, the relationship between mechanism and identification by electrophysiologic tests, and the relationship between mechanism and response to antiarrhythmic interventions. Reentry implies the continuous propagation of the impulse, as, for example, around an anatomic barrier of inexcitable tissues. This form of reentry is properly described as circus movement. However, circus movement need not take place around a finite inexcitable barrier, as suggested by computer models and demonstrated in studies on isolated rabbit atrium by Allessie et al.[17] If conditions are suitable, the propagating impulse can create a region of inexcitability around which the impulse circulates in a continuous manner. This type of circus movement has been called the leading circle mechanism. As a mechanism for reentrant excitation, it differs in many ways from reentry around an anatomic barrier. Boyden has developed a canine model of atrial tachyarrhythmia caused by leading circle reentry.[18] In this model partial pulmonary constriction and tricuspid insufficiency are used to create right atrial enlargement. The right atrial enlargement is associated with no significant changes in cellular electrophysiology or ultrastructure other than some hypertrophy of the atrial muscle fibers. In the model, atrial overdrive and premature stimulation initiate a regular sustained atrial tachycardia that resembles flutter. Maps of the atrial excitation sequence during the arrhythmia have shown that the rapid rhythm results from reentrant excitation of the leading circle type (FIG. 1). In the dog, this type of reentrant excitation shows distinctly different responses to electrophysiologic tests and standard antiarrhythmic drugs than does reentry around an anatomic barrier. In general, electrophysiologic tests fail to demonstrate a significant excitable gap, and reset by premature stimuli or entrainment by overdrive is difficult. Also, termination by a premature stimulus is unlikely. At the same time, the arrhythmia is much less stable than that resulting from circus movement around an anatomic barrier (see below) in that spontaneous termination is highly likely and terminations by standard local anesthetic-type antiarrhythmic drugs are almost invariable.

We also have studied atrial flutter in chronically "instrumented" dogs after creating a lesion similar to that employed by Rosenblueth and Garcia-Ramos.[19,20] To create the needed susceptibility to circus movement and arrhythmia, the inter-

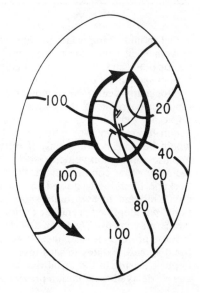

**FIGURE 1.** Excitation sequence of canine right atrium during atrial flutter in a dog with right atrial enlargement caused by chronic pulmonary constriction and tricuspid insufficiency. Map shows activation circulating around a normal area on the right atrial free wall. Activation times were determined from multiple simultaneous bipolar atrial electrograms.

caval tissue is incised and oversewn and then the incision extended toward the right atrial appendage. The induced arrhythmia in these dogs, termed RGR dogs, which has the electrocardiographic characteristics of flutter, satisfies all criteria for reentrant excitation due to circus movement (TABLE 2).

Several characteristics of this type of circus movement are of interest. Studies of atrial excitation sequence during the arrhythmia, both on the *in situ* heart and on the isolated supported heart, show that circus movement takes place in the tissues of the tricuspid ring and not around the cavae and the lesion between them. Recently, Page has studied the tricuspid ring isolated from the normal canine heart and shown that in it persistent circus movement can be initiated by burst-pacing or premature stimulation. The impulse propagates in fibers that are homogeneous in electrical characteristics and that generate typical fast-response atrial action potentials. This model of circus movement in the canine atrium thus permits characterization of a reentrant circuit with homogeneous electrophysiologic and anatomic properties. Preliminary studies on the *in situ* heart have demonstrated that there are reasonably predictable relationships between the effect of antiarrhythmic drugs on conduction velocity and the recovery of responsiveness, on one hand, and the rate of the arrhythmia, the duration of the excitable gap, and the likelihood of termination, on the other. Data obtained from studies on this

TABLE 2. Characteristics of Arrhythmia in RGR Dogs

1. Initiated by premature impulses
2. Initiated by rapid drive or burst pacing
3. Partially excitable gap demonstrable
4. Reset by premature impulses
5. Transient entrainment by overdrive
6. Fusion complexes during transient entrainment or with premature stimulation
7. Terminated by premature impulses
8. Terminated by overdrive or burst pacing
9. Demonstrable reentrant circuit with continuous activity

model should be important to our understanding of more complex paths for circus movement in which the tissues show electrophysiologic or anatomic abnormalities or both, and in which the impulse may be carried either by fast-response or slow-response action potentials or both.

For many years, the argument was presented that because of the reasonably rapid propagation of the cardiac impulse and the long duration of the cardiac refractory period, reentry due to circus movement could occur only if the path length for reentry was quite long. Circus movement around a very short path would become possible only if refractoriness were markedly abbreviated or if impulse conduction velocity were greatly decreased. Some years ago we studied the very slow conduction of slow responses in partially depolarized cardiac Purkinje fibers and showed that when the slow response carried the impulse, circus movement over quite short paths was possible.[21,22] In the same preparations, we identified reentrant excitation due to a mechanism quite distinct from circus movement. We termed this mechanism reflection.[2,4] With reflection the impulse propagates to an inexcitable site in the myocardium and, through electrotonic spread, excites tissues distal to the area of block after a delay. The new impulse arising in the distal tissues then generates an electrotonic potential that causes delayed reexcitation proximal to the area of inexcitability. Recent studies on isolated Purkinje fiber bundles in which a sucrose gap was used to cause an inexcitable segment[5] have provided a clear and detailed description of the nature and properties of reflected impulses.

These findings suggest that the behavior of a rhythm caused by reentry most likely will be influenced by the mechanism for reentry. In the case of circus movement, reentry due to the leading circle mechanism will differ from reentry due to circus movement around an anatomic barrier. Circus movement may result from the presence of tissues with unusual properties, as in reciprocating rhythms due to AV nodal reentry, anomalous AV pathways, or reentrant rhythms in the infarcted ventricle. Alternatively, the circus movement can take place in otherwise normal tissues with relatively uniform properties. Thus, an area of slow conduction and altered excitability may be present or absent. The circulating impulse may be a fast response, a slow response, or at times one and at times the other. An area of one-way block may be present only at the moment of initiation of the arrhythmia or at all times. Finally, reentry can result from reflection rather than from circus movement. Clearly studies designed to identify the cause of a particular reentrant rhythm in the *in situ* heart must take these problems into consideration. It seems likely that some of the apparently random differences in response to pacing protocols and antiarrhythmic and other drugs may in fact provide clues concerning the underlying mechanisms.

## AUTOMATIC RHYTHMS

Both normal and abnormal automaticity of cardiac fibers result from a similar change in the transmembrane potential of the automatic cells. In automatic cells, after completion of an action potential there is a slow depolarization that reduces the transmembrane potential towards the threshold value. This slow depolarization usually is called phase 4 depolarization. If, in given cell or in a group of cells, phase 4 depolarization brings the transmembrane potential to the threshold value with sufficient rapidity, a new response or action potential is initiated. Automaticity is a normal property of cells in the sinus node and of specialized cells in the atrium, AV junction, and His-Purkinje system. In contrast, atrial and ventricular muscle cells normally are not automatic. However, if atrial or ventricular muscle cells, or Purkinje fibers, are unable to repolarize fully, they may develop an abnormal form of automaticity. In this case, the maximum diastolic potential is reduced and each action potential is followed by slow depolarization during diastole that initiates spontaneous impulses at the threshold potential. It is very likely that the ionic bases for normal automaticity in Purkinje fibers and abnormal automaticity (in myocardial or Purkinje fibers) are quite different.[23] In spite of this, the time course of the change in the transmembrane potential is quite similar.

To demonstrate the presence of either normal or abnormal automatic activity in the *in situ* heart, it first was necessary to determine the nature and magnitude of the change in extracellular potential that resulted from the automatic activity of the pacemaker cells. This information was obtained some years ago through studies on the rabbit and canine sinus node.[24–26] The important consideration for these experiments was the realization that during the period of slow diastolic depolarization, and during the upstroke of the action potential in the pacemaker cells, electrical activity was not propagating. Under this condition one would expect the extracellular potential in the vicinity of the pacemaker cells to demonstrate a voltage–time course similar to that of the transmembrane potential of the

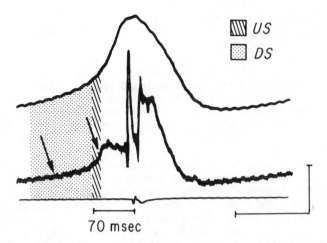

**FIGURE 2.** Transmembrane potential (**top trace**) and unipolar extracellular electrogram (**middle trace**) from the primary pacemaking area recorded simultaneously with a bipolar atrial electrogram (**bottom trace**). Diastolic slope (DS) and upstroke slope (US) are indicated by *arrows*. DS is within the *stippled area* and US is within the area indicated by *diagonal lines*. *Horizontal bar* is 150 msec and *vertical bar* corresponds to 35 mV for the transmembrane record and 25 $\mu$V for the unipolar electrogram. High-frequency components of the electrogram have been retouched for clarity.

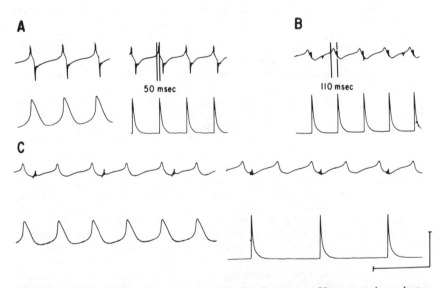

**FIGURE 3.** Effects of tetrodotoxin on the sinoatrial electrogram. **Upper trace** is an electrogram recorded at a fixed position over the sinoatrial pacemaker. **Bottom traces** are transmembrane potentials from either the sinoatrial pacemaker or an atrial trabeculum. *Horizontal bar* is 1000 msec and *vertical bar* corresponds to 100 mV for transmembrane potential and 200 $\mu$V for the electrogram.

pacemaker cells. In fact, as shown in FIGURE 2, high-gain, direct-coupled unipolar electrograms recorded from the vicinity of pacemaker cells in the rabbit or in the canine sinus node showed during normal sinus rhythm two distinct and characteristic deflections. During the diastolic interval there was a slow, negative-going deflection and then during the upstroke of the pacemaker cell action potential there was a more rapid negative-going deflection. This merged with a very large, rapid negative-going deflection when activity began to propagate in perinodal or atrial fibers. The two characteristic deflections in the unipolar electrogram were

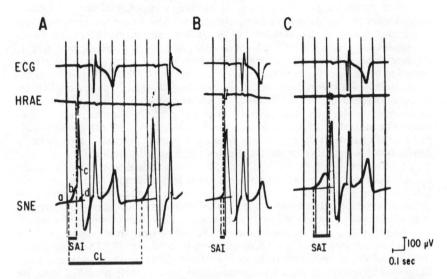

**FIGURE 4.** A record from a conscious dog showing, from *top to bottom,* inverted Z lead of the ECG, a high right atrial electrogram (HRAE), and sinus electrograms (SNE) recorded using AC amplifiers from site 7 (**A** and **C**) and site 8 (**B**). Each sinus electrogram in panel **A** shows a slow negative-going diastolic slope (a) and a slow negative-going upstroke slope (b) followed by rapid primary negativity (c). The sinoatrial interval (SAI) is measured from the point of departure of the upstroke slope from the line of trajectory of the diastolic slope (d) to the beginning of the primary negativity or the high right atrial electrogram. The cycle length (CL) of an automatic group is the interval between two consecutive points of departure of the upstroke slope from the trajectory of the diastolic slope. Note that with shorter (**B**) and longer (**C**) sinoatrial intervals, a less and more complete sinus potential can be seen. Voltage calibration is for sinus electrograms.

termed the diastolic slope and the upstroke slope. If the excitability of the atrium was abolished with tetrodotoxin, the unipolar electrogram recorded from the vicinity of sinus node pacemaker cells had the same configuration as the transmembrane action potential recorded from those cells (FIG. 3). The electrogram was much reduced in amplitude and opposite in polarity to the transmembrane potential. Under appropriate experimental conditions, electrograms recorded from Purkinje fiber bundles with abnormal automaticity showed similar diastolic and upstroke slopes. Subsequent studies (FIG. 4) showed that unipolar electrograms recorded from the *in situ* sinus node of canine[25,26] or human heart[27,28] also demonstrated the diastolic and upstroke slopes and that the presence of this typical electrogram configuration consistently identified automatic pacemakers.

Clinicians have experienced some difficulty in recording pacemaker activity from the sinus node through catheter electrodes for two reasons. First, the extracellular potential changes that result from phase 4 depolarization and phase 0 depolarization in the pacemaker cell group are small, in the range of 10 to 50 $\mu$V, and thus can easily be masked by larger changes in potential. At rapid heart rates, the masking potentials most likely will be the T and U deflections associated with the preceding cardiac cycle. Second, the extracellular potential changes characteristic of automatic pacemakers are slow changes in potential and must be recorded through amplifiers having an appropriately low frequency response. This requirement increases the likelihood of so-called baseline drift. Most clinical electrophysiologists have formed the habit of selectively filtering electrograms so as to eliminate undesired low-frequency components and to emphasize what are assumed to be the significant high-frequency components. Obviously this technique is not suitable for recording extracellular potential changes from automatic pacemakers. In spite of these difficulties, a number of groups have succeeded in identifying the diastolic and upstroke slopes in records from the human sinus node. The suitability of the technique to identify and localize ectopic automatic pacemakers has been shown through records of ectopic automatic activity in the canine heart recorded from atrium, His bundle, and AV junction.[29,30]

As stated earlier, the extracellular electrogram recorded from automatic pacemakers does not discriminate between normal and abnormal automaticity. For this reason, it is necessary to use additional tests to characterize the mechanism for an automatic rhythm in the *in situ* heart. Two means show reasonable promise of providing the necessary ability to discriminate. First, the responses of normally automatic foci to overdrive pacing differ quite consistently from responses of foci in which automaticity results from the abnormal mechanism.[23,31] The normal automaticity of either the sinus node or the His-Purkinje system[32] is significantly depressed by overdrive pacing at a suitable rate for a suitable period of time. We contrasted the response of automatic pacemakers with three levels of maximum diastolic potential to overdrive pacing, and have shown that whereas overdrive suppression of normal automaticity in canine Purkinje fibers bears a predictable relationship to the rate and duration of overdrive, abnormally automatic fibers with maximum diastolic potentials less than $-60$ mV almost never show overdrive suppression regardless of the duration or rate of overdrive.[31] Indeed, often minor enhancement of automaticity follows the period of overdrive. In fibers with intermediate levels of maximum diastolic potential, the response to overdrive is one of slight suppression of automaticity. These data are shown graphically in FIGURE 5.

Finally, the use of selected antiarrhythmic drugs probably can aid in differentiation between normal and abnormal automaticity as a cause of a sustained ectopic rhythm. Some local anesthetic antiarrhythmic drugs cause a clear dose-dependent suppression of normal phase 4 depolarization in specialized fibers.[33] Other drugs that exert similar effects on phase 0 and phases 2 and 3 of the action potential do not depress phase 4 depolarization in normally polarized Purkinje fibers.[34,35] The latter type of the drug may, however, be quite effective in slowing or suppressing abnormal automaticity regardless of its immediate cause. Ilvento et al. have used the response to overdrive and the responses to either ethmozin or lidocaine to characterize normally automatic and abnormally automatic ventricular rhythms in dogs with surgically induced heart block.[36] Rapid rhythms that did not show overdrive suppression were slowed significantly by ethmozin, but not by lidocaine. Slow rhythms that showed clear overdrive suppression were slowed significantly by lidocaine, but not by ethmozin. It seems likely that the actions of other selected antiarrhythmic drugs may provide a more consistent and precise separation between arrhythmias resulting from normal and abnormal automaticity. In general, abnormal automaticity is not markedly suppressed by the usual concentrations of drugs like lidocaine, procainamide, and quinidine. If maximum diastolic potential (MDP) in the abnormally automatic focus is positive to −60 mV, the slow-channel blocking drugs, like verapamil and nifedipine, should be effective in slowing or terminating the ectopic rhythm. These agents also would be

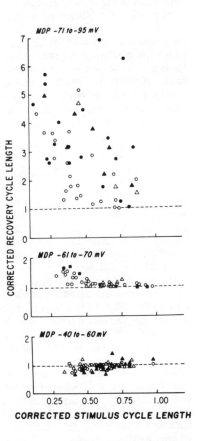

**FIGURE 5.** Effects of overdrive stimulation on the automatic activity of preparations with high potential automaticity (**upper panel**), intermediate potential automaticity (**middle panel**) and low potential automaticity (**lower panel**). Each symbol represents the results of one overdrive stimulus train on a preparation with a pacemaker maximal diastolic potential (MDP) in the range indicated. *Solid symbols* show results of 30-beat stimulus trains; *open symbols* show the results of 15-sec stimulus trains. *Circles* represent data from false tendon preparations; *triangles* represent data from infarct zone preparations; and *squares* represent data from right bundle branch preparations.

effective against some forms of triggered rhythms, which are discussed in the subsequent section.

One should not ignore the effects of the autonomic mediators, acetylcholine and norepinephrine, on normally and abnormally automatic foci. For the atrium, one would obviously expect the rhythm to slow dramatically under the influence of acetylcholine and to accelerate under the influence of norepinephrine, and thus to mimic the response of the normally automatic sinus rhythm. For the ventricle, however, some discrimination is provided in that acetylcholine typically slows and suppresses abnormally automatic rhythms in Purkinje fibers if MDP is positive to −60 mV. Since acetylcholine has only trivial effects on normal phase 4 depolarization in Purkinje fibers at normal resting potential, the response of the abnormally automatic focus most likely results from a decrease in slow inward current caused by the parasympathetic transmitter.

In summary, means are available to directly demonstrate automatic impulse origin in atrium or ventricle by recording suitable unipolar electrograms. The responses to overdrive stimulation differ between normally automatic and abnormally automatic foci as do the responses to selected antiarrhythmic agents. Use of these three techniques should permit the identification of automatic rhythms of both types in the *in situ* heart and the characterization of automaticity as resulting from a normal or abnormal mechanism. Limitations on the usefulness of these techniques will be imposed by the nature of the coupling between the automatic focus and the remainder of the heart. Exit block obviously will limit the degree to which the electrocardiogram can be used to determine the rate of the automatic focus and its response to interventions. Entry block necessarily will influence the effect of overdrive on the automatic focus. Finally, changes in coupling can modify the rate or rhythm of the automatic pacemaker cells. In spite of these difficulties it seems likely that means are available to characterize most cases of automatic rhythms.

## TRIGGERED ARRHYTHMIAS

The term "triggered activity" denotes a second type of spontaneous impulse initiation, distinct from automaticity, that may cause ectopic arrhythmias. "Triggering" is repetitive firing of the heart that occurs as a consequence of depolarizing afterpotentials.[3] Two types of depolarizing afterpotentials have been recognized: "early afterdepolarizations" (EAD) occur during phase 2 or 3 of the action potential, and "delayed afterdepolarizations" (DAD) occur during phase 4. Depolarizing afterpotentials, by definition, are not caused either by automatic activity or by reentrant activity (circus movement of conducted impulses). The action potentials occurring in a triggered fiber can resemble those of an automatic (pacemaker) cell in that, during triggered activity, rapid diastolic depolarization will occur and will gradually and smoothly lead to the upstroke of the next action potential. However, triggered activity differs from automaticity in that triggered cells can remain quiescent for protracted periods of time; triggered activity is initiated only by afterdepolarizations that occur when the cell has been activated one or more times. Triggered activity can resemble reentrant activity in that both can be initiated or terminated by premature stimuli or overdrive stimulation. Triggered and reentrant activity are different, however, in that triggering can be a focal event (occurring in a small group of cells). In contrast, reentry requires a site of unidirectional conduction block and an adjacent anatomic pathway over which slow conduction can occur to allow persistence of the initiating impulse until the end of the refractory period in the fibers proximal to the site of block. Thus, triggered activity in the *in situ* heart may functionally resemble reentrant activity, but each has different geometric requirements.

The existence of oscillatory (depolarizing) afterpotentials in isolated cardiac tissues was demonstrated more than 40 years ago,[37–41] and it has long been argued that many types of extrasystoles, both in experimental animals and humans, are in fact caused by such afterpotentials.[42] More recently, it has been suggested that afterdepolarizations are responsible for several types of arrhythmias: (1) Accelerated junctional escape rhythms may be produced by DADs after digitalis treatment[43]; (2) multifocal ventricular tachycardias in the canine heart 24 hours after coronary ligation have been attributed to DADs[44] occurring in the subendocardial Purkinje fibers surviving over the infarct zone; and (3) coupled ventricular extrasystoles in the dog with bradycardia can be induced by EADS engendered by treatment with N-acetyl procainamide[35] or by cesium chloride.[45]

However, at present, the causative role of afterdepolarizations in cardiac arrhythmias is still inferential. No direct evidence demonstrating the occurrence of delayed or early afterdepolarizations at the appropriate moments during arrhythmias in the *in situ* heart has yet been presented. It is quite feasible to record unipolar electrograms in the appropriate frequency range (0–1000 Hz) from isolated tissues producing early or delayed afterdepolarizations.[35,46] These unipolar electrograms indicate that distinct, low-amplitude extracellular potential changes occur as a consequence of the afterdepolarizations. The successful recording of such deflections in any of the experimental models of "triggered" arrhythmias that occur in the hearts of experimental animals has not yet been reported. Indeed, convincing evidence of this kind will be difficult to obtain in the intact heart. Because triggered beats presumably originate in ectopic foci of limited (anatomic) size, the likelihood of recording extracellular waveforms from "relevant" afterdepolarizations via a randomly placed recording lead is small. Ideally, it would be useful to first determine the activation sequence of the triggered beats and identify very precisely the ectopic focus. If the focus is found to be accessible, the unipolar recording lead would then have to be brought within a few millimeters of it to detect the afterpotentials. Then, the arrhythmia would have to be initiated and terminated. Presumably, the recording would reveal a "pacemaker slope" prior to the "upstroke slope" during sustained triggered activity, similar to the pattern seen in preparations with automatic activity.[24] Low-amplitude deflections characteristic of afterdepolarizations would presumably be detected at the end of a series of triggered beats or after a stimulus regime that was just under the "threshold" for eliciting triggered extrasystoles.

The experimental evidence outlined above would exclude macroscopic reentry as a cause of the arrhythmia on the basis of its genesis in a single focus and on the presence of a pacemaker slope in this focus during sustained activity. Moreover, the presence of afterdepolarizations (at the appropriate coupling intervals) when triggered beats did not occur would exclude automaticity with conduction block as a cause for these arrhythmias. However, it still might be difficult to exclude the possibility that these "triggered" arrhythmias could be arising as a result of reflection or microreentry. As shown by Antzelevitch *et al.*,[5] it is possible for the site of origin of a reflected beat (in the normal tissue on the proximal side of an inexcitable gap) to have apparent phase 4 depolarization induced by electrotonus. It was suggested that such sites of reflection can produce bursts of extrasystoles as well as single premature depolarizations. If so, this reflected activity might well appear to be triggered if recordings were taken from only one site (near the proximal side of the gap). During paroxysmal tachycardia, this site could show phase 4 depolarization, and after the termination of the arrhythmia, the final (electrotonic) reflection might appear in the recording as a subthreshold "afterpotential."

It might still be possible to discriminate between reflection and triggering as the cause of paroxysmal tachyarrhythmia. If the spread of the premature impulses were mapped, and it were found that activation spread radially from a discrete focus, it would have to be assumed that the arrhythmia was most likely triggered. If, on the other hand, a "dead" area or site of conduction block were found directly adjacent to the focus, this would suggest that microreentry or reflection could be the cause of the arrhythmia.

Further data will be needed before it will be possible to design tests to discriminate between triggering and reflection as the cause of an arrhythmia in the *in situ* heart. Such better tests might be based on the responses of triggered or reflected/microreentrant tachycardias to overdrive stimulation or to single premature stimuli.

## COMMENTS

A variety of experimental models of arrhythmias have been developed to mimic those that occur clinically. Insights into the electrophysiologic mechanisms of these arrhythmias are largely based on data from microelectrode studies on isolated, superfused cardiac tissues, or from theoretical considerations. Conclusive proof as to the causes of most of these experimental arrhythmias is still lacking. If it is possible to develop techniques to do detailed on-line mapping of the sequence of activation of the heart during extrasystoles, and to record local electrical activity from the ectopic foci of interest during these extrasystoles, it may be possible to generate appropriate evidence as to the causes of arrhythmias.

The main reason to determine the electrophysiologic mechanism of a given arrhythmia is, of course, to make pharmacotherapy less empiric, and more rational and predictable. We must recognize that ultimately it may not be necessary to determine the precise mechanism of the arrhythmia in order to provide rational drug treatment. This is so because it is quite likely that the ionic currents in the cells responsible for an arrhythmia, and thus the drugs to which the arrhythmia would respond, would be determined as much (or more) by the maximum diastolic potential of the "focus" or the "slow conduction pathway" as by the "electrophysiological mechanism of the arrhythmia." That is, we deem it likely that similar currents will be found to be involved in the generation of impulses in fibers with maximum diastolic potentials positive to $-60$ mV: this would include arrhythmias produced by abnormal automaticity, by triggered activity at the low level of membrane potential (by either early or delayed afterdepolarizations), or by slow conduction in partially depolarized tissues. It is likely that in arrhythmias caused by each of these mechanisms a drug that decreased slow inward current or enhanced outward current at this potential level would obtund or abolish the ectopic activity. Likewise, arrhythmias caused by similar mechanisms (automaticity, triggering, or reentry), in which the maximum diastolic potentials in the cells of the critical foci were more negative, could be expected to respond to different classes of agents (such as local anesthetics) due to the contribution, during the genesis of these impulses, of some "fast" sodium current.

Thus, it may prove most useful to determine the maximum diastolic potential at critical sites in the arrhythmic heart, and thereby the ionic currents that are supporting the arrhythmogenic (electrophysiologic) mechanisms. This may prove to be the essential information necessary for rational selection of an antiarrhythmic drug.

## REFERENCES

1. HOFFMAN, B. F. & M. R. ROSEN. 1981. Cellular mechanisms for cardiac arrhythmias. Circ. Res. **49:** 69–83.
2. CRANEFIELD, P. F. 1975. The Slow Response and Cardiac Arrhythmias. Futura Press. Mt. Kisco, NY.

3. CRANEFIELD, P. F. 1977. Action potentials, afterpotentials and arrhythmias. Circ. Res. 41: 415–423.
4. WIT, A. L., B. F. HOFFMAN & P. F. CRANEFIELD. 1972. Slow conduction and reentry in the ventricular conducting system. I. Return extrasystole in canine Purkinje fibers. Circ. Res. 30: 1–10.
5. ANTZELEVITCH, C., J. JALIFE & G. K. MOE. 1980. Characteristics of reflection as a mechanism of reentrant arrhythmias and its relationship to parasystole. Circulation 61: 182–191.
6. MINES, G. R. 1914. On circulating excitations in heart muscle and their possible relation to tachycardia and fibrillation. Trans. R. Soc. Can. Ser. 3, Sect IV 8: 43–52.
7. GARREY, W. E. 1914. The nature of fibrillary contraction of the heart. Its relation to tissue mass and form. Am. J. Physiol. 33: 397–414.
8. LEWIS, T., et al. 1918–1921. Observations upon flutter and fibrillation. Parts I–IX. Heart 7: 127–130, 191–346; 8: 37–58, 83–228.
9. ROSENBLUETH, A. & J. GARCIA RAMOS. 1947. Studies on flutter and fibrillation. II. The influence of artificial obstacles on experimental auricular flutter. Am. Heart J. 33: 677–684.
10. JANSE, M. J., F. J. L. VAN CAPELLE, G. E. FREUD & D. DURRER. 1971. Circus movement within the A-V node as a basis for supraventricular tachycardia as shown by multiple microelectrode recordings in the isolated rabbit heart. Circ. Res. 28: 403–414.
11. BIGGER, J. T., JR., & B. N. GOLDREYER. 1970. The mechanism of paroxysmal supraventricular tachycardia in man. Circulation 42: 673–688.
12. KOSOWSKY, B. D., J. I. HAFT, E. STEIN & A. N. DAMATO. 1968. The effects of digitalis on atrioventricular conduction in man. Am. Heart J. 75: 736–742.
13. LYONS, C. J. & M. J. BURGESS. 1979. Demonstration of re-entry within the canine specialized conduction system. Am. Heart J. 98: 595–603.
14. JANSE, M. J. J., F. J. L. VAN CAPELLE, H. MORSINK, et al. 1980. Flow of "injury" current and patterns of excitation during early ventricular arrhythmias in acute regional myocardial ischemia in isolated porcine and canine hearts: evidence for two different arrhythmogenic mechanisms. Circ. Res. 47: 151–165.
15. WIT, A. L., M. A. ALLESSIE, F. I. M. BONKE, W. LAMMERS, J. SMEETS & J. J. FENOGLIO, JR. 1982. Electrophysiologic mapping to determine the mechanism of experimental ventricular tachycardia initiated by premature impulses. Am. J. Cardiol. 49: 166–185.
16. HOROWITZ, L. N., M. E. JOSEPHSON & A. H. HARKEN. 1980. Epicardial and endocardial activation during sustained ventricular tachycardia in man. Circulation 61: 1227–1238.
17. ALLESSIE, M. A., F. I. M. BONKE & F. J. G. SCHOPMAN. 1977. The "leading circle" concept: A new model of circus movement in cardiac tissue without the involvement of an anatomical obstacle. Circ. Res. 41: 9–19.
18. BOYDEN, P. A. & B. F. HOFFMAN. 1981. The effects on atrial electrophysiology and structure of surgically induced right atrial enlargement in dogs. Circ. Res. 49: 1319–1331.
19. FRAME, L. H., R. L. PAGE, P. A. BOYDEN & B. F. HOFFMAN. 1983. A right atrial incision that stabilizes reentry around the tricuspid ring in dogs. Circulation 48(4): III–361.
20. FRAME, L. H., R. L. PAGE, & B. F. HOFFMAN. 1983. Characterization of a model for reentrant excitation around a fixed barrier. Circulation 48(4): III–219.
21. WIT, A. L., P. F. CRANEFIELD & B. F. HOFFMAN. 1972. Slow conduction and reentry in the ventricular conducting system. II. Single and sustained circus movement in networks of canine and bovine Purkinje fibers. Circ. Res. 30: 11–22.
22. WIT, A. L. & P. F. CRANEFIELD. 1978. Reentrant excitation as a cause of cardiac arrhythmias. Am. J. Physiol. 235: H1–H17.
23. HOFFMAN, B. F. & K. H. DANGMAN. 1982. Are arrhythmias caused by automatic impulse generation? In The Symposium on Normal and Abnormal Conduction of the Heart Beat. A. Paes de Carvalho, B. F. Hoffman & M. Lieberman, Eds.: 429–448. Futura Press. Mt. Kisco, NY.

24. CRAMER, M., M. SIEGAL, J. T. BIGGER & B. F. HOFFMAN. 1977. Characteristics of extracellular potentials from the sinoatrial pacemaker of the rabbit heart. Circ. Res. **41:** 292–300.
25. HARIMAN, R. J., B. F. HOFFMAN & R. E. NAYLOR. 1980. Electrical activity from the sinus node region in conscious dogs. Circ. Res. **47:** 775–791.
26. CRAMER, M., R. J. HARIMAN, R. BOXER, & B. F. HOFFMAN. 1978. Electrograms from the canine sinoatrial pacemaker recorded in vitro and in situ. Am. J. Cardiol. **42:** 939–946.
27. HARIMAN, R. J., E. KRONGRAD, R. A. BOXER, M. B. WEISS, C. N. STEEG & B. F. HOFFMAN. 1980. A method for recording electrical activity of the sinoatrial node and automatic atrial foci during cardiac catheterization in humans. Am. J. Cardiol. **45:** 775–780.
28. REIFFEL, J. A., E. GANG, J. GLIKLICH, M. B. WEISS, J. C. DAVIS, J. N. PATTON & J. T. BIGGER, JR. 1980. The human sinus node electrogram: A transvenous catheter technique and a comparison of directly measured and indirectly estimated sinoatrial conduction time in adults. Circulation **62:** 1324–1334.
29. HARIMAN, R. J., W. B. GOUGH, J. A. C. GOMES & N. EL-SHERIF. 1983. Recording of diastolic slope in a canine model of automatic and unifocal ventricular tachycardia. J. Am. Coll. Cardiol. **1:** 731.
30. HARIMAN, R. J. & C. M. CHEN. 1983. Recording of diastolic slope from the junctional area in dogs with junctional rhythm. Circulation **68:** 636–643.
31. DANGMAN, K. H. & B. F. HOFFMAN. 1983. Studies on overdrive stimulation of canine cardiac Purkinje fibers: Maximal diastolic potential as a determinant of the response. J. Am. Coll. Cardiol. **2:** 1183–1190.
32. VASSALLE, M. 1977. The relationship among cardiac pacemakers. Overdrive suppression. Circ. Res. **41:** 269–277.
33. BIGGER, J. T., JR., & B. F. HOFFMAN. 1980. Antiarrhythmic drugs. *In* The Pharmacological Basis of Therapeutics. A. G. Gilman, L. S. Goodman & A. Gilman, Eds.: 761–792. Macmillan. New York, NY.
34. DANGMAN, K. H. & B. F. HOFFMAN. 1980. Effects of nifedipine on electrical activity of cardiac cells. Am. J. Cardiol. **46:** 1059–1067.
35. DANGMAN, K. H. & B. F. HOFFMAN. 1981. In vivo and in vitro antiarrhythmic and arrhythmogenic effects of N-acetyl procainamide. J. Pharmacol. Exp. Ther. **217:** 851–862.
36. ILVENTO, J. P., J. PROVET, P. DANILO & M. R. ROSEN. 1982. Fast and slow idioventricular rhythms in the canine heart: A study of their mechanism using antiarrhythmic drugs and electrophysiologic testing. Am. J. Cardiol. **49:** 1909–1916.
37. SEEGERS, M. 1940. La réaction repetitive du coeur. C. R. Soc. Biol. **133:** 460–461.
38. SEEGERS, M. 1940. L'accommodation du rythme cardiaque. Arch. Int. Physiol. **50:** 277–308.
39. SEEGERS, M. 1941. Le rôle des potentiels tardifs du coeur. Mem. Acad. R. Med. Belg (series II) **1:** 1–30.
40. SEEGERS, M. 1947. Le battement auto-entretenu du coeur. Arch. Int. Pharmacodyn **75:** 144–156.
41. BOZLER, E. 1943. The initiation of impulses in cardiac muscle. Am. J. Physiol. **138:** 273–282.
42. SCHERF, D. & A. SCHOTT. 1953. Extrasystoles and Allied Arrhythmias. Heinemann Medical Books. Melbourne, Australia.
43. ROSEN, M. R., C. FISCH, B. F. HOFFMAN, P. DANILO, JR., D. E. LOVELACE & S. B. KNOEBEL. 1980. Can accelerated atrioventricular junctional escape rhythms be explained by delayed afterdepolarizations? Am. J. Cardiol. **45:** 1272–1284.
44. EL-SHERIF, N., W. B. GOUGH, R. H. ZEILER & R. MEHRA. 1983. Triggered ventricular rhythms in 1-day-old myocardial infarction in the dog. Circ. Res. **52:** 566–579.
45. BRACHMANN, J., B. J. SCHERLAG, L. V. ROSENSHTRAUKH & R. LAZZARA. 1983. Bradycardia-dependent triggered activity: Relevance to drug-induced multiform ventricular tachycardia. Circulation **68:** 846–856.
46. CRAMER, M., L. MARY-RABINE, A. WIT & B. F. HOFFMAN. 1977. Extracellular potentials produced by delayed afterdepolarizations. Circulation **56** (Suppl II): 302.

# The Cellular Mechanisms of Cardiac Antiarrhythmic Drug Action[a]

OFER BINAH[b] AND MICHAEL R. ROSEN[c,d]

[b]Departments of Physiology and Biophysics
Rappaport Institute for Research in Medical Sciences
Haifa, Israel

[c]Departments of Pharmacology and Pediatrics
College of Physicians & Surgeons
Columbia University
New York, New York 10032

In the following pages we will consider the actions of antiarrhythmic drugs in light of the mechanisms that are thought to be responsible for cardiac arrhythmias. It is not our purpose to provide an encyclopedic review of the effects of antiarrhythmic agents, but rather to use specific drugs to provide an example of the mechanisms of drug action. For more complete reviews of the actions of antiarrhythmic drugs, readers are referred to References 1–3.

As has been reviewed in the first two papers in this volume, cardiac arrhythmias may result from abnormalities of impulse initiation or impulse propagation.

## ABNORMALITIES OF IMPULSE INITIATION

The mechanisms for abnormal impulse initiation are automaticity and afterdepolarization.[4]

### Automaticity

We will use the ventricular specialized conducting system as an example here. In the normal specialized conducting system fibers may depolarize spontaneously during phase 4, or electrical diastole, thereby attaining threshold potential and inducing spontaneous action potentials.[5,6] In normal Purkinje fibers, at high levels of membrane potential (approximately −90 mV), automatic rhythms are characterized by a slow rate—usually less than 40 beats per minute—and by the ability to be "overdrive-suppressed."[4]

At very low levels of membrane potential ($\sim < -60$ mV) a more rapid automatic rhythm is seen. This can occur not only in specialized conducting fibers, but also in myocardial fibers, and appears to result from inward current that is carried by calcium and/or sodium during phase 4.[7,8] This automatic rhythm tends not to be suppressible after short periods of overdrive; however, after 3 or more minutes

[a] Certain of the studies referred to were supported by Grants HL28223, HL23358, and HL28958 from the National Heart, Lung, and Blood Institute of the National Institutes of Health, and by a grant from the Rothschild Foundation.
[d] To whom correspondence should be addressed.

31

of overdrive it may be suppressed. At intermediate levels of membrane potential the ability to suppress automatic rhythms through overdrive appears to vary between the two extremes mentioned above.[9,10]

It is reasonable to assume that many automatic tachyarrhythmias result from the form of automaticity that occurs at low membrane potentials. We state this because of the inability of normal Purkinje fibers to attain rates much faster than 40 beats per minute in the absence of catecholamines and much faster than 80 to 100 beats per minute in the presence of catecholamines. In contrast, abnormally automatic fibers at low membrane potentials can attain rates approaching 200 beats per minute in the presence of catecholamines. There are a number of means whereby antiarrhythmic drugs might modify such automatic rhythms; these are summarized in FIGURE 1. The rate at which the automatic focus fires (whether it is a normal or an abnormally automatic mechanism) is primarily dependent on three factors: (1) the level of maximum diastolic potential at which phase 4 depolarization is initiated; (2) the slope of phase 4 depolarization; and (3) the threshold potential that must be attained before the next action potential can be initiated.

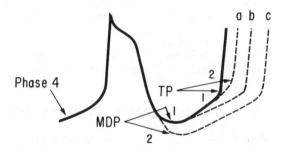

**FIGURE 1.** Schematic representation of the transmembrane potential of an automatic fiber (*solid line*) and the means (*broken line*) by which an antiarrhythmic drug can modify automaticity: **a** indicates a shift in threshold potential (TP$_1$) towards zero membrane potential (TP$_2$); **b** shows the effect of decreasing the slope of phase 4 depolarization; **c** shows displacement of the maximum diastolic potential (MDP1) to more negative values (MDP2).

Any intervention that moves membrane and threshold potentials closer to one another or increases the slope of phase 4 depolarization would tend to accelerate automatic rhythms. Any intervention that either (1) moves maximum diastolic potential in a more negative direction, (2) moves threshold potential in a more positive direction, and/or (3) decreases the slope of phase 4 depolarization would tend to decrease automatic rate and suppress an arrhythmia. We will now provide examples of each of these three interventions. Several drugs have been shown to increase the level of maximum diastolic potential of automatic fibers; these drugs include lidocaine, propranolol, and phenytoin.[11-13] During superfusion with any of these drugs, fibers at low levels of membrane potential and showing an abnormal automatic mechanism may be hyperpolarized and show a decrease in automatic rate or a cessation of the automatic rhythm altogether. An example of a drug that moves threshold potential to a more positive voltage is provided by quinidine.[3] As a result of quinidine's action on threshold potential, an automatic fiber will require more time to attain threshold, and spontaneous rate will be slowed. Finally, many antiarrhythmic drugs decrease the slope of phase 4 depolarization of normal cardiac fibers; such drugs include quinidine,[14] lidocaine,[15,16] and, if catecholamine is contributing to the slope of phase 4, beta blockers.[17] It is important to stress that the ability of beta blockers to modify automatic activity is dependent on the magnitude of preexisting catecholamine effects.

Even if a drug does not modify automatic impulse initiation by an effect on maximum diastolic potential, on threshold potential, or on the slope of phase 4, the drug still may modify the expression of the rhythm through its ability to alter propagation. For example, if the rate of firing of an automatic focus is unchanged by a drug, but the drug blocks conduction of the automatic impulses from the ectopic focus to the remainder of the heart, then it will have an antiarrhythmic effect. An example of this type of effect is provided by lidocaine,[18] which has been shown to induce conduction block even in instances where it does not appear to decrease the rate of the automatic focus. Similarly, any drug that increases the duration of refractoriness (such as quinidine[19]) would tend to increase the block of some very premature depolarizations induced by an automatic mechanism.

### Afterdepolarizations and Triggered Activity

Two types of afterdepolarizations have been described: early and delayed. Early afterdepolarizations are in some instances difficult to differentiate from automatic activity. They occur as oscillations interrupting phase 2 or phase 3 of repolarization and result in action potentials that fire at rapid rates. The resultant rhythms are referred to as "triggered." There are several ways in which early afterdepolarization-induced rhythms can be modified. Both lidocaine and procainamide[20] have been shown to repolarize fibers having early afterdepolarization-induced triggered activity, as shown in FIGURE 2. As a result of this repolarization, the membrane is returned to a normal level of membrane potential and the triggered activity ceases. Drugs that depress the slow inward current carried by calcium also can suppress early afterdepolarization-induced rhythms, as has been demonstrated with verapamil.

Delayed afterdepolarizations are oscillations in membrane potential that follow full repolarization.[21] When they attain threshold, they induce triggered arrhythmias whose rate tends to increase as the preceding drive rate increases. In studies of Purkinje fibers in which delayed afterdepolarizations and triggered activity were induced by digitalis, drugs that depress inward sodium current, such as lidocaine,[22] or that depress inward calcium current, such as verapamil,[22] were shown to depress the afterdepolarizations and the arrhythmia. In contrast, beta blockade has been shown to depress delayed afterdepolarizations and triggered activity only when the afterdepolarizations were induced by a combination of digitalis and catecholamine.[23] That agents having disparate mechanisms of action suppress the afterdepolarizations is not surprising given the mechanism for delayed afterdepolarizations. They are thought to result from an overload of intracellular calcium released from the sarcoplasmic reticulum.[24] This increases the monovalent cation conductance of the cell membrane, resulting in an oscillatory inward current carried in the main by sodium.[24] This information suggests that delayed afterdepolarizations might be suppressible by any agents that either decrease inward current carried by sodium or calcium and/or that increase repolarizing current that is carried by potassium.

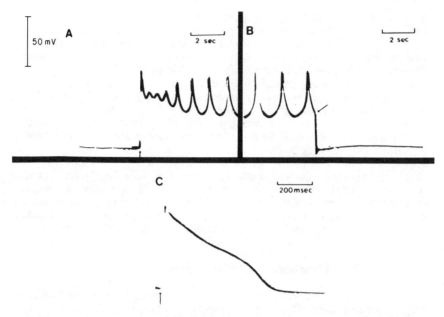

**FIGURE 2.** The effect of lidocaine on sustained rhythmic activity induced by early afterdepolarizations in a sheep cardiac Purkinje fiber. During control (panels **A** and **B**) a driven action potential is followed by an oscillatory activity, which gives rise to sustained nondriven action potentials (**A**). The rhythmic activity terminates only after an intracellular hyperpolarizing current pulse is applied (*arrow* in **B**). After lidocaine, 5 μg/ml, is added (panel **C**), the normal repolarization phase of the action potential is almost completely restored and oscillatory and triggered activity cease. (From Arnsdorf.[20] Reproduced by permission.)

## ABNORMALITIES OF IMPULSE PROPAGATION

FIGURE 3 shows the model for reentry described by Schmitt and Erlanger.[25] In this model there are several prerequisites for reentry. There must be a site of unidirectional conduction block and a pathway for retrograde propagation of the impulse. Moreover, the impulse must propagate sufficiently slowly along this pathway that refractoriness can terminate in those tissues into which the impulse is propagating. Hence, the crucial conditions are of timing, conduction velocity, and termination of refractoriness, and, if these are not met, there cannot be reentry.[26,27]

There are several means by which a drug might terminate such reentrant rhythms. One is by altering cardiac rate. If rate changes, several changes in the reentrant pathway can occur, as shown in FIGURE 4. In panel A, the fibers are undergoing phase 4 depolarization; there is slow conduction through a depressed segment and reentry. In panel B, as a result of drug effect sinus rate has slowed. Depending on the effect of the drug on phase 4 depolarization, one of two possible effects on conduction may be seen. If phase 4 is unchanged, the membrane may be further depolarized when the action potential is initiated, and as a result conduction may slow further or may fail completely. On the other hand, if the drug depresses phase 4 depolarization and hyperpolarizes the fiber, conduction velocity may increase. In either case, regardless of the effect of the drug on phase 4, the slowing of sinus rate will be followed by a prolongation of repolarization and refractoriness.[28] Hence, as sinus rate decreases, the determinants of both conduction velocity and refractoriness may change and the critical timing that is essential for reentry may no longer occur. The result is cessation of the arrhythmia.

Another possibility is shown in panel C of FIGURE 4. Here an increase in sinus rate occurs and repolarization is accelerated. Moreover, the action potential is initiated at an increased level of membrane potential and as a result it may propagate more rapidly. As a result, the timing requirements for reentry again may not be met and the arrhythmia may cease.

Considering the profound effects that changes in cardiac rate may have on the relationship of conduction velocity and refractoriness that is required for reentry, there are many ways in which pharmacologic agents can modify rate and as a result the reentrant rhythm. Beta blocking drugs such as propranolol, which reduce sympathetic effects on the sinus node, may decrease cardiac rate, thereby inducing cessation of reentrant rhythms.[28] Similarly, slow channel blockers, such as verapamil[29] or nifedipine,[30] can decrease the rate of impulse initiation through depression of phase 4 depolarization in the sinus node. Drugs such as edrophonium[14] which increase vagal effects on the heart may decrease the slope of phase 4 depolarization and the rate of impulse initiation in the sinus node, while vagolytic drugs such as atropine may speed sinus rate.

In addition, antiarrhythmic drugs may suppress reentry even if they do not change overall heart rate. To demonstrate how such drug actions may occur let us consider FIGURE 5. There are several assumptions that have to be made in reviewing this figure, the first of which is that in much of the heart there are normal action potentials, but in the depressed segment there are action potentials having characteristics of the slow response. Another assumption is that there are areas of

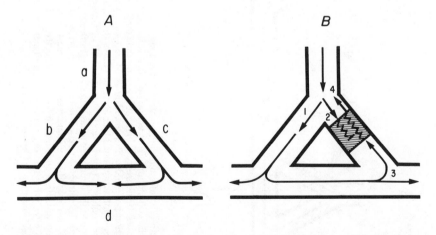

**FIGURE 3.** A model for reentry as suggested by Schmitt and Erlanger.[25] In panel **A**, a normal action potential propagates from the distal Purkinje system (a) through terminal Purkinje fiber branches (b and c) to activate the myocardium (d). In panel **B**, the conditions for reentrant excitation are shown. The antegrade propagation (2) in limb c encounters a depressed area (*crosshatching*) and is blocked. The normal propagation through limb b (1) activates the myocardium, invades the depressed area in a retrograde direction (3), and, after slowly propagating, reactivates the proximal conducting system (4).

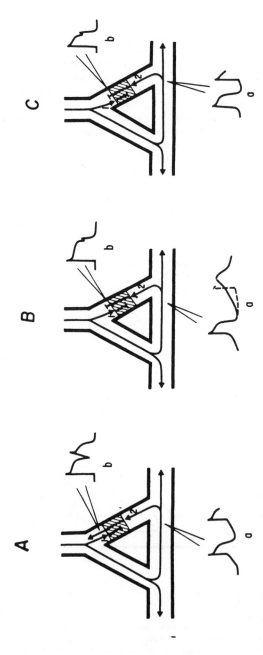

**FIGURE 4.** The means of modifying reentry by changing heart rate. In panel **A**, a model for reentry is shown (details are shown in FIGURE 3). Whereas antegrade conduction of the action potential is blocked in the depressed area (1), the impulse proceeding through the left limb and the myocardium crosses the depressed segment in a retrograde direction (2) and reexcites the proximal conducting system. At site a in the pathway is a nonautomatic action potential with marked phase 4 depolarization and at site b proximal to the depressed area an antegrade action potential followed by a reentrant action potential. Panel **B** shows the result of a slowing of cardiac rate. An antiarrhythmic drug can slow rate without affecting the slope of phase 4 (*solid trace*). This will result in a more positive activation voltage and slowed conduction which may lead to a block of further propagation to the depressed area. When a drug both slows rate and depresses the slope of phase 4 (*broken trace*), conduction velocity may increase such that the retrograde action potential will arrive at site b before its refractory period has terminated. In panel **C**, as heart rate is increased, conduction velocity is also increased as phase 4 is "overdrive-suppressed." Although the increase in heart rate is associated with an acceleration of repolarization and shortening of the effective refractory period, reentry will still terminate since the relationship between conduction velocity and effective refractory period is such that the retrograde impulse may arrive at site b before refractoriness is terminated. (From Rosen and Danilo.[60] Reproduced by permission.)

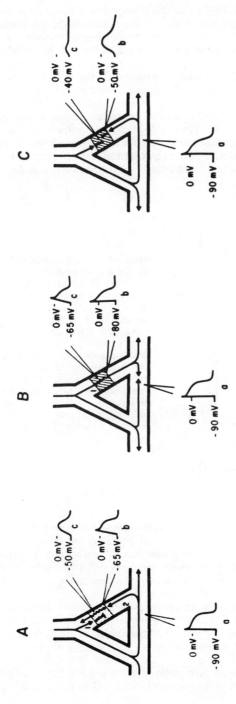

**FIGURE 5.** Mechanisms for suppressing reentry. In this model (panel **A**) three types of action potential are occurring. In most of the conducting system and the myocardium the action potential is a normal fast response (site a). In the depressed area (site c) there are slow responses and at intermediate sites (site b), depressed fast responses. In panel **B** a drug that hyperpolarizes the membrane at sites b and c suppresses reentry as a result of restoring the conduction in the antegrade direction. In panel **C** a drug suppresses reentry by further depolarizing the membrane potential at the depressed area, thereby inducing bidirectional conduction block. (From Rosen and Danilo.[60] Reproduced by permission.)

depressed fast responses; that is, action potentials are initiated at low levels of membrane potential, although they are still dependent on the fast inward current. FIGURE 5 shows two major means whereby reentry might be abolished. If the drug improves antegrade propagation—in effect removing the site of unidirectional block—then the normal activation pattern will be restored and the arrhythmia will cease (FIG. 5B). This effect would be expected if the drug hyperpolarized the depolarized tissues in the depressed segment, thereby providing a basis for the fast-response action potential to occur once again. Although there is no proof that any antiarrhythmic drug acts this way in the clinic, it has been suggested in experimental settings that phenytoin, lidocaine, and propranolol exert such an effect. Lidocaine has been shown to hyperpolarize cardiac fibers,[12,13] presumably as the result of a drug-induced decrease in steady-state sodium current,[31] and a similar effect is attributed to propranolol.[13] As for phenytoin, at low potassium

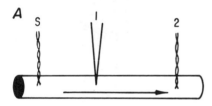

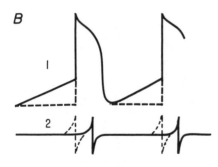

**FIGURE 6.** An experimental model showing the modification of conduction velocity as a result of depressing phase 4 depolarization. Panel **A** shows a Purkinje fiber stimulated at s, transmembrane potential recorded at 1, and surface electrogram recorded at 2. In panel **B**, in the control situation (*solid line*) there is marked phase 4 depolarization associated with slow conduction as measured between the upstroke of the action potential and the electrogram. Procainamide is added (*broken line*) and depresses phase 4. Activation voltage is therefore shifted to a more negative membrane potential, resulting in a faster conduction velocity.

concentrations, low concentrations of drug increase resting potential, upstroke velocity, and conduction velocity of atrial and Purkinje fibers. This has been especially prominent in experiments where mechanical trauma, low temperature, or digitalis have been used to depolarize the fibers.[32–35] The mechanisms responsible for these effects have not been determined, but nonetheless they would be associated with an improvement of conduction.

Another means for improving antegrade propagation is by decreasing the slope of phase 4 depolarization. This has been demonstrated for procainamide[36] (FIG. 6): Fibers having a marked degree of phase 4 depolarization showed an increased propagation velocity as procainamide decreased the slope of phase 4 and hyperpolarized the fibers.

A more common means for terminating reentry is the induction of bidirectional conduction block. The site of bidirectional block will be influenced in part by the mechanism of action of the drug as suggested in FIGURE 5C. A drug such as quinidine, which depresses the fast inward current in fibers having either the normal fast response[14,37] or the depressed fast-response action potential,[38] would block conduction at both sites a and b in FIGURE 5. Quinidine also displaces threshold potential to more positive voltages, reducing cardiac excitability.[39] In addition, quinidine has minor effects on the slow-response action potential,[40] which might suppress conduction at site c in FIGURE 5 as well. Summarizing the effects of quinidine, then, we see that it has a rather nonspecific action on conduction, depressing this in normal and depolarized tissues. This is reflected in the ECG, which shows that therapeutic concentrations of quinidine prolong the P-R interval and QRS complexes, thus indicating widespread depression of conduction in the heart.

Quinidine also prolongs repolarization and refractoriness.[19] This provides another means for suppressing reentry as it modifies the critical timing relationship between repolarization and conduction that permits reentry to occur. Once repolarization is prolonged and the refractory period is similarly prolonged, then an impulse arising at a time shortly after the refractory period during control would—in the presence of quinidine—arrive before refractoriness is terminated and fail to propagate further.

Lidocaine, also a local anesthetic compound, has a very different effect on conduction and repolarization. Nonetheless it, too, can terminate reentrant rhythms. Unlike quinidine, lidocaine has only small effects on the maximum rate of rise of phase 0 ($\dot{V}_{max}$) of normal cardiac fibers and does not modify threshold potential or conduction in the normal ventricular specialized conducting system or myocardium.[15,16] This is reflected in the fact that lidocaine routinely does not have effects on normal electrocardiographic complexes. However, lidocaine markedly depresses the $\dot{V}_{max}$ of fibers having depressed fast responses.[41] The mechanism for this action of lidocaine appears to be its increased binding affinity for inactivated sodium channels that occur at low levels of membrane potential.[42,43] This effect is enhanced at low pH because lidocaine is increasingly ionized as pH decreases.[44,45] As a result, whenever ischemia results in reduced membrane potential and acidosis, lidocaine would be expected to depress $\dot{V}_{max}$ and conduction to a greater extent than in normal tissues. The effect of lidocaine also is enhanced at elevated potassium concentrations. An elevated potassium concentration is also seen in myocardial ischemia, and this, too, may contribute to the effect of lidocaine.

In contrast to quinidine, lidocaine accelerates repolarization and the duration of the effective refractory period. Nonetheless, the duration of refractoriness is prolonged relative to that of the action potential. This appears to result from block of sodium entry through sodium channels that remain open during the plateau.[31,46] Lidocaine, then, is much more specific than quinidine in its actions in that it modifies repolarization and refractoriness in normal as well as diseased tissues, but depresses conduction only in fibers having already depressed fast responses.

## USE-DEPENDENCE

As mentioned earlier, antiarrhythmic agents that are also local anesthetics, such as quinidine and lidocaine, exert some of their antiarrhythmic action by blocking the fast (sodium) channel. It is generally accepted that the block they induce is not a simple plugging of the channel. Moreover, the depressant effect on $\dot{V}_{max}$ is influenced by variables such as the firing rate,[42,47–50] the number of action potentials at any particular rate,[51] extrasystoles and their time relation to the basic firing rate,[52–54] the membrane potential,[52,55] and the pH.[44]

This action of drugs is referred to as "frequency"- or "use"-dependent. The meaning of the term "use-dependent" is that the depression of the fast inward current, as measured by the reduction in $\dot{V}_{max}$, is dependent on the rate of firing or "use" of the fiber; that is, the depression is greater after an action potential has occurred than after a rest period. Furthermore, the recovery from the use-dependent depression in $\dot{V}_{max}$ occurs with a time constant that may vary considerably from drug to drug.[56,57] The use-dependent depression and the recovery process are illustrated schematically in FIGURE 7: When drug application is followed by a rest interval long enough for drug equilibration, $\dot{V}_{max}$ of the first action potential after the rest interval is only slightly reduced compared to the drug-free value. However, after several driven action potentials, $\dot{V}_{max}$ gradually decreases to a steady-state level that is markedly lower than the control value. Furthermore, recovery from depression is also use-dependent; the longer the rest period after steady-state depression has been attained, the more closely $\dot{V}_{max}$ returns to the pre-drug level.

The phenomenon of use-dependent depression of $\dot{V}_{max}$ by local anesthetics in cardiac tissues has attracted a great deal of interest both from the theoretical and the practical points of view, and attempts have been made to design a model that simulates the interactions between local anesthetics (antiarrhythmic drugs) and the sodium channel. The model must not only simulate the block of the sodium channel under "normal conditions," but it should also be powerful enough to account for the depression of $\dot{V}_{max}$ under abnormal conditions.

The model we review here was developed by Hondeghem and Katzung[56] as an extension of the Strichartz-Courtney model that was proposed for the action of local anesthetics in nerve.[58,59] In FIGURE 8, R represents the resting channel; A, the activated channel; and I, the inactivated channel. R', A' and I' represent the

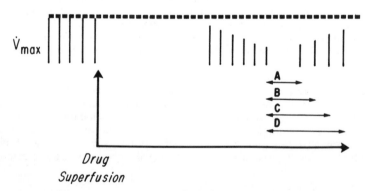

**FIGURE 7.** A schematic illustration of the use-dependent depression of $\dot{V}_{max}$ and the recovery process. After drug superfusion coupled with a rest interval, the $\dot{V}_{max}$ of the first upstroke is smaller than the predrug level (*broken line*) and gradually declines towards a steady state as the number of driven beats increases. When stimulation is discontinued, the depression of $\dot{V}_{max}$ is gradually removed as the rest interval is progressively prolonged (D > C > B > A).

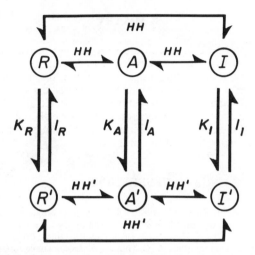

**FIGURE 8.** Diagram illustrating the mechanism of action of antiarrhythmic drugs in a sodium channel undergoing transitions between three states. R = resting (closed), A = activated (open), and I = inactivated (closed) drug-free fractions of the population of sodium channels. R', A', and I' are the respective drug-associated fractions. The transition between the states follows Hodgkin and Huxley first-order kinetics with voltage-dependent rate constants (HH). HH' are the same rate constants shifted on the voltage axis for the drug-associated channels. $K_R$, $K_A$, and $K_I$ are the association rate constants for the antiarrhythmic drug and $I_R$, $I_A$, and $I_I$ are the dissociation rate constants. (From Hondeghem and Katzung.[56] Reproduced by permission.)

resting, active, and inactivated channels that are drug-associated. In addition, $K_R$, $K_A$, and $K_I$ are the association rate constants between the drug-free and the drug-associated channels. The transition from one channel state to the other is governed by Hodgkin and Huxley kinetics, where HH' denotes the same type of kinetics, but with the h parameter shifted on the voltage axis.

That $\dot{V}_{max}$ will be increasingly depressed as the driving rate increases is explained by the much higher affinity of the drug for open channels than for closed channels. In this connection, the affinity of the drug to the sodium channel will determine the post-stimulation recovery rate of $\dot{V}_{max}$ and the interstimulus interval during which a considerable decrease in $\dot{V}_{max}$ will occur. In the case of quinidine, which exhibits a very slow post-stimulation recovery, the interstimulus interval will be much longer than in the case of lidocaine, which is characterized by fast removal of drug-induced depression of $\dot{V}_{max}$. With respect to the greater depression of $\dot{V}_{max}$ in depolarized or diseased fibers, the model can account for such selective depression in several ways, such as higher affinity of the drug for the depolarized than for polarized channels, or a slower drug dissociation rate constant from the depolarized than from polarized channels. According to this model, the rate constants are not directly voltage-dependent, but depend on the state of the channel. However, on the basis of their voltage clamp experiments, Weld et al.[55] concluded that the rate constants are in fact voltage-dependent and can therefore explain the selective effects of antiarrhythmic drugs in depolarized tissue.

## SUMMARY

In the preceding pages we have considered a number of mechanisms whereby drugs may modify arrhythmias and we also have demonstrated that certain types of action are specific to individual drugs. In addition, through the description of the use-dependence of drug effects, we have shown that the specificity of a drug's action often is attributable to its interactions with specific channels. As we learn more about the specificity of individual drug effects we should be better able not only to understand the actions of presently available drugs, but also to discover compounds that promise to be of use in the future.

## REFERENCES

1. DANILO, P., JR. & M. R. ROSEN. 1981. Antiarrhythmic drugs. In Cardiac Pharmacology. R. D. Wilkerson, Ed.: 275–303. Academic Press. New York, NY.
2. BIGGER, J. T., JR. & B. F. HOFFMAN. 1980. Antiarrhythmic drugs. In The Pharmacological Basis of Therapeutics. A. G. Gilman, L. Goodman & A. Gilman, Eds.: 729–766. Macmillan. New York, NY.
3. BOYDEN, A. B. & A. L. WIT. 1983. Pharmacology of the antiarrhythmic drugs. In Cardiac Therapy. M. R. Rosen & B. F. Hoffman, Eds.: 171–234. Martinus Nijhoff. Boston, MA.
4. HOFFMAN, B. F. & M. R. ROSEN. 1981. Cellular mechanisms for cardiac arrhythmias. Circ. Res. 49: 1–15.
5. DIFRANCESCO, D. 1981. A new interpretation of the pacemaker current in calf Purkinje fibers. J. Physiol. 314: 359–376.
6. NOBLE, D. 1975. The Initiation of the Heart Beat. Clarendon Press. Oxford.
7. DANGMAN, K. & B. F. HOFFMAN. 1980. Effects of nifedipine on electrical activity of cardiac cells. Am. J. Cardiol. 46: 1059–1067.
8. TODA, N. 1970. Barium-induced automaticity in relation to calcium ions and norepinephrine in the rabbit left atrium. Circ. Res. 27: 45–57.
9. HOFFMAN, B. F. & K. DANGMAN. 1982. Are arrhythmias caused by automatic impulse generation? In Normal and Abnormal Conduction in the Heart. P. Paes de Carvalho, M. Lieberman & B. Hoffman, Eds.: 429–448. Futura. Mount Kisco, NY.
10. VASSALLE, M. 1977. The relationship among cardiac pacemakers: Overdrive suppression. Circ. Res. 41: 269–277.
11. BIGGER, J. T., H. C. STRAUSS, A. L. BASSETT & B. F. HOFFMAN. 1968. Electrophysiological effects of diphenylhydantoin on canine Purkinje fibers. Circ. Res. 22: 221–236.
12. GADSBY, D. C. & P. F. CRANEFIELD. 1977. Two levels of resting potential in cardiac Purkinje fibers. J. Gen. Physiol. 70: 725–746.
13. ARNSDORF, M. F. & D. J. MEHLMAN. 1978. Observations on the effects of selected antiarrhythmic drugs on mammalian cardiac Purkinje fibers with two levels of steady-state potential: Influences of lidocaine, phenytoin, propranolol, disopyramide and procainamide on repolarization, action potential shape and conduction. J. Pharmacol. Exp. Ther. 207: 983–991.
14. HOFFMAN, B. F. 1958. The action of quinidine and procainamide on single fibers of dog ventricle and specialized conducting system. An. Acad. Bras. Cienc. 29: 365—368.
15. DAVIS, L. D. & J. V. TEMTE. 1969. Electrophysiological actions of lidocaine on canine ventricular muscle and Purkinje fibers. Circ. Res. 24: 639–655.
16. BIGGER, J. T. & W. T. MANDEL. 1970. Effect of lidocaine on transmembrane potentials of ventricular muscle and Purkinje fibers. J. Clin. Invest. 49: 63–77.
17. TSIEN, R. W. 1974. Effects of epinephrine on the pacemaker potassium current of cardiac Purkinje fibers. J. Gen. Physiol. 64: 293–319.

18. ARAVINDAKSHAN, V., C.-S. KUO & L. S. GETTES. 1977. Effect of lidocaine on escape rate in patients with complete atrioventricular block. Am. J. Cardiol. **40:** 177–183.
19. VAUGHAN WILLIAMS, E. M. 1958. The mode of action of quinidine on isolated rabbit atria interpreted from intracellular potential electrodes. Br. J. Pharmacol. **13:** 276–287.
20. ARNSDORF, M. F. 1977. The effect of antiarrhythmic drugs on triggered sustained rhythmic activity in cardiac Purkinje fibers. J. Pharmacol. Exp. Ther. **201:** 689–700.
21. CRANEFIELD, P. F. 1977. Action potentials, afterpotential, and arrhythmias. Circ. Res. **41:** 415–423.
22. ROSEN, M. R. & P. DANILO. 1980. Effects of tetrodotoxin, lidocaine, verapamil, and AHR-2666 on ouabain-induced delayed afterdepolarization in canine Purkinje fibers. Circ. Res. **46:** 117–124.
23. HEWETT, K. & M. R. ROSEN. 1982. β-adrenergic modulation of digitalis-induced delayed afterdepolarizations and triggered activity. Am. J. Cardiol. **49:** 913.
24. TSIEN, R. W. & D. O. CARPENTER. 1978. Ionic mechanisms of pacemaker activity in cardiac Purkinje fibers. Fed. Proc. **37:** 2127–2131.
25. SCHMITT, F. O. & J. ERLANGER. 1967. Directional differences in the conduction of the impulse through heart muscle and their possible relation to extrasystolic and fibrillary contractions. Am. J. Physiol. **87:** 326–347.
26. MOE, G. K. 1975. Evidence for reentry as a mechanism for cardiac arrhythmias. Rev. Physiol. Biochem. Pharmacol. **72:** 56–66.
27. WIT, A. L. & P. F. CRANEFIELD. 1978. Reentrant excitation as a cause of cardiac arrhythmias. Am. J. Physiol. **235:** H1–H17.
28. ROSEN, M. R. 1979. Cardiac drugs. In Current Cardiology. M. I. Ferrer, Ed.: 259–303. Houghton Mifflin. Boston, MA.
29. WIT, A. L. & P. CRANEFIELD. 1974. Effect of verapamil on the sinoatrial and atrioventricular nodes of the rabbit and the mechanism by which it arrests reentrant atrioventricular nodal tachycardia. Circ. Res. **35:** 413–425.
30. NING, W. & A. L. WIT. 1983. Comparison of the direct effects of nifedipine and verapamil on the electrical activity of the sinoatrial and atrioventricular nodes of the rabbit heart. Am. Heart J. **106:** 345–355.
31. COLATSKY, T. 1982. Mechanisms of action of lidocaine and quinidine on action potential duration in rabbit cardiac Purkinje fibers: An effect on steady-state sodium currents? Circ. Res. **50:** 17–27.
32. ROSEN, M. R., P. DANILO, JR., M. B. ALONSO & C. E. PIPPENGER. 1974. Effects of therapeutic concentrations of diphenylhydantoin on transmembrane potentials of normal and depressed Purkinje fibers. J. Pharmacol. Exp. Ther. **197:** 594–604.
33. BIGGER, J. T., H. C. STRAUSS, A. L. BASSETT & B. F. HOFFMAN. 1968. Electrophysiological effects of diphenylhydantoin on canine Purkinje fibers. Circ. Res. **22:** 221–236.
34. STRAUSS, H. C., J. T. BIGGER, A. L. BASSETT & B. F. HOFFMAN. 1968. Actions of diphenylhydantoin on the electrical properties of isolated rabbit and canine atria. Circ. Res. **23:** 463–477.
35. BASSETT A. L., J. T. BIGGER JR. & B. F. HOFFMAN. 1970. "Protective" action diphenylhydantoin on canine Purkinje fibers during hypoxia. J. Pharmacol. Exp. Ther. **173:** 336–343.
36. SINGER, D. H., H. C. STRAUSS & B. F. HOFFMAN. 1967. Biphasic effects of procainamide on cardiac conduction. Bull. N.Y. Acad. Med. **43:** 1194–1195.
37. VAUGHAN WILLIAMS, E. M., & L. SZEKERES. 1961. A comparison of tests of antifibrillatory action. Br. J. Pharmacol. **17:** 424–432.
38. HONDEGHEM, L. M. 1976. Effects of lidocaine, phenytoin and quinidine on ischemic canine myocardium. J. Electrocardiol. **9:** 203–209.
39. HOFFMAN, B. F., M. R. ROSEN & A. L. WIT. 1975. Electrophysiology and pharmacology of cardiac arrhythmias. VII. Cardiac effects of quinidine and procainamide. Am. Heart J. **90:** 117–122.
40. NAWRATH, H. 1981. Action potential, membrane currents and force of contraction in

mammalian heart muscle fibers treated with quinidine. J. Pharmacol. Exp. Ther. **216:** 176–182.
41. BRENNAN, F. J., P. F. CRANEFIELD & A. L. WIT. 1978. Effects of lidocaine on slow response and depressed fast response action potentials of canine cardiac Purkinje fibers. J. Pharmacol. Exp. Ther. **204:** 312–324.
42. HONDEGHEM, L. M. & B. G. KATZUNG. 1980. Test of a model of antiarrhythmic drug action: Effects of quinidine and lidocaine on myocardial conduction. Circulation **61:** 1217–1224.
43. GINTANT, G. A., B. F. HOFFMAN & R. E. NAYLOR. 1983. The influence of molecular form of local anesthetic-type antiarrhythmic agents on reduction of the maximum upstroke velocity of canine cardiac Purkinje fibers. Circ. Res. **52:** 735–746.
44. NATTEL, S., V. ELHARRAR, D. ZIPES & J. C. BAILEY. 1981. pH-dependent electro-physiological effects of quinidine and lidocaine on canine cardiac Purkinje fibers. Circ. Res. **48:** 55–61.
45. GRANT, A. O., L. STRAUSS, A. G. WALLACE & H. C. STRAUSS. 1980. The influence of pH on the electrophysiologic effects of lidocaine on guinea pig ventricular myocardium. Circ. Res. **47:** 542–550.
46. CARMELIET, E. & T. SAIKAWA. 1982. Shortening of the action potential and reduction of pacemaker activity by lidocaine, quinidine, and procaineamide in sheep cardiac Purkinje fibers: An effect on Na or K currents? Circ. Res. **50:** 257–272.
47. WEST, T. C. & D. N. AMORY. 1960. Single fiber recording of the effect of quinidine at atrial and pacemaker sites in the isolated right atrium of the rabbit. J. Pharmacol. Exp. Ther. **130:** 183–193.
48. JENSEN, R. A. & B. G. KATZUNG. 1970. Electrophysiological actions of diphenylhydantoin on rabbit atria. Circ. Res. **26:** 17–27.
49. TRITTHART, H., B. FLECKENSTEIN & A. FLECKENSTEIN. 1971. Some fundamental actions of antiarrhythmic drugs on the excitability and contractility of single myocardial fibers. Naunyn Schmiedebergs Arch. Pharmakol. **269:** 212–218.
50. CHEN, C. M. & L. S. GETTES. 1976. Combined effects of rate, membrane potential and drugs on maximum rate of use ($\dot{V}_{max}$) of action potential upstroke of guinea pig papillary muscle. Circ. Res. **38:** 464–469.
51. HEISTRACHER, P. 1971. Mechanism of action of antifibrillatory drugs. Naunyn Schmiedebergs Arch. Pharmakol. **269:** 199–212.
52. CHEN, C. M., L. S. GETTES & B. G. KATZUNG. 1975. Effect of lidocaine and quinidine on steady-state characteristics and recovery kinetics of $(dV/dT)_{max}$ in guinea pig ventricular myocardium. Circ. Res. **37:** 20–29.
53. WELD, F. M. & J. T. BIGGER, JR. 1975. Effect of lidocaine on the early inward transient current in sheep cardiac Purkinje fibers. Circ. Res. **37:** 630–639.
54. DRIOT, P. & D. GARNIER. 1972. Analyse en courant et voltage impose des propriétés anti-arythmiques de la quinidine appliquée au myocarde de la grenouille. C. R. Acad. Sci. (Paris) **274:** 3421–3424.
55. WELD, F. M. J. COROMILAS, J. N. ROTTMAN & J. T. BIGGER, JR. 1982. Mechanisms of quinidine-induced depression of maximum upstroke velocity in ovine cardiac Purkinje fibers. Circ. Res. **50:** 369–376.
56. HONDEGHEM, L. M. & B. G. KATZUNG. 1977. Time and voltage-dependent interactions of antiarrhythmic drugs with cardiac sodium channels. Biochem. Biophys. Acta **474:** 373–398.
57. COURTNEY, K. R. 1980. Interval dependent effects of small antiarrhythmic drugs on excitability of guinea pig myocardium. J. Mol. Cell Cardiol. **12:** 1273–1286.
58. STRICHARTZ, G. R. 1973. The inhibition of sodium currents in myelinated nerve by quaternary derivatives of lidocaine. J. Gen. Physiol. **62:** 37–57.
59. COURTNEY, K. R. 1975. Mechanism of frequency-dependent inhibition of sodium currents in frog myelinated nerve by the lidocaine derivative. GEA 968. J. Pharm. Exp. Ther. **195:** 225–236.
60. ROSEN, M. R. & P. DANILO, JR. Cellular electrophysiologic mechanisms of antiarrhythmic drug action. A. N. Richards Symposium. In press.

# Clinical Consequences of the Lipophilicity and Plasma Protein Binding of Antiarrhythmic Drugs and Active Metabolites in Man

DENNIS E. DRAYER

*Department of Pharmacology*
*Cornell University Medical College*
*New York, New York 10021*

There are two important physical constants of a drug: octanol/buffer (pH 7.4) partition coefficient $K_p$, which defines lipophilicity (lipid solubility), and ionization constant $K_a$; and two important biological constants: percent plasma protein binding and percent tissue binding. Octanol is usually chosen for $K_p$ determination since it is thought to represent rather well the physical properties of biological cell membranes, which are considered lipoprotein barriers. Together these constants determine the rate and extent that a drug will move from one biological compartment in the body to another separated by cell membranes. Generally, as the number of nonpolar groups such as aliphatic, unsubstituted aromatic, or halogens in a drug molecule increases, so do the following: lipophilicity, the affinity for the lipid portion of cell membranes, and the rate of diffusion across them. Drug lipophilicity and affinity for and rate of diffusion across cell membranes decrease as the number of polar groups such as hydroxyl (OH), acetamido (NHCCH₃),

$$\overset{\parallel}{O}$$

sulfonamido ($RSO_2NH$), amino ($NH_2$), methoxy ($OCH_3$), carboxy ($CO_2H$), or nitro ($NO_2$) in a drug increase. Although eleven of the currently marketed beta blockers differ only in the substituents in the aromatic ring (FIG. 1), there is a marked difference in lipophilicity with the partition coefficient ranging from 0.16 for sotalol to 4467 for propranolol.[1]

Beta-adrenoceptor blocking drugs (beta blockers) have several structural features in common with the beta-receptor agonist, isoproterenol (FIG. 1). A hydrogen on the amine and hydroxyl group on the beta-carbon of the side chain are essential for beta-receptor activity. This aliphatic hydroxyl group gives the molecule optical activity, and the *levo* or (−) isomers of both beta-receptor agonists and antagonists are much more potent than the *dextro* or (+) isomers. A conspicuous structural difference between beta agonists and beta blockers is that the latter have an oxymethylene bridge between the aromatic nucleus and the ethanolamine side chain.

The purpose of this manuscript is to describe a relationship between structure and lipophilicity and between lipophilicity and several pharmocokinetic properties of eleven beta blockers (taken as a group) and ten antiarrhythmic drugs (treated as a separate group). An overview of the pharmacokinetic properties influenced by the lipophilicity of beta blockers is presented in FIGURE 2. Also, the concept of bioisosterism (which involves structural modification of a drug for the purpose of developing a new drug that shows a similar spectrum of therapeutic

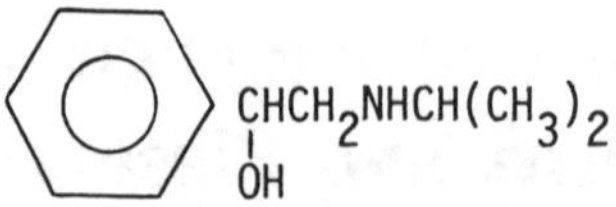

$$CHCH_2NHCH(CH_3)_2$$
$$\mid$$
$$OH$$

ISOPROTERENOL

$$ArOCH_2CHCH_2NHCH(CH_3)_2$$
$$\mid$$
$$OH$$

**FIGURE 1.** Chemical structure for isoproterenol and general chemical formula for beta blockers where Ar is a substituted aromatic group. An exception is sotalol, which does not contain an oxymethylene bridge between the aromatic moiety and the ethanolamine side chain. Also, nadolol and timolol contain a *tert*-butyl group instead of an isopropyl group.

activities but, it is hoped, less undesirable effects) will be illustrated with practolol versus atenolol and procainamide versus its *p*-hydroxy analogue.

In the beta blocker series, propranolol, alprenolol, oxprenolol, and metoprolol are considered highly lipophilic beta blockers. Propranolol is lipophilic since it contains two aromatic rings, while alprenolol, oxprenolol, and metoprolol are lipophilic by virtue of the presence of many aliphatic carbons. Practolol, nadolol, atenolol, and sotalol are considered highly hydrophilic (having an affinity for water) because of the presence of polar functional groups. For practolol, the polar functional group is the acetylamino group; for nadolol, the two hydroxyl groups on the cyclohexyl ring; for atenolol, the acetamido group; and for sotalol the sulfonamido group. The partition coefficients for these drugs are indicated in FIGURE 3.

In the antiarrhythmic drug series, verapamil, lidocaine, quinidine, and aprindine are considered highly lipophilic by virtue of the presence of many aliphatic and/or aromatic groups which negate the hydrophilicity caused by the presence of two or more polar groups. Conversely, procainamide and *N*-acetylprocainamide

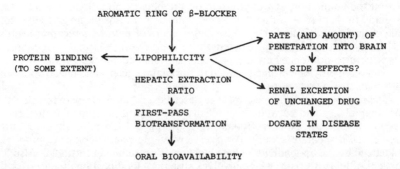

**FIGURE 2.** Pharmacokinetic properties influenced by lipophilicity of beta blockers. *Arrows* indicate influence.

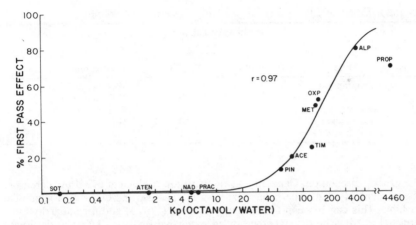

**FIGURE 3.** Relationship between partition coefficient $K_p$ and percent first-pass biotransformation of beta blockers. Abbreviations: PROP, propranolol; ALP, alprenolol; OXP, oxprenolol; MET, metoprolol; TIM, timolol; ACE, acebutolol; PIN, pindolol; PRAC, practolol; NAD, nadolol; ATEN, atenolol; SOT, sotalol. Partition coefficients were taken from Cruickshank.[1]

(which have three polar groups without an extensive nonpolar backbone) and bretylium, which is a quaternary ammonium salt, are highly hydrophilic compounds. Very strangely, disopyramide, which contains two unsubstituted aromatic rings and two isopropyl groups but only two polar groups, is hydrophilic ($K_p = 0.66$). The partition coefficients for these drugs are indicated in FIGURE 4.

First-pass effect refers to biotransformation of an orally administered drug during passage through intestinal mucosal cells and liver cells prior to reaching

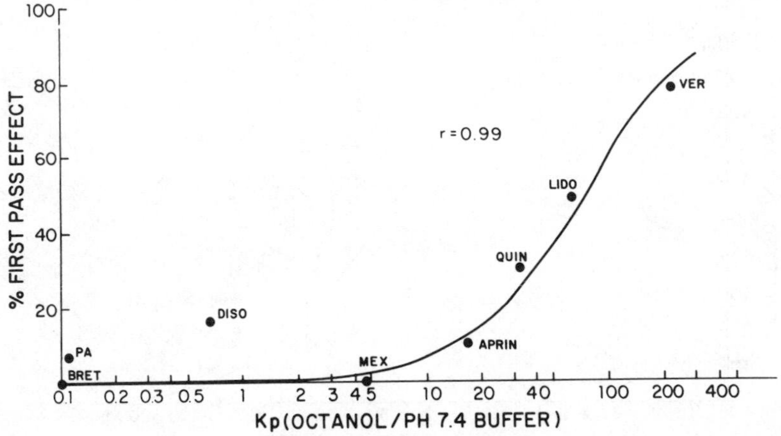

**FIGURE 4.** Relationship between partition coefficient $K_p$ and percent first-pass biotransformation of antiarrhythmic drugs. Abbreviations: VER, verapamil; LIDO, lidocaine; QUIN, quinidine; APRIN, aprindine; MEX, mexiletine; DISO, disopyramide; PA, procainamide; BRET, bretylium.

**TABLE 1.** Effect of Liver Cirrhosis on Drug Systemic Availability

| Drug | Systemic Availability (%) Controls | Patients | Reference |
|------|----------|----------|-----------|
| Propranolol | 38 | 54 | Wood et al.[20] |
| Labetalol | 33 | 63 | Homeida et al.[21] |
| Metoprolol | 50 | 84 | Regardh et al.[22] |
| Lidocaine | 39 | 91 | Huet et al.[18] |
| Verapamil | 22 | 52 | Somogyi et al.[23] |

the general circulation. Generally, as the partition coefficient of a drug increases, the percent of drug undergoing first-pass metabolism increases in a sigmoidal fashion. This can be seen for the beta blockers (FIG. 3) and for antiarrhythmic drugs (FIG. 4). The disadvantage of an extensive first-pass effect is the lower bioavailability after oral administration, which may necessitate, as indicated with lidocaine, changing the route of administration from the oral to the intravenous.

Changes in the patient's condition also influence the bioavailability of orally administered drugs. Severe liver disease, for example, acts both to decrease the metabolic clearance of some drugs by the liver, and to produce portal-systemic shunting of blood away from the liver. Both changes tend to decrease the first-pass effect for oral drugs and hence to increase bioavailability (TABLE 1). In some individuals with severe cirrhosis, portal hypertension, and portal-systemic shunting, the oral bioavailability of lidocaine may be markedly increased from the usual value of 30–40% to well over 90%. In this situation oral lidocaine therapy may be a realistic possibility.[18]

Generally, as the partition coefficient of a drug increases, the percent of drug excreted unchanged in the urine decreases in a sigmoidal fashion. This can be seen for the beta blockers (FIG. 5) and the antiarrhythmic drugs (FIG. 6). Since

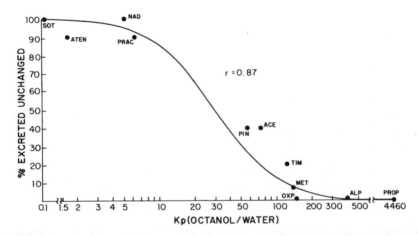

**FIGURE 5.** Relationship between partition coefficient $K_p$ and percent of beta blocker excreted unchanged in urine. Abbreviations are listed in legend of FIGURE 3.

lipophilic beta blockers and antiarrhythmic drugs are eliminated mainly by bio-transformation (excreted unchanged only to a minor extent), dosage reduction may be necessary in patients with liver, but not renal, disease. Conversely, the hydrophilic drugs are eliminated mainly by renal excretion of unchanged drug, necessitating dosage reduction in patients with poor renal function. This topic will be discussed elsewhere in this volume.

Drug dissolved in plasma is in equilibrium between that fraction which is reversibly bound to plasma proteins and that which is unbound in plasma water (FIG. 7). The latter fraction is thought to be related to the intensity of a drug's action since this establishes the diffusion gradient for the drug to get to the receptor site (FIG. 7). Alpha$_1$-acid glycoprotein is the plasma protein that mainly binds the basic beta blockers and the other antiarrhythmic drugs, whereas albumin mainly binds acidic drugs. Usually, in a series of drugs, increasing lipophilicity is associated with increased protein binding.[2] This, however, is not com-

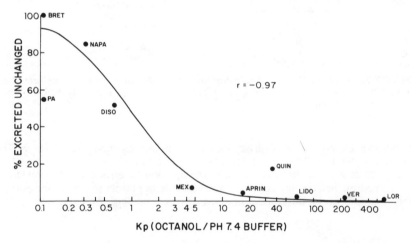

**FIGURE 6.** Relationship between partition coefficient $K_p$ and percent of antiarrhythmic drug excreted unchanged in urine. Abbreviations are listed in legend of FIGURE 4.

pletely the case for the beta blockers (FIG. 8) or the antiarrhythmic drugs (FIG. 9) since only some of the lipophilic drugs are highly protein-bound and only some of the hydrophilic drugs are poorly protein-bound.

One last point should be made about protein binding: Drug metabolites are generally more polar (that is, they have lower partition coefficients) and are less protein-bound than are their respective parent drugs (FIG. 10). For instance, lidocaine is more lipophilic ($K_p = 65$) than its two dealkylated metabolites, mono-ethylglycinexylidide (MEGX) and glycinexylidide (GX), and is 50% bound to plasma proteins in normal subjects. GX is the least lipophilic ($K_p = 1.3$) of these three compounds and is only 5% bound to plasma proteins. MEGX is of intermediate polarity and protein binding. Similarly, quinidine is more lipophilic ($K_p = 36$) than two of its oxidized metabolites [2'-oxoquinidinone and (3S)-3-hydroxy-quinidine] and is 89% bound to plasma proteins in normal subjects. 2'-Oxoquinidinone is the least lipophilic of these three compounds ($K_p = 21$) and

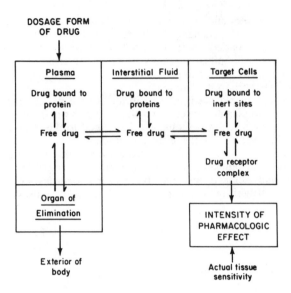

**FIGURE 7.** Representation of the diffusion equilibria that occur to relate the concentration of drug in plasma to the drug concentration at the receptor site. (From Reidenberg.[11] Reprinted by permission.)

is only 46% bound. (3S)-3-Hydroxyquinidine is of intermediate polarity ($K_p = 31$) and protein binding (74%). Therefore, the contribution of the active drug metabolites listed in FIGURE 10 to parent drug therapy will be erroneously estimated if one compares the concentration of the metabolite in plasma to that of the parent drug and ignores the differences in plasma protein binding. An exception to this

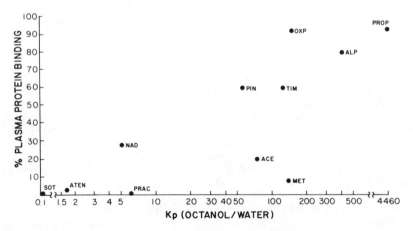

**FIGURE 8.** Relationship between partition coefficient $K_p$ and percent plasma protein binding of beta blockers. Abbreviations are listed in legend of FIGURE 3.

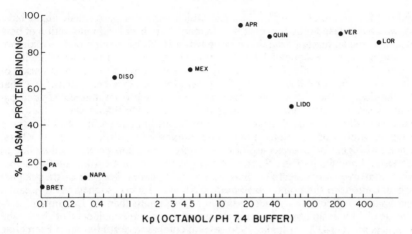

**FIGURE 9.** Relationship between partition coefficient $K_p$ and percent plasma protein binding of antiarrhythmic drugs. Abbreviations are listed in legend of FIGURE 4.

generalization is that $N$-acetylprocainamide ($K_p = 0.31$) is slightly more lipophilic than is procainamide ($K_p = 0.11$), but is slightly less protein-bound than the parent drug (11% versus 16%).

Beta blockers have been detected in both cerebrospinal fluid (CSF) and brain in man.[4,10] In single-dose studies in animals, after distribution equilibrium between brain and plasma had occurred (1 hr for the lipophilic propranolol and 12–24 hr for the hydrophilic practolol), the brain/plasma ratio was 7 for propranolol

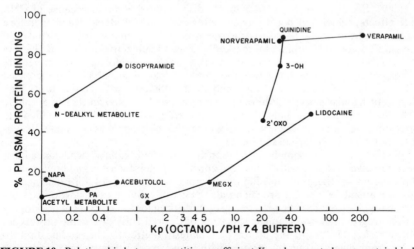

**FIGURE 10.** Relationship between partition coefficient $K_p$ and percent plasma protein binding of antiarrhythmic drugs and their pharmacologically active drug metabolites. Abbreviations: 3-OH, (3S)-3-hydroxyquinidine; 2'OXO, 2'-oxoquinidinone; MEGX, monoethylglycinexylidide; GX, glycinexylidide; PA, procainamide; NAPA, $N$-acetylprocainamide.

and 0.8 for practolol.[3] Chronic studies, which were not performed, might have shown an increased ratio for practolol. In man after chronic administration of beta blockers, the amount of drug in the brain was as follows: propranolol > oxprenolol, metoprolol >> atenolol.[4] This order is closely related to the lipophilicity of the drugs. A flaw in this study is that atenolol was given for the shortest period of time (an average of 6 days versus 10–13 days for the other beta blockers) and at 0.6 the dose of the other drugs. Also, the brain tissue from atenolol-treated patients was taken at a somewhat longer time after dosing than it was in the other patients. Although both of these studies are somewhat flawed, it seems that there is higher brain concentrations of lipophilic compared to hydrophilic beta blockers. Since this higher brain concentration may only reflect nonspecific binding due to increased lipophilicity (FIG. 7), the following question can be asked on this somewhat controversial subject: Do lipophilic beta blockers, because of their higher concentrations in the brain, cause more CNS side effects (such as vivid dreams, nightmares, hallucinations, depression, and insomnia) than do hydrophilic beta blockers? This is an important clinical question since the incidence of these side effects is about 1–3%[7] or higher, and several comparative studies have been done to answer it. For example, nine patients had a prior history of CNS side effects (nightmares, hallucinations or both) while receiving beta blockers. These symptoms were confirmed in six as drug-related during rechallenge with atenolol (100 mg) and either propranolol (80–160 mg twice a day) or metoprolol (100–200 mg twice a day). These six patients entered into a double-blind crossover study for two 4-week periods. Thirty-one episodes of nightmares or hallucinations were reported. 30 during treatment with the lipophilic propranolol or metoprolol and only one during treatment with hydrophilic atenolol.[5] In another study involving 104 patients receiving atenolol, thirty-three were started on atenolol because of CNS side effects (insomnia, mild depression, nightmares, or hallucinations) during previous treatment with other beta blockers (mainly propranolol). In 24 of these 33 patients, these CNS side effects either disappeared or were markedly diminished. Mean duration of atenolol therapy was 16 months (mean dose, 163 mg/day). Six of the original 104 patients discontinued atenolol because of CNS side effects, which did not disappear after cessation of atenolol and therefore were thought to be unrelated to drug therapy.[6] Finally, in a short-term study (10 days), pindolol and propranolol markedly affected subjective reports of sleep in terms of both increased dreaming and awakening. Metoprolol had an intermediate effect, while that of atenolol was the same as that of placebo.[8] The increased effect of pindolol, which is of intermediate lipophilicity, may be due to its high degree of agonist activity. Although other studies have shown that hydrophilic beta blockers such as atenolol do cause CNS effects in man,[9] they are difficult to interpret since a comparison with lipophilic beta blockers was not done. Therefore they will not be discussed further.

So far structure–lipophilicity relationships and their clinical significance have been reviewed. Next I will discuss the concept of bioisosterism and how it alters the structure–activity relationship for practolol versus atenolol, for procaine versus procainamide, and for procainamide versus its *p*-hydroxy analogue. Bioisosterism involves the modification of a prototype drug for the purpose of developing a new drug that shows a similar spectrum of desired activities as the prototype, but, it is hoped, less of the prototype's undesired effects. The modification involves replacing a group in question with an isostere. Isosteres are groups that have identical peripheral layers of electrons and are similar sterically. Thus, oxygen atom, NH and $CH_2$ groups of atoms are isosteric (six valence electrons);

and fluorine atom, hydroxyl (OH), amino ($NH_2$) and methyl ($CH_3$) groups of atoms are isosteric (seven valence electrons).

Practolol was developed by Imperial Chemical Industries (ICI) Limited in the United Kingdom in 1966 followed by atenolol in 1968. Practolol and atenolol are isosteric compounds. The NH group of atoms in practolol is replaced with the isosteric $CH_2$ group of atoms, and the $CH_3$ group in practolol is replaced by the isosteric $NH_2$ group of atoms (FIG. 11). The resulting atenolol is about three times more potent a beta blocker on a milligram basis. Therefore, the beta-receptor has been "fooled." However, there is a marked difference in toxicity. Practolol causes the clinical syndrome of keratoconjunctival scarring, sclerosing peritonitis, psoriatic skin lesion, and serous otitis. This was found to occur in at least 1300 patients receiving practolol and led to its withdrawal from use. Patients developing this syndrome also had a high incidence of antinuclear antibody. Presently, no validated examples of this syndrome have been reported for atenolol after about 3 million patient–years of exposure. In fact, atenolol (for 2–6 yr) was substituted for

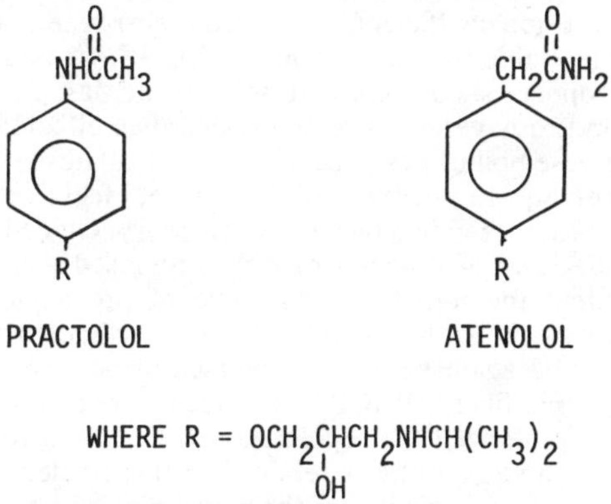

FIGURE 11. Chemical structures for practolol and atenolol, which are isosteric compounds.

practolol in 30 patients with this syndrome and all of these patients either lost their symptoms completely or were markedly improved.[12] Practolol also has been reported to cause systemic lupus erythematosus in some patients and antinuclear antibody in from 30–64% of patients receiving it. To my knowledge, this has not been reported after atenolol administration. These facts, I think, conclusively prove that the beneficial beta blocking effects of practolol therapy can be disassociated from some serious side effects by the slight structural modifications made in converting practolol to atenolol. Since atenolol came into clinical use after practolol, and was developed by the same drug company, it is possible that this structural modification of the practolol molecule was done under the guidance of the theory of bioisosterism. In any case, it is a marvelous triumph for this concept.

Another isosteric pair that I think is of interest is procaine and procainamide. The only difference between these two drugs is that procaine contains an ester functional group and procainamide contains an amide functional group which are isosteric. In 1936, Mautz demonstrated that direct application of procaine to the myocardium elevated the threshold of ventricular muscle to electrical stimulation. Extension of this observation by numerous workers has established that the cardiac actions of procaine resemble those of quinidine. However, the therapeutic value of procaine as an antiarrhythmic agent is limited by rapid enzymatic hydrolysis (half-life of 0.7 min in normal subjects) and prominent adverse effects on the CNS. It was these undesirable properties that led to the synthesis of procainamide and to clinical trials in 1951.[16,19] Since then, the pharmacologic actions of procainamide were shown to be qualitatively similar to those of procaine. The advantages of procainamide are as follows: procainamide is not hydrolyzed by plasma esterases and therefore possesses a more satisfactory duration of action (half-life of 3–4 hr in normal subjects); and it is effective after oral administration. In addition, it may have a more favorable ratio between cardiac and CNS activities.[19] All these benefits were obtained simply by replacing an oxygen atom in procaine with the isosteric NH group of atoms. A possible explanation of the greater disassociation of CNS side effects from antiarrhythmic effects during procainamide therapy is that procainamide has 0.1 the lipophilicity, as defined by a membrane/buffer partition coefficient, compared to procaine,[17] and therefore procainamide may be less able to penetrate into the CNS.

This story, I propose, should not end here. In the last 20 years or so, procainamide was found to have undesirable extracardiac effects, the most serious being a syndrome resembling systemic lupus erythematosus in approximately 25% of patients receiving chronic therapy. Therefore, I feel that further structural modification of the procainamide molecule is necessary. Guided by bioisosterism, the aromatic amino group of procainamide was replaced with the isosteric hydroxyl group to yield the p-hydroxy analogue of procainamide (abbreviated PHOPA). PHOPA was shown by us to have antiarrhythmic activity comparable to that of procainamide against aconitine-induced atrial arrhythmia in dogs. In isolated canine Purkinje fibers, PHOPA significantly reduced the rate of phase zero depolarization, prolonged the repolarization time, and reduced automaticity.[13] Thus, antiarrhythmic activity is retained in this isostere of procainamide. The probable explanation for this is that these two bioisosteres have very similar electron densities on respective carbons, as indicated by nearly identical respective [13]C nuclear magnetic resonance chemical shifts.[13] It is of interest that a compound similar to PHOPA, but having a propyl rather than ethyl bridge between the amide nitrogen and the tertiary amine nitrogen, has antiarrhythmic activity slightly less than that of procainamide against ouabain-induced and coronary artery ligation-induced arrhythmias in dogs.[14]

The aromatic amino group on the procainamide molecule is suspected of being causally related to the induction of antinuclear antibodies and a systemic lupus erythematosus-like syndrome.[15] The reasons for this will be given in a paper by Reidenberg in this volume. Since PHOPA does not contain an aromatic amino group, it should not cause these toxicities as readily (if at all) as does procainamide, and this was the main reason for PHOPA's synthesis. Clinical trials will be necessary to prove whether this is indeed the case.

## SUMMARY

1. In two series of antiarrhythmic drugs tested, as the octanol/water partition coefficient increases so do the following: elimination from the body by biotrans-

formation, first-pass biotransformation in the liver and gastrointestinal tract after oral administration, protein binding to some extent, and penetration into brain tissue.

2. Patients receiving lipophilic beta-adrenoreceptor blocking drugs may experience more central nervous system side effects than those receiving hydrophilic beta blockers.

3. Structural modification of a drug, guided by the concept of bioisosterism, may allow the disassociation of therapeutic from toxic activities.

4. Alpha-1 acid glycoprotein is the major plasma protein that binds the basic antiarrhythmic drugs. Antiarrhythmic drug metabolites are generally more polar (less lipophilic) and less plasma protein-bound than the parent drugs.

## ACKNOWLEDGMENT

I greatly appreciate the gracious assistance of Diann Glickman of the Pharmacy Department of New York Hospital for gathering some of the information presented here.

## REFERENCES

1. CRUICKSHANK, J. M. 1980. The clinical importance of cardioselectivity and lipophilicity in beta blockers. Am. Heart J. **100:** 160–178.
2. JUSKO, W. J. & M. GRETCH. 1976. Plasma and tissue protein binding of drugs in pharmacokinetics. Drug Metab. Rev. **5:** 43–140.
3. JOHNSSON, G. & C. G. REGARDH. 1976. Clinical pharmacokinetics of $\beta$-adrenoreceptor blocking drugs. Clin. Pharmacokinetics **1:** 233–263.
4. NEIL-DWYER, G., J. BARTLETT, J. MCAINSH & J. CRUICKSHANK. 1981. $\beta$-Adrenoceptor blockers and the blood-brain barrier. Br. J. Clin. Pharmacol. **11:** 549–553.
5. WESTERLUND, A. & V. FROLUNDA. 1982. Letter to the editor. N. Engl. J. Med. **307:** 1343–1344.
6. HENNINGSEN, N. C. & I. MATTIASSON. 1979. Long-term clinical experience with atenolol—a new selective $\beta$-1-blocker with few side effects from the central nervous system. Acta Med. Scand. **205:** 61–66.
7. SIMPSON, F. O. 1974. $\beta$-adrenergic receptor blocking drugs in hypertension. Drugs **7:** 85–105.
8. BETTS, T. A. & C. ALFORD. 1983. $\beta$-blocking drugs and sleep. A controlled trial. Drugs **25** (Suppl. 2): 268–272.
9. SALEM, S. A. & D. G. MCDEVITT. 1983. Central effects of beta-adrenoceptor antagonists. Clin. Pharmacol. Ther. **33:** 52–57.
10. TAYLOR, E. A., D. JEFFERSON, J. D. CARROLL & P. TURNER. 1981. Cerebrospinal fluid concentrations of propranolol, pindolol and atenolol in man: Evidence for central actions of $\beta$-adrenoceptor antagonists. Br. J. Clin. Pharmacol. **12:** 549–559.
11. REIDENBERG, M. M. 1981. Is protein binding important? In Therapeutic Drug Monitoring. A. Richens & V. Marks, Eds.: 23–30. Churchill Livingstone. New York, NY.
12. CRUICKSHANK, J. M. 1983. How safe are $\beta$-blockers? Drugs **25** (Suppl. 2): 331–340.
13. DRAYER, D. E., B. H. SLAVEN, M. M. REIDENBERG, E. E. BAGWELL & M. CORDOVA. 1977. Antiarrhythmic activity of p-hydroxy-N-(2-diethylaminoethyl) benzamide (the p-hydroxy isostere of procainamide) in dogs and mice. J. Med. Chem. **20:** 270–274.
14. REYNOLDS, R. D., W. E. BURMEISTER, S. V. CALZADILLA, R. J. LEE, M. M. REIDENBERG & D. E. DRAYER. 1982. Comparison of antiarrhythmic effects of procainamide, N-acetylprocainamide and p-hydroxy-N-(3-diethylaminopropyl) benzamide (41325). Proc. Soc. Exp. Biol. Med. **169:** 156–160.

15. KLUGER, J., D. E. DRAYER, M. M. REIDENBERG & R. LAHITA. 1981. Acetylprocainamide therapy in patients with previous procainamide-induced lupus syndrome. Ann. Int. Med. **95:** 18–22.
16. MOE, G. K. & J. A. ABILDSKOV. 1975. Antiarrhythmic drugs. *In* Pharmacologic Basis of Therapeutics, 5th ed., L. S. Goodman & A. Gilman, Eds.: 683–704. Macmillan. New York, NY.
17. CIOFALO, F. R. 1981. Effects of some membrane perturbers on alpha$_1$-adrenergic receptor binding. Neurosci. Lett. **21:** 313–318.
18. HUET, M., J. LELORIER, G. POMIER & D. MARLEAU. 1979. Bioavailability of lidocaine in normal volunteers and cirrhotic patients. Clin. Pharmacol. Ther. **25:** 229–230.
19. MARK, L. C., H. J. KAYDEN, J. M. STEELE, *et al.* 1951. The physiological disposition and cardiac effects of procainamide. J. Pharmacol. Exp. Ther. **102:** 5–15.
20. WOOD, A. J., D. M. KORNHAUSER, G. R. WILKINSON, D. G. SHAND & R. A. BRANCH. 1978. The influence of cirrhosis on steady-state blood concentration of unbound propranolol after oral administration. Clin. Pharmacokinetics **3:** 478–487.
21. HOMEIDA, M., L. JACKSON & C. J. ROBERTS. 1978. Decreased first-pass metabolism of labetalol in chronic liver disease. Br. Med. J. **2:** 1048–1050.
22. REGARDH, C. G., L. JORDO & M. ERVIK *et al.* 1981. Pharmacokinetics of metoprolol in patients with hepatic cirrhosis. Clin. Pharmacokinetics **6:** 375–388.
23. SOMOGYI, A., M. ALBRECHT, G. KLIEMS, K. SCHAFER & M. EICHELBAUM. 1981. Pharmacokinetics, bioavailability and ECG response of verapamil in patients liver cirrhosis. Br. J. Clin Pharmacol. **12:** 51–60.

# Metabolism and Excretion of Antiarrhythmic Drugs

P. A. ROUTLEDGE

*Department of Pharmacology and Therapeutics*
*Welsh National School of Medicine*
*Cardiff, Wales*

In order to be able to enter cells, and to exert pharmacologic effects, drugs must normally possess some degree of lipid solubility. Such agents are difficult to eliminate from the body, however, since they also readily diffuse back through the renal tubular cell membranes to reenter the plasma and would thus be likely to persist in the body for long periods. This is why the ability of the body to metabolize drugs is so important. It has been calculated, for example, that a highly lipid-soluble drug that is distributed widely throughout tissue, but is not metabolized, would have an elimination half-life of around 100 years.[1]

The primary goal of metabolism is therefore to obtain compounds with lower lipid/water partition coefficients; these are termed "polar" compounds. Not only is it more difficult for such drugs to be passively resorbed in the renal tubule, but they are also more susceptible to the active secretory mechanisms for anions and cations in the proximal renal tubule.

## METABOLISM

### Sites and Mechanisms

Metabolism of antiarrhythmic compounds may involve two major phases (TABLE 1). Phase I processes normally involve the substitution of one chemical group by another to obtain a more polar compound, and this can be achieved by oxidation, reduction, and hydrolysis. Phase II reactions, on the other hand, entail the addition of a small molecule (for example, glucuronic acid or acetate) to the drug to form a more polar conjugate and are therefore also called conjugation reactions. Any one drug may undergo metabolism by either phase I or phase II reactions or by both in turn or concurrently before the metabolites can be excreted in the urine.

Several organs possess enzyme systems capable of metabolizing drugs. If the drug is administered orally, the first such organ it meets is the gut. This has enzymes not only in the mucosal cells, but also in the microorganisms inhabiting the lumen. These organisms can metabolize digoxin in the rat cecum for example[2]; and in man, if digoxin is given as enteric-coated granules or is introduced into the jejunum, more dihydrodigoxin is excreted in the urine than after conventional administration.[3] The mucosal cells are rich in enzyme activity, particularly in the tips of the villi, and phase I and II reactions have been described there. Enzyme activity is greatest in the jejunum and decreases progressively both distally and proximally, although some activity is still present in the buccal and rectal mucosa. The gut appears to be particularly rich in conjugation reactions (for example, sulfation and glucuronidation), although they appear to be easily satu-

TABLE 1. Pathways and Sites of Hepatic Drug Metabolism[a]

| Pathway | Site |
|---|---|
| **Phase I** | |
| *Oxidations* | |
| Aliphatic oxidation | Smooth endoplasmic reticulum |
| Aromatic hydroxylation | Smooth endoplasmic reticulum |
| N-dealkylation | Smooth endoplasmic reticulum |
| O-dealkylation | Smooth endoplasmic reticulum |
| N-oxidation | Smooth endoplasmic reticulum |
| N-hydroxylation | Smooth endoplasmic reticulum |
| S-oxidation | Smooth endoplasmic reticulum |
| Deamination | Smooth endoplasmic reticulum/mitochondria |
| *Reduction* | Smooth endoplasmic reticulum/cytosol |
| *Hydrolysis* | Smooth endoplasmic reticulum/cytosol |
| **Phase II** | |
| *Conjugations* | |
| Glucuronidation | Smooth endoplasmic reticulum |
| Acetylation | Cytosol |
| Mercapturic Acid | Cytosol |
| Sulfation | Cytosol |
| Methylation | Cytosol |
| Amino acids | Cytosol |

[a] Modified from Hager et al.[45]

rated by the presence of excess substrate, and their role in the metabolism of antiarrhythmic drugs is probably small.

The lung also possess metabolic potential and all drugs, irrespective of their mode of administration, must pass through it before entering the systemic circulation. Not only are the lungs much lighter than the liver (850 g versus 1500 g) but they also contain a more heterogeneous cell population, having more than 40 different cell types. Of these, only four cell types appear to contain enzymes capable of metabolizing drugs. These are the capillary endothelial cells, the pulmonary macrophages, the type II pneumocytes (alveolar cells), and the nonciliated bronchiolar epithelial cells (Clara cell).[4] There is evidence of some metabolism of propranolol in the rabbit isolated perfused lung preparation,[5] but the role of the lung in the metabolism of antiarrhythmic drugs in man is presently unclear. Metabolism in the lung should be distinguished from the uptake of basic drugs (such as lidocaine and propranolol) by the organ in concentrations much greater than in the blood. These agents are subsequently released to be metabolized elsewhere.

By far the most important organ for drug metabolism is the liver. Implicit in the term "hepatic-portal system" is the understanding that orally administered drug must pass through this "gateway" before entering the systemic circulation. If the ability of the liver to metabolize the drug is great, it may therefore undergo presystemic metabolism on its first pass through the liver so that, despite complete absorption, its bioavailability may be low and variable.[6] Some antiarrhythmic compounds undergoing extensive presystemic metabolism in man are alprenolol, lidocaine, methyldigoxin, metoprolol, propranolol, and verapamil. Only small changes in the proportion of these drugs removed on the first pass through the liver (extraction ratio) may cause marked changes in bioavailability, so that the plasma levels attained after oral administration of the same dose may vary markedly among individuals. These agents must, of course, undergo subsequent passes through and metabolism by the liver, but by this time they have been distributed through the body tissues so that, although the proportion of drug extracted is the same, the amount metabolized is much less.

The principal site of drug metabolism in the liver is the hepatocyte. Drug entering the liver by either the hepatic artery or portal vein must pass between or through these cells before leaving through the hepatic vein into the inferior vena cava. Metabolism can occur in the smooth endoplasmic reticulum, cytosol, or in mitochondria. The most important of these sites is the smooth endoplasmic reticulum, which is abundant and contains hemoproteins collectively known as cytochromes P-450. Similar cytochromes are also present in the intestinal mucosa and the pulmonary cells previously described.

The major pathways for phase I and II reactions are listed in TABLE 1. Some examples of drugs metabolized by this route are alprenolol and apridine, which undergo aromatic hydroxylation. Lorcainide and verapamil are metabolized by N-dealkylation, while mexiletine undergoes N- and D-dealkylation, for example. Tocainide undergoes oxidative deamination to lactoxylidide, although a small proportion is also glucuronidated. Many other antiarrhythmic drugs are metabolized by one or more of these routes.

### Factors Affecting the Metabolism of Antiarrhythmic Drugs

The ability to metabolize antiarrhythmic as well as other drugs varies among individuals as well as within individuals, and some of the factors responsible for this variance are listed in TABLE 2. Pharmacogenetic factors will be discussed elsewhere in this volume. Metabolism may also be affected at the extremes of age, for metabolism of some drugs is reduced in the elderly. This is not universal, however, and although the metabolic clearance of propranolol[7] and phenytoin[8] decreases in the elderly, the metabolic clearance of lidocaine is probably unchanged.[9]

In the neonate, phase I reactions, particularly hydroxylation, appear to be immature, but some phase II reactions also appear to be underdeveloped. While sulfation is often normal at birth, acetylation may be reduced for a month or so and glucuronidation and glycine conjugation may take 2 to 3 months to develop

TABLE 2. Factors Affecting the Metabolism and Excretion of Antiarrhythmic Drugs

| Factors Affecting Drug Metabolism | Factors Affecting Drug Excretion |
|---|---|
| Pharmacogenetic factors | Extremes of age |
| Extremes of age | Environmental factors |
| Environmental factors | Other drugs |
|  | Disease states |
| Enzyme inducers |   Cardiac disease |
| Enzyme inhibitors |   Renal disease |
| Continued drug administration |  |
|  |  |
| Disease states |  |
|   Liver disease |  |
|   Cardiac disease |  |
|   Renal disease |  |

normally.[10] Unfortunately, few data concerning metabolism of antiarrhythmic drugs are available, partly because of the associated technical and ethical difficulties.

Several factors can increase the metabolic clearance of drugs by the liver by the process of enzyme induction, in which increased synthesis of cytochrome P-450 gradually occurs on exposure to a variety of drugs or other substances. The major drugs responsible include the barbiturates and some nonbarbiturate hypnotics and tranquilizers and the antiepileptic drugs, carbamazepine and phenytoin. Recently the antituberculosis agent rifampicin has been shown to be a powerful enzyme-inducing agent and can increase the metabolism of mexiletine,[11] for example. Phenytoin similarly increases mexiletine clearance.[12] The other enzyme-inducers involved include polycyclic hydrocarbons in the diet and cigarette smoke, and some of the chlorinated insecticides. The magnitude of the effects of these substances upon the metabolic clearance of any particular drug will depend upon the route of administration of the drug as well as the initial ability of the liver to metabolize the drug. If the drug is normally efficiently metabolized by the liver, the clearance will depend predominantly on the rate of delivery of the drug to the organ (that is, upon hepatic blood flow), and the effect of enzyme induction will be small after the drug is delivered intravenously. After oral administration, however, the drug will undergo extensive presystemic metabolism by the induced enzymes since this process is not markedly flow-dependent and the amount reaching the systemic circulation (that is, bioavailability) will be markedly reduced.[4] This differential effect is illustrated by the 100% difference in plasma concentrations when the same dose of lidocaine was given orally to normal individuals and patients receiving anticonvulsant drugs and the 10% difference between the groups when lidocaine was given intravenously[13] (FIG. 1). A similar effect has been shown with the beta blocking agent, alprenolol.[14] Other drugs which normally undergo marked presystemic metabolism and would be expected to show this route-dependent phenomenon are metoprolol, propranolol, and verapamil. If the initial metabolic clearance of a drug is low and therefore not dependent on hepatic blood flow, the effect of induction is likely to be similar, irrespective of the route of administration. It is also important to note that induction may take 10–14 days to occur after initiation of therapy and a similar time to regress after the inducing agent is withdrawn. This may cause the offending agent's effect to be missed and can result in serious interactions if not anticipated.

Other agents can impair the metabolism of drugs by a variety of mechanisms, including substrate competition and competitive or noncompetitive inhibition. One example of inhibition caused by concomitant drug therapy is the reduction in the metabolic clearance of lidocaine,[15] metoprolol,[16] propranolol,[17] phenytoin[18] and labetalol[19] caused by cimetidine, a histamine-2 receptor antagonist. This appears to be related in part to a reduction in activity of the cytochrome P-450 system responsible for the metabolism of these drugs, caused by the histamine-2 receptor antagonist binding to the cytochrome. In general, the effects are greatest with cimetidine, which possesses an imidazoline ring structure, and less with ranitidine, which contains a furan ring structure. Glucuronidation pathways appear to be less affected than phase I reactions.[20,21]

Since, as previously described, the intravenous clearance of drugs that are normally efficiently cleared by the liver is dependent on organ blood flow as well as enzyme activity, agents that reduce hepatic blood flow may reduce the clearance of these drugs. This is the suggested mechanism for the reduction in intravenous lidocaine clearance associated with concomitant propranolol administration.[22] It has also been suggested that histamine-2 receptor antagonists may interact with intravenously administered highly cleared drugs, at least in part, by causing a reduction in hepatic blood flow, although these conclusions are based on indirect estimates of blood flow.[17]

Continued administration of some antiarrhythmic drugs may also be associated with accumulation of the agent to plasma concentrations greater than expected from the initial pharmacokinetic profile, and this can occur after chronic oral administration of propranolol[23] and verapamil[24] and intravenous administra-

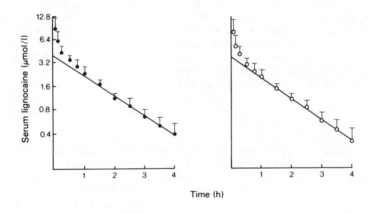

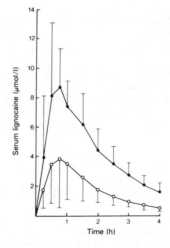

**FIGURE 1.** Mean serum lidocaine concentration (±S.D.) after lidocaine hydrochloride, 100 mg intravenously (*top*) and 750 mg orally (*right*) in six healthy subjects (●) and in six epileptic patients (○). (From Perucca and Richens.[13] Reproduced by permission.)

tion of lidocaine.[25] It has been postulated that intermediate products of metabolism may inhibit metabolism of the parent compound (product inhibition) to cause this effect, but the precise mechanism is unknown.

Finally, disease states may be associated with altered drug metabolism. The most important of these is liver disease, in which clearance may be reduced both by a reduction in viable hepatocytes and by a reduced hepatic blood flow. Thus, the intravenous clearance of lidocaine is decreased markedly (by about 40%) in patients with hepatic cirrhosis.[26] The effect of liver disease on the clearance of highly cleared drugs is also likely to be greater when the drug is given orally rather than intravenously, and this illustrated by verapamil.[27,28]

Drug metabolism may also be impaired in heart failure, a not uncommon problem in patients who require antiarrhythmic drugs. One mechanism for this is the reduction in hepatic blood flow so that the clearance of lidocaine, a flow-dependent drug, is reduced in heart failure in direct proportion to the cardiac output.[26] There may also be changes in hepatocyte function because some agents that do not show flow-dependent metabolic clearance (such as aprindine[29]) may also be more slowly cleared after acute myocardial infarction. It is important to remember, however, that several antiarrhythmic drugs (for example, propranolol and lidocaine) bind to the acute-phase protein alpha-1 acid glycoprotein (AAG),[30–32] which rises shortly after myocardial infarction. Increases in total plasma drug concentration may therefore occur by virtue of redistribution, while the change in free (active) plasma drug concentration may be much less. Although these redistributional changes may have effects on the subsequent metabolism of the drug, they may not therefore reflect a primary derangement in the metabolism of the drug after myocardial infarction.

Although renal failure is more likely to be associated with changes in disposition of drugs primarily excreted unchanged in the urine, drugs that are metabolized may also show altered kinetics of the parent compound. There is some evidence, for example, that the total body clearance of quinidine may be reduced in renal disease.[33] Although the metabolism of some other noncardiac drugs is affected, the evidence for antiarrhythmic agents indicates no effect of renal disease on the metabolism of the parent compound in the case of propranolol and lidocaine.[26,34] Data for other antiarrhythmic drugs are scant. It is important to remember that changes in plasma protein binding associated with renal disease may result in changes in total plasma drug concentration, as previously described in cardiac and liver disease. The plasma protein binding of many drugs (for example, phenytoin) may be markedly reduced because of both hypoalbuminemia and reduced affinity of the albumin for the drugs.[35] In contrast, the plasma protein binding of other agents, chiefly those that bind substantially to alpha-1 acid glycoprotein (for example, propranolol and lidocaine), may be increased because of an increase in this protein in renal disease.[30,36] This reinforces the importance of measurement of free as well as total plasma drug concentration in future studies of the metabolism of substantially protein-bound antiarrhythmic drugs in disease states.

### Markers for Drug Metabolism

Since so many factors can affect drug metabolism, it is not surprising that the plasma drug concentration after any given dose of drug may vary markedly among individuals. This is particularly important in the case of antiarrhythmic drugs because the plasma drug concentration is often related to the pharmacologic effect. The use of standard doses of the drug may therefore result in inadequate response in some patients and toxicity in others. How can the practicing clinician estimate the likely changes in drug metabolism in an individual and adjust the dose accordingly?

Unfortunately, none of the easily measured patient variables (age, sex, body weight or body surface area), alone or in combination, are closely related to the individual's ability to metabolize drugs. The plasma albumin and prothrombin time may give some rough indication of the derangement in drug metabolism associated with liver disease, and the severity of heart failure may also give some indication of the reduction in metabolism of drugs in which liver blood flow is an important determinant of this process.[26]

The use of model compounds (for example, antipyrine and indocyanine green)[37] has also been advocated, but not all authors have agreed concerning their value, and at best they are indirect measures of the metabolism of the drug in question.[38] Because rapid methods now exist to measure drug concentration directly, therapeutic drug monitoring of several antiarrhythmic agents is becoming an increasingly important tool with which the physician can predict[39] and compensate for variability in the metabolism of some antiarrhythmic compounds, although rapid and reliable methods to measure free as distinct from total drug are still needed.

## EXCRETION

### Sites and Mechanisms

There are several potential sites for excretion of drugs from the body. Saliva, sweat, milk, and lacrimal and vaginal secretions do contain drugs, but the amounts excreted by these are negligible. Several drugs can be excreted in the bile, but the role of this route in antiarrhythmic drug excretion is largely unexplored.

The kidney is the major organ for elimination of water-soluble drugs and drug metabolites, and although the two kidneys are only 1% of body weight, they receive around 25% of the cardiac output. Three major processes determine the excretion of drugs by the kidney. These are glomerular filtration, tubular reabsorption, and tubular secretion.

Glomerular filtration is a passive process of ultrafiltration of plasma through the glomerular capillaries. The clearance of drug by this route will depend on the rate of delivery to the organ as well as the degree of plasma protein binding of the drug. If a drug (gentamicin, for example) is not protein-bound and is not reabsorbed or actively secreted, its clearance will approach the glomerular filtration rate. Reabsorption of drug occurs primarily from the proximal tubule by a passive process, dependent on the relative solubilities of the drug in urine or plasma water, the ability of the drug to cross the tubular cell membrane, and the urine flow rate. Finally, active tubular secretion, which also occurs in the proximal tubule, is a process by which weak acids or bases may be secreted by the separate transport process into the tubular fluid in a way not considered to be limited by protein binding.[40]

### Factors Affecting the Excretion of Antiarrhythmic Agents and Their Metabolites

Situations that affect any of the three processes involved in renal drug excretion may alter renal clearance (TABLE 2). Glomerular filtration rate may be reduced by conditions causing reduced renal perfusion (such as shock or cardiac failure) as well as by intrinsic disease of the kidney. Thus, the dose of procainamide, which is 50% or more excreted unchanged in the urine, should be reduced in patients with cardiac failure as well as in those with chronic renal failure. The glomerular filtration rate, when expressed as a function of body surface area, is lower in the newborn infant, but reaches adult proportions after about a month. The glomerular filtration rate also rises in pregnancy, until at 36 weeks it is 50% greater than normal. Increasing age is also associated with a roughly linear decline in glomerular filtration rate from the age of 40, and this rate decreases in men from 125 ml/min at age 40 to 60 ml/min at the age of 90. These changes should be taken into account when prescribing drugs excreted by these mechanisms, but it must be stressed that there is wide variability among individuals in the magnitude of these changes. The total clearance of drug will also increase if protein binding of the drug is reduced; but, under first-order conditions, the concentration of free drug in the plasma will be unaffected (although the total plasma drug concentration will be reduced) and drug effect should remain the same.

Tubular reabsorption of drugs may be markedly affected by changes in the degree of ionization of the drug in urine, since nonionized drug can pass down a concentration gradient back into the plasma. Thus, there is an exponential relationship between the renal clearance of mexiletine and urine pH so that only small reductions in urine pH will produce marked increase in renal drug clearance.[11] Since the renal route normally contributes only 14% towards the total clearance of the drug, such changes are unlikely to cause clinical changes in mexiletine disposition. Such changes may be potentially more important in the case of tocainide, in which 40% of the total elimination is from the kidneys and for which a rise in urine pH can reduce renal drug excretion.[41] Although it is difficult to determine the influence of active tubular secretion upon the renal excretion of specific drugs, the importance of this route can be inferred from the fact that the renal clearance of many drugs exceeds the glomerular filtration rate. This is true of the renal clearance of disopyramide,[42] which accounts for 40% of the total clearance of this drug. Procainamide and N-acetylprocainamide excretion by the kidney also involves active secretion by the mechanism for organic bases.[43] The renal tubular secretory mechanism is immature in neonates, particularly if they are premature, and drugs in which this pathway contributes substantially to drug clearance should be used with care. The efficiency of the renal tubular secretory mechanism may also decline in elderly individuals and be partly responsible for the reduced clearance of procainamide in this age group.[43] Digoxin, although neither a base or acid compound, may also be actively secreted in the nephron possibly in the distal convoluted tubule.[44] Several drugs (quinidine[45] and spironolactone,[46] for example) may compete for this excretory route and reduce renal digoxin clearance. Verapamil may also interact with digoxin by the same mechanism,[47] although it also reduces the nonrenal component of digoxin clearance.[48]

## Markers for Renal Excretion of Antiarrhythmic Drugs

The factors that have been discussed can be seen to cause variability among individuals in the renal clearance of drugs, which, although not as great as in hepatic clearance, contributes substantially to variability in pharmacologic response. Fortunately, in the case of renal excretion, however, a relatively useful and easily measured index of renal function is available. This is the endogenous creatinine clearance, which can either be determined directly by measurement of serum and 24-hour urine creatinine concentration or be calculated using the serum creatinine concentration and the patient's sex, age, and body weight.[49] This marker reflects primarily the process of glomerular filtration rather than tubular reabsorption or secretion, so its greatest value would be expected to be in predicting the renal excretion of drugs in which glomerular filtration is the principal pathway of elimination. It is thus particularly useful in predicting the clearance of aminoglycoside antibiotics (such as gentamicin). It also appears, however, to be related to the clearance of digoxin, which undergoes glomerular filtration, tubular reabsorption, and active secretion. This may be because the decline in these processes tends to occur in parallel in renal disease (the phenomenon of "glomerulotubular balance").[50] Unfortunately, measurement of endogenous creatinine clearance has several disadvantages. First, the reproducibility of measurement is poor and it may be necessary to make several collections to allow for this. Second, it is inaccurate in the presence of rapidly changing renal function. Finally, only a very few antiarrhythmic agents are predominantly excreted unchanged by the kidney, and so it is of limited value in antiarrhythmic therapy. Of those drugs that are excreted predominantly by this route, bretylium has not been studied extensively and N-acetylprocainamide clearance is relatively poorly related to creatinine clearance in normal individuals, although it does serve as a rough guide to the adjustment of the latter drug as well as to adjustment of disopyramide and procainamide dosage.[43,51,52] Fortunately, it is now possible to measure directly the plasma concentration of several drugs in which renal excretion is an important factor. Among the antiarrhythmic drugs are included digoxin, procainamide, N-acetylprocainamide, and disopyramide, and by judicious determination of plasma drug concentration, it is possible to compensate for interpatient variability in renal clearance mechanisms.

## CONCLUSIONS

Subjects vary markedly in their ability to metabolize and excrete antiarrhythmic compounds. This variability can lead to marked differences in response at any given dosage so that some subjects may be nonresponsive and others may show signs of drug toxicity. By a knowledge of the routes and mechanisms of metabolism and/or excretion of a particular compound, as well as the factors affecting these processes, it is possible to increase the effectiveness of these agents and to reduce the incidence of adverse effects. For several agents, this goal can be achieved by the use of therapeutic drug monitoring to supplement clinical findings, but the possible role of unmeasured but active metabolites must also be considered. Because of the difficulty in discovering more effective antiarrhythmic agents, it is not possible to discard new agents on the basis of variability in their metabolic handling.[53] It is important, however, that studies of the metabolism and excretion of new drugs in man go hand in hand with studies of efficacy. Such studies can be best carried out by collaboration between cardiologist, clinical pharmacologist, and clinical pharmacist in the early stages of the drug's development so that agents can be subsequently optimally used in the clinical setting.

## REFERENCES

1. BRODIE, B. B. 1964. Distribution and fate of drugs: Therapeutic implications. *In* Absorption and Distribution of Drugs. T. B. Binns, Ed.: 199–251. Churchill Livingstone. Edinburgh and London.
2. SCHELINE, R. R. 1973. Metabolism of foreign compounds by gastrointestinal microorganisms. Pharmacol. Rev. **25**: 451–523.

3. MAGNUSSON, J. O., B. BERGDAHL, C. BOGENTOFT & U. JONSSON. 1982. Metabolism of digoxin and absorption site. Br. J. Clin. Pharmacol. **14:** 284–285.
4. ROUTLEDGE, P. A. 1982. Presystemic drug metabolism of exogenous compounds by the lung. *In* Presystemic Drug Elimination. C. F. George, D. G. Shand & A. G. Renwick, Eds. Butterworth. Boston.
5. KORNHAUSER, D. M., R. E. VESTAL & D. G. SHAND. 1980. Uptake of propranolol by the lung and its displacement by other drugs: Involvement of the alveolar macrophage. Pharmacology **20:** 275–283.
6. ROUTLEDGE, P. A. & D. G. SHAND. 1979. Presystemic drug elimination. *In* Annual Review of Pharmacology and Toxicology. R. George, R. Okun and A. K. Cho, Eds. Vol. **19:** 447–468. Annual Reviews Inc. Palo Alto, CA.
7. CASTLEDEN, C. M. & C. F. GEORGE. 1979. The effect of aging on the hepatic clearance of propranolol. Br. J. Clin. Pharmacol. **7:** 49–54.
8. BAUER, L. A. & R. A. BLOUIN. 1982. Age and phenytoin kinetics in adult epileptics. Clin. Pharmacol. Ther. **31:** 301–304.
9. NATION, R. L., E. J. TRIGGS & M. SELIG. 1977. Lignocaine kinetics in cardiac patients and aged subjects. Br. J. Clin. Pharmacol. **4:** 439–448.
10. GLADTKE, E. & G. HEIMANN. 1975. The rate of development of elimination functions in kidney and liver of young infants. *In* Basic and Therapeutic Aspects of Perinatal Pharmacology. P. L. Morselli, S. Garattini & F. Seren, Eds. Raven Press. New York, NY.
11. PENTIKÄINEN, P. J., I. H. KOIVULA & H. A. HILTUNEN. 1982. Effect of rifampicin treatment on the kinetics of mexiletine. Eur. J. Clin. Pharmacol. **23:** 261–266.
12. BEGG, E. J., P. M. CHINWAH, C. WEBB, R. O. DAY & D. N. WADE. 1982. Enhanced metabolism of mexiletine after phenytoin administration. Br. J. Clin. Pharmacol. **14:** 219–223.
13. PERUCCA, E. & A. RICHENS. 1979. Reduction of oral bioavailability of lignocaine by induction of first pass metabolism in epileptic patients. Br. J. Clin. Pharmacol. **8:** 21–31.
14. ALVAN, G., K. PIAFSKY, M. LIND & C. BAHR. 1977. Effect of pentobarbital on the disposition of alprenolol. Clin. Pharmacol. Ther. **22:** 316–321.
15. FEELY, J., G. R. WILKINSON, C. B. MCALLISTER & A. J. J. WOOD. 1982. Increased toxicity and reduced clearance of lidocaine by cimetidine. Ann. Intern. Med. **96:** 592–594.
16. KIRCH, W., H. KÖHLER, H. SPAHN & E. MUTSCHLER. 1981. Interactions of cimetidine with metoprolol, propranolol or atenolol. Lancet **2:** 531–532.
17. FEELY, J., G. R. WILKINSON & A. J. J. WOOD. 1981. Reduction of liver blood flow and propranolol metabolism by cimetidine. New Engl. J. Med. **304:** 692–695.
18. NEUVONEN, P. J., R. A. TOKOLA & M. KASTE. 1981. Cimetidine-phenytoin interaction: Effect on serum phenytoin concentration and antipyrine test. Eur. J. Clin. Pharmacol. **21:** 215–220.
19. DANESHMEND, T. K. & C. J. C. ROBERTS. 1981. Cimetidine and bioavailability of labetalol. Lancet **1:** 565.
20. KLOTZ, U. & I. REIIMANN. 1980. Influence of cimetidine on the pharmacokinetics of desmethyldiazepam and oxazepam. Eur. J. Clin. Pharmacol. **18:** 517–520.
21. PATWARDHAN, R. V., G. W. YARBOROUGH, P. V. DESMOND, R. F. JOHNSON, S. SCHENKER & K. V. J. R. SPEEG. 1980. Cimetidine spares the glucuronidation of lorazepam and oxazepam in man. Gastroenterology **79:** 912–916.
22. OCHS, H. R., G. CARSTENS & D. J. GREENBLATT. 1980. Reduction in lidocaine clearance during continuous infusion and by coadministration of propranolol. N. Engl. J. Med. **303:** 373–377.
23. WOOD, A. J. J., K. CARR, R. E. VESTAL, S. BELCHER, G. R. WILKINSON & D. G. SHAND. 1978. Direct measurement of propranolol bioavailability during accumulation to steady-state. Br. J. Clin. Pharmacol. **6:** 345–350.
24. SHAND, D. G., S. C. HAMMILL, L. AANONSEN & E. L. C. PRITCHETT. 1981. Reduced verapamil clearance during long-term administration. Clin. Pharmacol. Ther. **30:** 701–703.

25. BAUER, L. A., T. BROWN, M. GIBALDI, L. HUDSON, S. NELSON, V. RAISYS & J. P. SHEA. 1982. Influence of long term infusions on lidocaine kinetics. Clin. Pharmacol. Ther. **31:** 433–437.
26. THOMSON, D. D., K. L. MELMON, J. A. RICHARDSON, K. COHN, W. STEINBRUNN, R. CUDIHEE & M. ROWLAND. 1973. Lidocaine pharmacokinetics in advanced heart failure, liver disease and renal failure in humans. Ann. Intern. Med. **78:** 499–508.
27. SOMOGYI, A., M. ALBRECHT, G. KLIEMS, K. SCHÄFER & M. EICHELBAUM. 1981. Pharmacokinetics, bioavailability and E.C.G. response of verapamil in patients with liver cirrhosis. Br. J. Clin. Pharmacol. **12:** 51–60.
28. WOODCOCK, B. G., I. RIETBROCK, H. F. VÖHRINGER & N. RIETBROCK. 1981. Verapamil disposition in liver disease and intensive care patients. Kinetics, clearance and apparent blood flow relationships. Clin. Pharmacol. Ther. **29:** 27–34.
29. HAGEMEIJER, F. 1975. Absorption, half life and toxicity of oral aprindine in patients with acute myocardial infarction. Eur. J. Clin. Pharmacol. **9:** 21–25.
30. PIAFSKY, K. M., O. BORGA, I. ODAR-CEDERLOF, C. JOHANSSON & F. SJOQVIST. 1978. Increased plasma protein binding of propranolol and chlorpromazine mediated by disease-induced elevations of plasma alpha-1-acid glycoprotein. N. Engl. J. Med. **299:** 435–439.
31. ROUTLEDGE, P. A., W. W. STARGEL, G. S. WAGNER & D. G. SHAND. 1980. Increased plasma propranolol binding in myocardial infarction. Br. J. Clin. Pharmacol. **9:** 438–439.
32. ROUTLEDGE, P. A., W. W. STARGEL, G. S. WAGNER & D. G. SHAND. 1980. Increased alpha-1-acid glycoprotein and lidocaine disposition in myocardial infarction. Ann. Intern. Med. **93:** 701–704.
33. DRAYER, D. E., D. T. LOWENTHAL, K. M. RESTIVO, A. SCHWARTZ, C. E. COOK & M. M. REIDENBERG. 1978. Steady-state serum levels of quinidine and active metabolites in cardiac patients with varying degrees of renal function. Clin. Pharmacol. Ther. **24:** 31–39.
34. WOOD, A. J. J., R. E. VESTAL, C. SPANNATH, W. J. STONE, G. R. WILKINSON & D. G. SHAND. 1979. Propranolol disposition in renal failure. Clin. Res. **27:** 239A.
35. SHOEMAN, D. W. & D. L. AZARNOFF. 1972. The alterations of plasma proteins in uremia as reflected in their ability to bind digitoxin and diphenylhydantoin. Pharmacology. **7:** 169–177.
36. GROSSMAN, S. H., D. DAVIS, B. B. KITCHELL, D. G. SHAND & P. A. ROUTLEDGE. 1982. Diazepam and lidocaine plasma protein binding in renal disease. Clin. Pharmacol. Ther. **31:** 350–357.
37. ZITO, R. A. & P. R. REID. 1978. Lidocaine kinetics predicted by indocyanine green clearance. N. Engl. J. Med. **298:** 1160–1163.
38. BAX, N. D. S., G. T. TUCKER & H. F. WOODS. 1980. Lignocaine and indocyanine green kinetics in patients following myocardial infaction. Br. J. Clin. Pharmacol. **10:** 356–361.
39. ROUTLEDGE, P. A., W. W. STARGEL, A. BARCHOWSKY, G. S. WAGNER & D. G. SHAND. 1982. Control of lidocaine therapy: New perspectives. Ther. Drug Monit. **4:** 265–270.
40. HEWITT, W. R. & J. B. HOOK. 1983. The renal excretion of drugs. *In* Progress in Drug Metabolism, vol. 7. J. W. Bridges & L. F. Chasseaud, Eds. Wiley. New York, NY.
41. LALKA, D., M. B. MEYER, B. R. DUCE & A. T. ELVIN. 1976. Kinetics of the oral antiarrhythmic lidocaine congener, tocainide. Clin. Pharmacol Ther. **19:** 757–766.
42. CUNNINGHAM, J. L., D. D. SHEN, I. SHUDO & D. L. AZARNOFF. 1977. The effects of urine pH and plasma protein binding on the renal clearance of disopyramide. Clin. Pharmacokinet. **2:** 373.
43. REIDENBERG, M. M., M. CAMACHO, J. KLUGER & D. E. DRAYER. 1980. Aging and renal clearance of procainamide and acetyl procainamide. Clin. Pharmacol. Ther. **28:** 732–735.
44. BRATER, D. C. 1980. The pharmacological role of the kidney. Drugs **19:** 31–48.
45. HAGER, W. D., P. FENSTER, M. MAYERSOHN, D. PERRIER, P. GRAVES, F. I. MARUS &

S. GOLDMAN. 1979. Digoxin-quinidine interaction: Pharmacokinetic evaluation. N. Engl. J. Med. **300:** 1238–1241.

46. WALDORFF, S., J. D. ANDERSON, N. HEEBOLL-NIELSEN, N. O. G. NEILSEN, E. MOLTKE, U. SORENSEN & E. STEINESS. 1978. Spironolactone-induced changes in digoxin kinetics. Clin. Pharmacol. Ther. **24:** 162–167.

47. KLEIN, H. O., K. LANG, E. D. SEGNI & E. KAPLINSKY. 1980. Verapamil-digoxin interaction. N. Engl. J. Med. **303:** 160.

48. PEDERSEN, K. E., A. DORPH-PEDERSEN, N. A. KLITGAARD & F. NIELSEN-KUDSK. 1981. Digoxin-verapamil interaction, a single-dose pharmacokinetic study. Clin. Pharmacol. Ther. **30:** 311–316.

49. COCKROFT, D. W. & M. H. GAULT. 1976. Prediction of creatinine clearance from serum creatinine. Nephron **16:** 31–41.

50. BRICKER, N. S. 1979. The pathophysiology of chronic renal disease. *In* Cecil's Textbook of Medicine, 15th ed. P. B. Beeson, W. McDermott & J. B. Wyngaarden, Eds.: 1346–1351. W. B. Saunders. Philadelphia, PA.

51. LUDDEN, T. M. & M. H. CRAWFORD. 1982. N-Acetylprocainamide kinetics after single and repeated oral doses. Clin. Pharmacol. Ther. **31:** 343–349.

52. WHITING, B. & H. L. ELLIOT. 1977. Disopyramide in renal impairment. Lancet **2:** 1363.

53. IDLE, J. R., N. S. OATES, R. R. SHAH & R. L. SMITH. 1983. Protecting poor metabolisers, a group at high risk of adverse drug reactions. Lancet **1:** 1388.

54. HUNTER, J. & L. F. CHASSEAUD. 1976. Clinical aspects of microsomal enzyme induction. *In* Progress in Drug Metabolism. J. W. Bridges & L. F. Chasseaud, Eds. Vol. **1:** 129–191. Wiley. New York, NY.

# The Pharmacogenetics of Antiarrhythmic Drugs

MARCUS M. REIDENBERG

Department of Pharmacology and Medicine
Cornell University Medical College
New York, New York 10021

One of the fundamental questions of clinical pharmacology is: Why do different persons respond differently to the same dose of the same drug? Pioneers in this field, such as Dr. B. B. Brodie, discovered that different persons had different plasma concentrations of drugs when given identical doses and that these differences in concentrations were often due to individual differences in the rates of metabolism of these drugs. Drug metabolism and disposition then became a legitimate area for medical research. Other pioneers, such as Dr. R. T. Williams, began a study of the chemical reactions of drug metabolism and identified reaction pathways by which drugs were biotransformed. Then investigators began to study the factors controlling the rates of these pathways to learn some of the reasons for the individual differences in rates of drug metabolism. A person's inheritance appeared to be one of the important factors controlling the rate of drug metabolism and, through this, the drug concentration in the body and the intensity of drug effects.

## ACETYLATION

Knight, Selin, and Harris in 1959 and Evans, Manley, and McKusick in 1960 presented data to show that a major reason for the individual differences in the rate of isoniazid metabolism was genetic.[1,2] They observed, by studying families, that this trait was inherited by simple Mendelian laws involving a single gene locus. The slow metabolizer was homozygous for the slow gene, while the rapid metabolizer was either homozygous for the rapid gene or the heterozygote. Additional studies gave further support to this single-gene Mendelian inheritance concept for isoniazid acetylation.[3-5] Other drugs such as sulfamethazine, dapsone, and hydralazine are also acetylated by the same enzyme that acetylates isonazid, with individuals having either rapid or slow phenotypes, the phenotype proportion in a population varying from one ethnic group to another.[6-8]

Peters et al.[9] were the first to observe the polymorphic acetylation of dapsone, with the ratio of monoacetyldapsone concentration to dapsone concentration in plasma higher in rapid than in slow acetylators, an observation we subsequently confirmed.[10] These studies demonstrated that dapsone could be used as a probe to identify the genetic acetylator phenotype of an individual.

Procainamide is an aromatic amine that could be acetylated (FIG. 1) and was considered a potential substrate for this genetically controlled polymorphic acetylation pathway of drug metabolism. Dreyfuss et al. observed N-acetylprocainamide (NAPA) in the pooled urine of four patients receiving procainamide,[11]

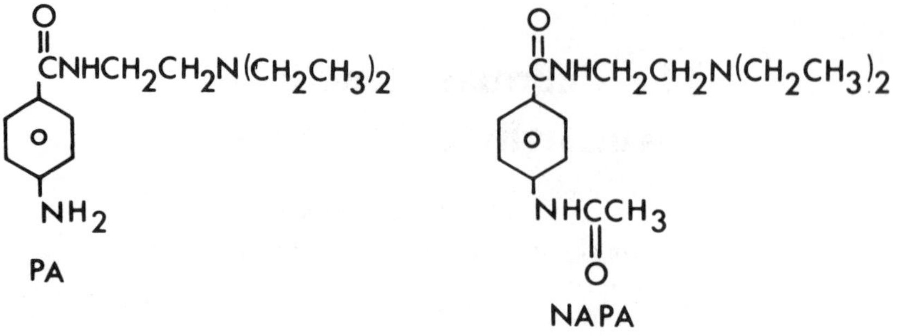

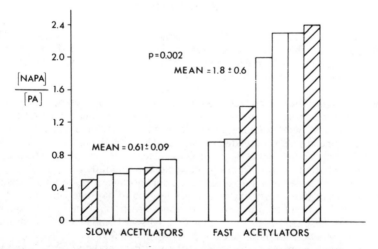

**FIGURE 1.** Chemical structures of procainamide (PA) and *N*-acetylprocainamide (NAPA).

and we observed NAPA in the plasma from each of four patients receiving procainamide orally.[12]

The next question was: Is procainamide acetylation carried out by the genetic polymorphic acetylation pathway? For this study, subjects had their acetylator phenotypes determined with dapsone and then had the NAPA and procainamide levels in plasma measured 3 hours after administration of a dose of procainamide after a minimum of 3 days at constant dose so that a steady state with respect to procainamide and NAPA could be presumed to exist. The subjects who were rapid acetylators of dapsone had higher NAPA to procainamide concentration ratios in their plasma samples than did the subjects who were slow acetylators (FIG. 2). Renal clearance of procainamide was similar in slow and rapid acetylators. NAPA clearance was also the same for each acetylator phenotype. Thus, procainamide was found to be subject to this genetically controlled acetylation.[13]

**FIGURE 2.** Ratio of *N*-acetylprocainamide concentration to procainamide concentration (3 hours after last dose of procainamide) in serum from subjects receiving procainamide orally. The acetylator phenotypes of the subjects were identified with dapsone. The *open bars* represent arrhythmia patients; the *hatched* bars are for obese but otherwise normal volunteers.

Two consequences of this polymorphic acetylation have been observed. Patients receiving procainamide who are slow acetylators develop antinuclear antibody after a shorter period of procainamide therapy than do rapid acetylators.[14] More important, slow acetylators appear to develop the procainamide-induced lupus syndrome after a shorter duration of procainamide therapy than do rapid acetylators. This was observed in the early study[14] and recently updated by Dr. Dennis E. Drayer to include additional cases[15,16] (FIG. 3). (This research led to the trials of NAPA as an antiarrhythmic drug, demonstrating its very weak potency, if any, as an inducer of antinuclear antibody (ANA) and lupus, and suggesting that it is the amino group on procainamide that "incites" the lupus.[17]) Thus, one of the reasons some persons develop the procainamide-induced lupus syndrome earlier than others is that they have the susceptible phenotype (slow) of this genetically controlled rate of procainamide acetylation.

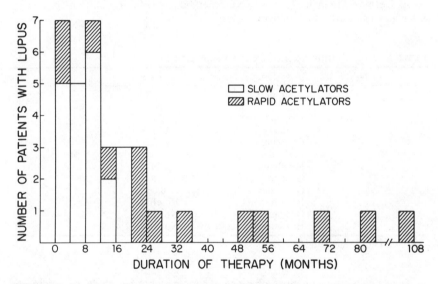

FIGURE 3. Frequency histogram showing the relationship between acetylation phenotype and the duration of procainamide therapy prior to the onset of procainamide-induced lupus.

## OXIDATION

Since oxidation is the major pathway of metabolism of most drugs, many studies have been done to learn the factors that control its rate in different persons. Studies by Vesell and others in the 1960s comparing differences between identical and fraternal twins showed that there was substantial genetic control of drug oxidation rates, but the genetic mechanisms remained obscure[18] since the measurements of the drug half-life values that were done had unimodal distributions. In the mid 1970s, the large variation was noted in dose of the antihypertensive drug, debrisoquine, to achieve blood pressure control. This dose variation was noted to be due to individual variation in the rate of metabolism of this drug. Poor metabolizers of debrisoquine had a much greater intensity of effect of this drug at standard dose than did normal metabolizers. Then in 1977, Mahgoub *et al.*, in

England, demonstrated a biomodal distribution of the urinary debrisoquine/4-hydroxydebrisoquine concentration ratio and another single-gene polymorphism in drug metabolism, now for a pathway of drug oxidation, was discovered.[19-21]

In 1975, Dengler and Eichelbaum were studying sparteine, a drug with antiarrhythmic and uterus-stimulating activity. Two subjects developed adverse effects and were found to have very high concentrations of this drug in their plasma samples. Subsequent studies found a bimodal distribution of the oxidized metabolites of sparteine in urine, and family studies showed that the inheritance was by two alleles on a single locus. The poor metabolizer was homozygous for the recessive allele.[22,23] Inaba et al., in Canada, have recently shown that the same persons who are poor metabolizers of debrisoquine are also poor metabolizers of sparteine,[24] so that a clear defect in a specific drug oxidation pathway has been demonstrated. This deficiency is inherited as an autosomal recessive gene for poor metabolism. About 3-8% of those populations studied (British, Swedish, Swiss, German, Ghanaian) are very poor metabolizers of drugs biotransformed by this pathway of drug metabolism.

TABLE 1. *In Vitro* Inhibition of Dehydrosparteine Formation[a]

| Drug | $K_i$ ($\mu$M) |
|---|---|
| Alprenolol | 15-20 |
| Metoprolol | 15-20 |
| Propranolol | 15-20 |
| Timolol | 15-20 |
| Oxprenolol | 15-20 |
| Lidocaine | 80 |
| Mexiletine | 30 |
| Quinine | 10 |
| Quinidine | 0.06 |
| Isoproterenol | No effect |
| Ouabain | No effect |
| Hexamethonium | No effect |

[a] From Otton, Inaba, and Kalow.[29]

The clinical consequences of being a poor metabolizer of debrisoquine are beginning to be observed. Many beta blockers appear to be metabolized by this pathway of drug metabolism. Four patients with very high plasma levels of alprenolol, metoprolol, or timolol were found to be poor metabolizers of debrisoquine.[25] A 25-mg dose of metoprolol caused a more intense and prolonged beta blockade in a poor debrisoquine metabolizer than in a normal metabolizer.[26] Another beta blocker, bufuralol, had much higher levels and an increased risk of side effects in poor debrisoquine metabolizers than in normal metabolizers.[27] Thus, many beta blockers are metabolized by the debrisoquine pathway, and poor metabolizers achieve high levels at usual doses and are at increased risk for drug toxicity.

Poor metabolism of encainide has also been correlated with poor metabolism of debrisoquine.[28]

Recently, Otton, Inaba, and Kalow presented data on the *in vitro* inhibition of sparteine oxidation by a variety of drugs (TABLE 1).[29] Their demonstration of $K_i$ values of 15-20 $\mu$M for the beta blockers correlates well with the clinical observations just summarized. From their *in vitro* data in TABLE 1, one could predict that lidocaine, mexiletine, and quinidine might accumulate in poor sparteine/debriso-quine metabolizers.

Our observations of the ratio of serum levels of 3-hydroxyquinidine/quinidine in serum from 67 patients did not indicate a small "outlier" group of poor metabolizers.[30] If anything, there may have been a small number of outliers at the rapid metabolism end of the frequency histogram. This, along with many observations by many investigators, suggests that there are other genetically controlled pathways of drug oxidation that are of importance for the metabolism of antiarrhythmic drugs. Recently, Penno and Vesell published their observations indicating monogenic control of pathways of antipyrine oxidation.[31] This appears to be under different genetic control than the debrisoquine/sparteine metabolic pathway.[32] It remains for future research to identify whether there is relevance of this work to the pharmacogenetics of antiarrhythmic drugs.

## CONCLUSION

Genetic factors exist that account for some of the variation between individuals in the dose–response relationships or time–action characteristics of antiarrhythmic drugs. The inheritance of enzyme systems that metabolize drugs slowly accounts for some of the apparent sensitivity of certain individuals to adverse reactions or toxicity. As greater understanding of clinical pharmacology and pharmacogenetics develops and is applied to antiarrhythmic therapeutics, responses to drugs in this class should become more predictable, and in this way, therapeusis will become both safer and more effective.

## REFERENCES

1. KNIGHT, R. A., M. J. SELIN & H. W. HARRIS. 1959. Cited in Evans et al.[2]
2. EVANS, D. A. P., K. A. MANLEY & V. A. MCKUSICK. 1960. Genetic control of isoniazid metabolism in man. Brit. Med. J. 2: 485–491.
3. EVANS, D. A. P. & T. A. WHITE. 1964. Human acetylation polymorphism. J. Lab. Clin. Med. 63: 394–403.
4. EVANS, D. A. P. 1968. Genetic variations in the acetylation of isoniazid and other drugs. Ann. N.Y. Acad. Sci. 151: 723.
5. LUNDE, P. K. M., K. FRISLID & V. HANSTEEN. 1977. Disease and acetylation polymorphism. Clin. Pharmacokinetics 2: 182–197.
6. DRAYER, D. E. & M. M. REIDENBERG. 1977. Clinical consequences of polymorphic acetylation of basic drugs. Clin. Pharmacol. Ther. 22: 251–258.
7. WEBER, W. W. & D. W. HEIN. 1979. Clinical pharmacokinetics of isoniazid. Clin. Pharmacokinetics 4: 401–422.
8. UETRECHT, J. P. & R. L. WOOSLEY. 1981. Acetylator phenotype and lupus erythematosus. Clin. Pharmacokinetics 6: 118–134.
9. PETERS, J. H., G. R. GORDON, D. C. GHOUL, J. G. TOLENTINO, G. P. WALSH & L. LEVY. 1972. The disposition of the antileproic drug dapsone (DDS) in Philippine subjects. Am. J. Trop. Med. Hyg. 21: 450–457.
10. REIDENBERG, M. M., D. DRAYER, A. L. DEMARCO & C. T. BELLO. 1973. Hydralazine elimination in man. Clin. Pharmacol. Ther. 14: 970–977.
11. DREYFUSS, J., J. T. BIGGER, A. I. COHEN & E. C. SCHREIBER. 1972. Metabolism of procainamide in Rhesus monkey and man. Clin. Pharmacol. Ther. 13: 366–371.
12. DRAYER, D. E., M. M. REIDENBERG & R. W. SEVY. 1974. N-acetylprocainamide: an active metabolite of procainamide. Proc. Soc. Exp. Biol. Med. 146: 358–363.

13. REIDENBERG, M. M., D. E. DRAYER, M. LEVY & H. WARNER. 1975. Polymorphic acetylation of procainamide in man. Clin. Pharmacol. Ther. **17:** 722–730.
14. WOOSLEY, R. L., D. E. DRAYER, M. M. REIDENBERG, A. S. NIES, K. CARR & J. A. OATES. 1978. Effect of acetylator phenotype on the rate at which procainamide induces antinuclear antibodies and the lupus syndrome. N. Engl. J. Med. **298:** 1157–1159.
15. KLUGER, J., D. E. DRAYER, M. M. REIDENBERG & R. LAHITA. 1981. Acetylprocainamide therapy in patients with previous procainamide-induced lupus syndrome. Ann. Int. Med. **95:** 18–23.
16. EHRLICK, G. C., M. FREEMAN-NARROD & G. S. WINEBURGH. 1979. Predominance of slow acetylators among patients with rheumatoid arthritis. Eur. J. Rheumatol. Inflammation **2:** 196–198.
17. REIDENBERG, M. M. 1983. Aromatic amines and the pathogenesis of lupus erythematosus. Am. J. Med. **75:** 1037–1042.
18. VESELL, E. S. 1974. Polygenic factors controlling drug response. Med. Clin. N. Amer. **58:** 951–963.
19. MAHGOUB, A., L. G. DRING, J. R. IDLE, R. LANCASTER & R. L. SMITH. 1977. The polymorphic hydroxylation of debrisoquine in man. Lancet **2:** 584–586.
20. EVANS, D. A. P., A. MAHGOUB, T. P. SLOAN, J. R. IDLE & R. L. SMITH. 1980. A family and population study of the genetic polymorphism of debrisoquine oxidation in a white British population. J. Med. Genet. **17:** 102–105.
21. WOOLHOUSE, N. M., B. ANDOH, A. MAHGOUB, T. P. SLOAN, J. R. IDLE & R. L. SMITH. 1979. Debrisoquine hydroxylation polymorphism among Ghanaians and Caucasians. Clin. Pharmacol. Ther. **26:** 584–591.
22. EICHELBAUM, M., N. SPANNBRUCKER, B. STEINCKE & H. J. DENGLER. 1979. Defective N-oxidation of sparteine in man: A new pharmacogenetic defect. Eur. J. Clin. Pharmacol. **16:** 183–187.
23. EICHELBAUM, M. 1982. Defective oxidation of drugs. Clin. Pharmacokinet. **7:** 1–22.
24. INABA, T., A. VINKS, S. V. OTTON & W. KALOW. 1983. Comparative pharmacogenetics of sparteine and debrisoquine. Clin. Pharmacol. **33:** 394–399.
25. ALVAN, G., C. VON BAHR, P. SEIDEMAN & F. SJOQVIST. 1982. High plasma concentrations of β-receptor blocking drugs and deficient debrisoquine hydroxylation. Lancet **i:** 333.
26. SHAH, R. R., N. S. OATES, J. R. IDLE & R. L. SMITH. 1982. Beta-blockers and drug oxidation states. Lancet **i:** 508–509.
27. DAYER, P., F. COURVOISIER, L. BALANT & J. FABRE. 1982. Beta-blockers and drug oxidation states. Lancet **i:** 509.
28. WOOSLEY, R. L., D. M. RODEN, H. J. DUFF, E. L. CAREY, A. J. J. WOOD & G. R. WILKINSON. 1981. Co-inheritance of deficient oxidative metabolism of encainide and debrisoquine. Clin. Res. **29:** 501A.
29. OTTON, S. V., T. INABA & W. KALOW. 1983. Some cardiovascular drugs subject to the hepatic oxidation defect. Second World Conference on Clinical Pharmacology, Abstract No. 623.
30. DRAYER, D. E., M. HUGHES, B. LORENZO & M. M. REIDENBERG. 1980. Prevalence of high (3S)-3-hydroxyquinidine/quinidine ratios in serum, and clearance of quinidine in cardiac patients of varying ages. Clin. Pharmacol. Ther. **27:** 72–75.
31. PENRO, M. B. & E. S. VESELL. 1983. Monogenic control of variations in antipyrine metabolite formation. J. Clin. Invest. **71:** 1698–1709.
32. EICHELBAUM, M., L. BERTILSSON & J. SAIVC. 1983. Antipyrine metabolism in relation to polymorphic oxidations of sparteine and debrisoquine. Br. J. Clin. Pharmacol. **15:** 317–321.

# Metabolites of Cardiac Antiarrhythmic Drugs: Their Clinical Role

ROBERT E. KATES

*Division of Cardiology*
*Stanford University School of Medicine*
*Stanford, California 94305*

In recent years considerable attention has been focused on the metabolism of administered chemical substances. While historically metabolism was viewed primarily as a process of detoxification whereby drugs are deactivated and converted to more rapidly eliminated substrates, it is now well recognized that metabolic alteration of administered drugs may lead to the production of compounds with enhanced or new pharmacologic properties; subsequent accumulation of these metabolites may be substantial.

The metabolism of drugs used to treat and prevent cardiac rhythm abnormalities deserves special attention. Antiarrhythmic drugs are highly toxic compounds and metabolic transformation leading either to their deactivation or to the production of active metabolites strongly affects their clinical efficacy. In those cases where significant metabolites are produced, it is essential to elucidate their pharmacologic properties and disposition characteristics. Without such information, the safe and optimal use of these drugs is not possible.

While the metabolic profiles of most antiarrhythmic drugs are not fully elucidated, the extent of metabolism is known for most. The extent of metabolism is generally determined by analysis of drug excreted into the urine after intravenous administration. The difference between the dose administered and the amount excreted unchanged in the urine is assumed to be due to metabolism. As illustrated in TABLE 1, most antiarrhythmic drugs are extensively metabolized, the notable exception being bretylium. Also listed in TABLE 1 are the major reported metabolites of these drugs. The chemical structures of these metabolites, along with their parent drug, are shown in FIGURE 1. The metabolites listed have been reported either to accumulate in plasma of patients after administration of parent drug or to be pharmacologically active. Some of these metabolites are both cardioactive and accumulate extensively.

Since most antiarrhythmic drugs are tertiary amines, N-dealkylation is a major route of metabolism for these compounds. It has been shown[1] that the rate of demethylation of tertiary amines is greater than for secondary amines. Therefore, it is not too surprising that the secondary amine metabolites of several of these drugs are eliminated slowly and accumulate extensively. Other routes of metabolism which produce active metabolites also involve minor structural modifications, such as aromatic hydroxylation, O-demethylation, and N-acetylation.

Two factors need to be considered in assessing the clinical role of metabolites of antiarrhythmic drugs. The first is their intrinsic pharmacologic activities, and the second is the extent to which they accumulate in the body. Listed in TABLE 1 are the relative plasma concentrations and relative potencies of these metabolites. The relative concentrations are expressed as fractions of the concentration of their respective parent drugs, and represent steady-state conditions. The manner by which relative potency is determined for these metabolites is described below. In almost all cases, these are evaluated in animal arrhythmia models.

## Metabolites of Antiarrhythmic Drugs

Compound                     Structure

| Compound | R | R' | Structure |
|---|---|---|---|
| 1. Amiodarone | $C_2H_5$ | – | 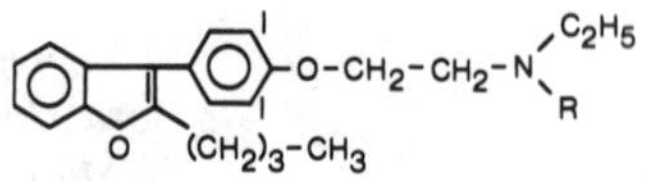 |
|    desethylamiodarone | H | – | |
| 2. Disopyramide | $CH(CH_3)_2$ | – | 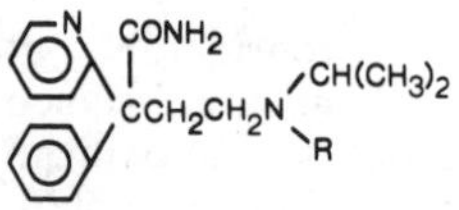 |
|    mono-N-dealkylated disopyramide | H | – | |
| 3. Encainide | $CH_3$ | H | 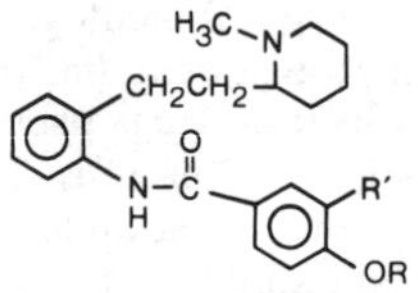 |
|    O-demethyl encainide | H | H | |
|    3-methoxy-O-demethyl encainide | H | $OCH_3$ | |
| 4. Lidocaine | $CH_2CH_3$ | $CH_2CH_3$ | 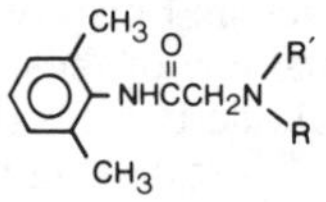 |
|    monoethylglycine xylidide | $CH_2CH_3$ | H | |
|    glycine xylidide | H | H | |
| 5. Lorcainide | $CH_2(CH_3)_2$ | – | 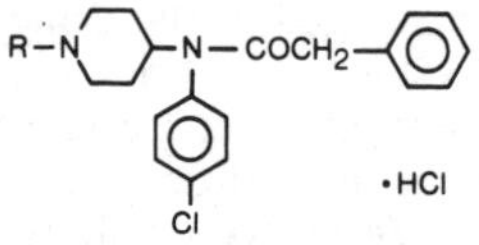 |
|    norlorcainide | H | – | |
| 6. Procainamide | H | – | 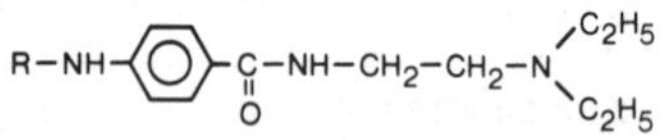 |
|    N-acetylprocainamide | $CH_3\overset{O}{\overset{\|}{C}}$ | – | |
| 7. Quinidine | H | – | 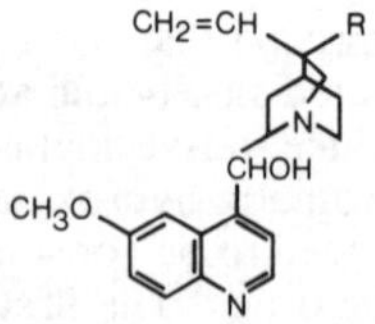 |
|    3-hydroxyquinidine | OH | – | |

**FIGURE 1.** Chemical structures of antiarrhythmic drugs and their major active metabolites.

## INDIVIDUAL DRUGS

This paper considers the currently available data on the primary antiarrhythmic drugs in use today. For each drug the metabolic profile (if known), the extent of accumulation and pharmacologic properties of significant metabolites, and the clinical relevance of these metabolites are discussed.

### Amiodarone

The metabolism of amiodarone has not been characterized completely, but data from Andreasen et al.[2] and Riva et al.[3] suggest that amiodarone is extensively metabolized. In both of these investigations urine was collected from patients during chronic oral amiodarone therapy, and analysis of the urine indicated that no unmetabolized amiodarone was present. Studies by Broekhuysen et al.,[4]

TABLE 1. Metabolites of Antiarrhythmic Drugs

| Drug | % Metabolized | Major Metabolites | Relative Potency | Relative Plasma Concentration |
|------|---------------|-------------------|------------------|-------------------------------|
| Amiodarone | 99 | N-desethylamiodarone | — | 1 |
| Bretylium | 20 | — | — | — |
| Disopyramide | 40–60 | N-desisopropyl diso- | <.5 | .5 |
| Encainide | — | O-demethyl encainide | >1 | 5 |
| | | 3-methoxy-O-demethyl encainide | ≥1 | 5 |
| Lidocaine | 95 | Monoethylglycine xylidide | .83 | .5–2 |
| | | glycine xylidide | .1 | .1–1 |
| Lorcainide | 97 | Norlorcainide | 1 | .5–4 |
| Mexiletine | 80 | — | — | — |
| Procainamide | 50 | N-acetylprocainamide | <1 | .5–2.5 |
| Propafenone | 99 | 5-hydroxypropafenone | 2 | — |
| Quinidine | 85 | 3-hydroxyquinidine | 1 | .2–.8 |
| Tocainide | 50–70 | — | — | — |

utilizing radioiodinated drug, found that amiodarone is deiodinated to a small extent. Their data suggest that about 20% of an administered dose undergoes deiodination. However, the deiodinated metabolites are probably not cardioactive. Several potential metabolites have been analyzed,[5] but only the mono-N-desethyl derivative has been positively identified in the blood of patients during chronic oral treatment. Harris and coworkers[6] reported accumulation of this metabolite in the plasma of 70 patients during chronic amiodarone therapy. They reported a range of steady-state desethylamiodarone trough levels of 0.3 to 4.7 $\mu$g/ml. For comparison, the range of amiodarone levels was 0.2 to 5.2 $\mu$g/ml. These data indicate that this metabolite accumulates in the plasma to levels comparable with those of the parent drug, amiodarone. The di-desethyl metabolite has been identified in the blood and myocardium of chronically treated dogs, but does not appear to accumulate in man.[7]

Whether N-desethylamiodarone is pharmacologically active or not is presently unknown. If experience with N-dealkylated metabolites of other antiarrhythmic drugs can be used as a reference, there is good justification to speculate that this metabolite of amiodarone is cardioactive.

Harris and coworkers[6] reported that both amiodarone and N-desethylamiodarone were detectable in the plasma of patients 12 months after discontinuation of therapy, and they estimated an elimination half-life for N-desethylamiodarone of 60 days. This is longer than their reported half-life for amiodarone of 52 days.

While the clinical significance of the accumulation of N-desethylamiodarone is not clearly defined, clinical data do exist which suggest that it does have an effect on myocardial conduction. Wellens and coworkers[8] reported that both atrial and ventricular refractory periods and the H-V interval change after chronic oral, but not single intravenous bolus, doses of amiodarone. Other measured electrophysiologic effects showed similar changes after both intravenous and chronic oral administration. These differences have been interpreted to suggest qualitative differences between amiodarone and its N-dealkylated metabolite. This conclusion is based on the observation that little to no metabolite is present following single intravenous bolus doses of amiodarone, but significant accumulation does occur after chronic oral therapy. The difference in electrophysiologic effects after oral and intravenous amiodarone may be due to this metabolite.

### Disopyramide

While disopyramide is predominantly excreted unchanged in the urine (TABLE 1), approximately 15–25% of an administered dose is metabolized via N-dealkylation.[9,10]

The most extensive report dealing with the accumulation of the mono-N-dealkylated metabolite of disopyramide is that of Aitio,[11] who measured plasma levels of disopyramide and mono-N-dealkylated disopyramide in 118 patients who were receiving disopyramide chronically for control of cardiac rhythm abnormalities. Three categories of patients were studied: patients with renal impairment, patients with normal renal function who were taking known enzyme-inducing drugs, and patients with normal renal function who were not taking enzyme-inducing agents. In the patients with renal impairment (serum creatinine = 181 ± 16 $\mu$mol/liter), the mean trough concentration of the metabolite was 1.41 ± 0.19 $\mu$g/ml. The ratio of metabolite/disopyramide was 0.52 ± 0.15. In patients with normal renal function, the trough levels of the mono-N-dealkylated disopyramide were 1.67 ± 0.38 $\mu$g/ml and 2.85 ± 0.14 $\mu$g/ml for the patients taking, and not taking, enzyme-inducing drugs, respectively. The ratios of metabolite/disopyramide were 0.34 ± 0.03 and 1.21 ± 0.26 for the two groups, respectively. Despite the availability of numerous analytical methods for measuring the mono-N-dealkylated metabolite of disopyramide, very few other reports have appeared in the literature describing the accumulation of this metabolite in patients.

Mono-N-dealkylated disopyramide does have significant cardiac effects. Grant and coworkers[12] studied the relative effects of disopyramide and this metabolite in guinea pig atria and found that mono-N-dealkylated disopyramide is about 20 to 25% as potent as disopyramide in regard to prolonging the refractory period. These investigators also reported that this metabolite produces a transient positive inotropic effect before producing a negative inotropic effect at doses three to four times those of disopyramide. Baines and coworkers[13] also studied the comparative pharmacologic actions of disopyramide and this metabolite. Using an isolated guinea pig ilium preparation these investigators found that mono-N-dealkylated disopyramide had 24 times the anticholinergic potency as the parent drug. These data suggest that the anticholinergic side effects of disopyramide may be due, in large part, to this metabolite.

Other than the above mentioned plasma level data for mono-$N$-dealkylated disopyramide, little else has been reported. There are currently no reported pharmacokinetic data for this metabolite.

On the basis of the data of Baines and coworkers,[13] it appears that the clinical significance of the major metabolite of disopyramide is due to its striking anticholinergic effects. Its effect would be most prominent in individuals who are fast metabolizers of disopyramide or who are taking drugs known to induce hepatic microsomal enzymes,[11] since induction of hepatic enzymes leads to a greater production of this metabolite. Under these conditions, the accumulation of metabolite can produce plasma levels greater than those of the parent drug and thus presumably enhance the anticholinergic effects. The role of mono-$N$-dealkylated disopyramide appears to be one of limiting the usefulness of the parent drug.

## Encainide

At least two metabolites of encainide have been identified. These are $O$-demethyl encainide (ODE) and 3-methoxy-$O$-demethyl encainide (MODE). A third metabolite, $N$-demethyl encainide, also has been identified in serum from some patients.

The accumulation of $O$-demethyl- and 3-methoxy-$O$-demethyl encainide has been documented in patients treated chronically with encainide for ventricular arrhythmias.[14] Mean steady-state concentrations of these two metabolites were both greater than five times the mean steady-state level of the parent drug. While the mean concentration ratios (metabolite/encainide) were greater than 5, there was substantial interpatient variability. One individual in the group studied produced very minor amounts of these metabolites and had concentration ratios of 0.7 and 0.06 for $O$-demethyl and 3-methoxy-$O$-demethyl encainide, respectively.

The pharmacologic effects of these two metabolites have been reported by Gomoll and coworkers,[15] Dresel,[16] and Elharrar and Zipes.[17] Gomoll and coworkers reported that in the ouabain-induced arrhythmia model in dogs, 3-methoxy-$O$-demethyl encainide was about equipotent to the parent drug, while $O$-demethyl encainide was considerably more potent in suppressing ouabain-induced arrhythmias. However, in conscious dogs who had previously undergone two-stage coronary ligation, the minimal antiarrhythmic doses of encainide, $O$-demethyl encainide and 3-methoxy-$O$-demethyl encainide were 1.0, 0.5 and 0.25 mg/kg, respectively. These data suggest that 3-methoxy-$O$-demethyl- and $O$-demethyl encainide are both more effective antiarrhythmic agents in this model than the parent drug. Dresel[16] studied these compounds in a rabbit Langendorff preparation. The concentration of the two metabolites required to slow atrial and His-Purkinje conduction was 10% of the molar concentration of encainide required to produce the same effect. The concentration of metabolites required to slow AV nodal conduction was 1% of that required for encainide.

Elharrar and Zipes[17] reported that $O$-demethyl encainide was nine times as potent as, and 3-methoxy-$O$-demethyl encainide equipotent to, the parent drug when evaluated with a canine Purkinje and ventricular fiber preparation. They concluded that these metabolites had electrophysiologic profiles similar to the parent drug, but that the $O$-demethyl metabolite was far more potent.

Further data relating to the activity of these metabolites have been reported by Jackman and coworkers.[18] These investigators reported that after chronic administration of encainide, prolongation of the ventricular refractory period occurs.

Acute studies carried out following administration of single doses of encainide have failed to show this effect.[19] This difference has been attributed to the metabolites. After single doses of encainide, the plasma levels of these metabolites are low, but they accumulate during chronic administration of the drug and accrue to levels in the plasma that are sufficient to produce electrophysiologic effects. The effect on the ventricular refractory period probably represents a qualitative difference between the effects of these metabolites and their parent drug.

Carey and coworkers[20] evaluated the antiarrhythmic response after both an acute intravenous dose and chronic oral administration of encainide to groups of patients who were rapid and slow metabolizers of encainide. These investigators found a correlation between the concentration of encainide and antiarrhythmic efficacy only in the slow metabolizers (concentrations from 250–600 ng/ml). In those with rapid metabolisms, who produced the O-demethyl metabolite, the best correlation between concentration and efficacy was with O-demethyl encainide and not the parent drug.

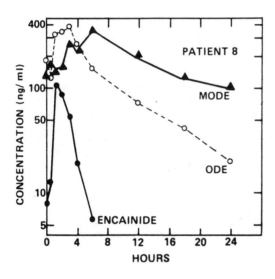

FIGURE 2. Plasma concentration–time curves for encainide (●), ODE (○), and MODE (▲) in a patient after discontinuation of long-term oral encainide administration. (From Kates *et al.*[14] Reprinted by permission.

The O-demethyl and 3-methoxy-O-demethyl metabolites of encainide accumulate extensively due to their slow elimination from the body. After discontinuation of encainide administration, the time course of disappearance of these metabolites from the plasma has been studied in patients.[14] FIGURE 2 illustrates the disappearance time course of encainide, ODE, and MODE in one patient after discontinuation of long-term oral encainide therapy. It can be readily appreciated that ODE and MODE are eliminated much more slowly than encainide itself. O-demethyl encainide was reported to decay with a half-life of 11.41 ± 9.58 hr and the disappearance of 3-methoxy-O-demethyl encainide was too slow to determine an elimination half-life during the blood-sampling period. At the time of the last blood sample (24 hr), the mean plasma concentration of this metabolite was still 59.8 ± 39.9% of the mean steady-state level.

These two metabolites of encainide are clearly of clinical importance. They have been shown to be similar to encainide in the electrophysiologic effects they produce, and O-demethyl encainide is by far the more potent compound. In addition to being cardioactive, these metabolites accumulate extensively in the plasma. During chronic oral therapy with encainide, these metabolites are the dominant species in the plasma, with encainide almost completely cleared from the body during each dosing interval. The slow disappearance of these metabolites is a major factor to consider when designing studies of the clinical efficacy of encainide, especially if a crossover design is employed.

## Lidocaine

The metabolism of lidocaine has been studied extensively, and several metabolites of lidocaine identified.[21-24] The two metabolites that have generated the most interest are the mono- and di-N-desethylated compounds; these are monoethylglycinexylidide and glycinexylide, respectively.

Concentrations of glycinexylidide (GX) and monoethylglycinexylidide (MEGX) during constant infusion of lidocaine have been reported for patients with renal failure, congestive heart failure, and arrhythmias without other complicating problems.[25-27] Accumulation of MEGX is not different between arrhythmia patients with and without congestive heart failure. The mean (± S.D.) concentration ratio (MEGX/lidocaine) was 0.23 ± 0.26. After a 12-hr infusion of lidocaine to four patients with renal failure, the levels of both metabolites ranged from 20 to 60% of those of lidocaine.

Drayer and coworkers[28] also recently evaluated the plasma levels of lidocaine, MEGX and GX in 33 patients who were infused with lidocaine for a period of at least 1 day. The ratios of the serum concentrations of MEGX/lidocaine and GX/lidocaine were 0.36 ± 0.26 and 0.11 ± 0.11, respectively.

These metabolites of lidocaine have been studied in regard to their effects on both myocardial conduction and the central nervous system.[29-32] Blumer and coworkers[29] evaluated the convulsant potencies of lidocaine and these two metabolites in rats. These investigators concluded that lidocaine and MEGX are equally potent with respect to convulsant properties, but that GX did not produce convulsions. Burney and coworkers[30] evaluated lidocaine and these two metabolites in a ouabain-induced arrhythmia model employing guinea pig atria. The potency of MEGX was reported to be 83% that of the parent drug, and GX was reported to be only 10% as potent as lidocaine. Studies by Strong and coworkers[32] were carried out in mice with chloroform-induced ventricular tachycardia to evaluate the antiarrhythmic potency of these metabolites. Normalizing their results for plasma levels, these investigators concluded that MEGX was 99%, and GX was 26%, as potent as lidocaine.

Similar results have been reported by Freedman and coworkers.[31] These investigators studied the antiarrhythmic potency of lidocaine and MEGX in dogs after coronary artery ligation. They reported that lidocaine and MEGX are equipotent, but that at high plasma levels, lidocaine has a greater negative inotropic effect than does this metabolite.

Drayer and coworkers[28] noted that on the average, MEGX levels were higher in patients who exhibited signs of toxicity. They suggested that MEGX contributes to toxicity during lidocaine therapy.

Limited data exist regarding the disposition time course of these two metabolites of lidocaine. Strong and coworkers[32] administered GX intravenously to two normal subjects and collected blood samples for a period of 24 hr. They reported disappearance half-lives of 9.6 and 10 hr. They also reported that between 40 to

60% of the administered GX was eliminated unchanged in the urine. Halkin and coworkers[26] measured lidocaine and MEGX concentrations in three patients after termination of lidocaine that had been infused for 11 hr. They reported disappearance half-lives for MEGX ranging from 1.2 to 3.3 hr.

The clinical implications of the two major metabolites of lidocaine have been discussed by several investigators, but no consensus appears to have been reached. In most cases, GX does not exert an appreciable clinical effect because of its low potency and relatively minor accumulation. MEGX, however, does warrant further consideration. It is a potent antiarrhythmic and convulsant agent which has been shown to accumulate to plasma levels that approach or even exceed those of lidocaine. While GX has a long elimination half-life, the half-life of MEGX is similar to that of lidocaine. After discontinuation of a lidocaine infusion, the time course of dissipation of effect should parallel that of the decay of lidocaine, and the monoethyl metabolite, from the plasma.

### Lorcainide

The complete metabolism of lorcainide has not been reported, but one major metabolite has been identified. Lorcainide undergoes $N$-dealkylation, producing the important active metabolite, norlorcainide. This metabolite is a product of the first-pass clearance of orally administered lorcainide and is not produced in significant amounts after intravenous administration.

The first report documenting the accumulation of norlorcainide in patients treated with lorcainide was that of Meinertz and coworkers.[33] Trough steady-state plasma concentrations of lorcainide and norlorcainide were evaluated in five patients who were being treated chronically with lorcainide. The concentration of norlorcainide was $2.01 \pm 0.93$ times the simultaneously measured lorcainide concentration. In another report[34] similar results were obtained. In this study mean steady-state concentrations of lorcainide and norlorcainide were calculated. The concentration ratios of norlorcainide/lorcainide were $2.2 \pm 0.9$ and $2.7 \pm 1.5$ after 2 and 4 weeks of therapy, respectively.

The pharmacologic activity of norlorcainide has been studied in the dog,[35] and norlorcainide has been administered intravenously to one patient.[33] Studies in anesthetized dogs showed that the electrophysiologic effects of norlorcainide are both qualitatively and quantitatively similar. Administration of norlorcainide to one patient with frequent ventricular extrasystoles demonstrated that this compound has significant antiarrhythmic effects. This metabolite produced widening of the QRS and prolongation of the P-Q interval. In a recent study[36] it was reported that the electrophysiologic effects of intravenous and oral lorcainide differ. The differences noted were prolongation of the A-H interval and the atrial and ventricular refractory periods. These effects were only observed following oral administration. The difference was attributed to the presence of norlorcainide after oral but not after intravenous administration.

Norlorcainide is slowly cleared from the body and has an elimination half-life that is approximately three times as long as that of the parent drug. The disappearance half-life of norlorcainide was reported to be $26.8 \pm 8.2$ hr.[37] FIGURE 3 illustrates the disappearance time course of lorcainide and norlorcainide in one patient after discontinuation of oral lorcainide after 1 week of therapy. It can be appreciated that significant concentrations of norlorcainide remain in the plasma for days after lorcainide has been essentially cleared from the body.

Norlorcainide has been shown to still be present in the plasma of one patient as late as 1 week following his last dose.

The accumulation of norlorcainide is of considerable clinical importance. It has definite antiarrhythmic effects, and in some respects is equipotent with lorcainide. It also appears to possess some properties that make it qualitatively different from its parent drug. The accumulation of norlorcainide, when considered along with its potency, argues for its major role as a contributor to the clinical efficacy of lorcainide. The long half-life of norlorcainide must be considered when designing a clinical study involving a crossover design. Further studies are needed to elucidate more fully the role of this important metabolite. At present, it appears that norlorcainide is itself a unique and potentially valuable antiarrhythmic agent.

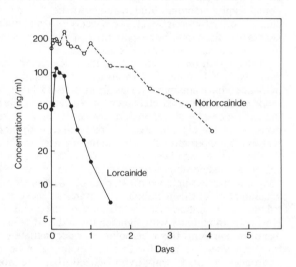

**FIGURE 3.** Plasma concentration–time curves for lorcainide (●) and norlorcainide (○) in a patient after discontinuation of lorcainide therapy. Lorcainide had been administered for 1 week. The last dose was administered at time = 0.

## Procainamide

The metabolism of procainamide has been studied extensively and its major metabolite, N-acetylprocainamide, is well known. It is generally accepted that the enzyme (N-acetyltransferase) involved in the metabolism of procainamide is bimodally distributed, some individuals being fast "acetylators" and others slow.

The accumulation of N-acetylprocainamide in patients receiving procainamide depends on both the acetylator status of the patient and his or her renal function. Reidenberg and coworkers[38] measured the plasma concentrations of N-acetylprocainamide and procainamide in 16 patients of known acetylator phenotype who were receiving chronic procainamide therapy. The ratio of the plasma concentrations (N-acetylprocainamide/procainamide) was higher in the rapid acetylator group (1.8) than in the slow acetylator group (0.61). The highest N-acetylprocainamide level in the slow acetylators was 5.0 μg/ml and in the fast acetylators it was 15.1 μg/ml.

N-acetylprocainamide accumulates extensively in patients with impaired renal function, since it is eliminated primarily by the kidneys. Drayer and coworkers[39] studied six patients with renal function impairment, four of whom were on chronic dialysis. N-acetylprocainamide concentrations were found to be between 14 and 28 μg/ml, while the mean concentration of the parent drug was only 6.2 μg/ml.

The cardiovascular effects of N-acetylprocainamide have been studied extensively, and clinical trials have been carried out to evaluate this metabolite as a unique antiarrhythmic agent. These studies have provided data relative to the actions of this metabolite in the absence of the confounding influence of the parent drug. N-acetylprocainamide is highly cardioactive, but its electrophysiologic effects are both quantitatively and qualitatively different from those of procainamide.[40] In the absence of procainamide, plasma levels of N-acetylprocainamide between 15 and 25 μg/ml are required to produce an antiarrhythmic effect. These data would suggest that N-acetylprocainamide is about one-third as potent as procainamide. Roden and coworkers[41] have reported, however, that the clinical antiarrhythmic spectra of N-acetylprocainamide and procainamide are not necessarily the same. Some patients respond to N-acetylprocainamide, but not to the parent drug. The reverse is also true.

The disposition kinetics of N-acetylprocainamide have recently been reviewed extensively.[42] In patients with normal renal function, the disappearance half-life of N-acetylprocainamide varies from 5 to 15 hr.[43] Stec and coworkers[44] have reported that the renal clearance of N-acetylprocainamide is directly related to the clearance of endogenous creatinine. Reidenberg and coworkers[45] reported a decrease in the clearance of this metabolite with increasing age. This decrease was evident even after the age-related changes in renal function are considered.

The clinical significance of the N-acetyl metabolite of procainamide has received a considerable amount of attention, partly because of its potential as a unique antiarrhythmic agent. In patients without renal function impairment, the accumulation of this metabolite, even in fast acetylators, is not sufficient to contribute to the antiarrhythmic efficacy or the cardiac toxicity of procainamide. However, in patients with significantly reduced renal function, due to either old age or impairment, this metabolite may accumulate extensively and be contributory. An alternate role for this metabolite of procainamide was suggested by Schroeder et al.,[46] who hypothesized that the concentrations of N-acetylprocainamide that normally accrue are not sufficient to contribute to the antiarrhythmic efficacy of the parent drug, but are sufficient to compete with procainamide for myocardial binding sites, and that subsequently N-acetylprocainamide is a competitive antagonist. Further studies are needed to fully evaluate this possibility.

### Quinidine

Several metabolites of quinidine have been identified and at least two of these are cardioactive. Quinidine undergoes oxidation in the liver, producing 3-hydroxyquinidine, 2'-oxoquinidine, O-desmethylquinidine, and possibly an N-oxide rearrangement product.[47-49] These products of metabolic oxidation are known to be subsequently conjugated and are eliminated primarily as glucuronide conjugates. Horning and coworkers[50] recently reported isolating significant quantities of the diastereoisomers of 10, 11-dihydroxy-10, 11-dihydroquinidine in the urine of patients taking quinidine.

The steady-state accumulation of 3-hydroxy- and 2'-oxoquinidine has been studied by Drayer and coworkers[48] in patients with normal and impaired renal function. In patients with normal renal function, the steady-state trough concentrations of the 3-hydroxy and 2'-oxo metabolites of quinidine were 38% ± 24% and 4% ± 1% of the quinidine concentration, respectively. These ratios do not change substantially in azotemic patients. Kewitz and coworkers[51] reported steady-state levels of quinidine, 3-hydroxy quinidine, and quinidine N-oxide in patients during chronic oral therapy. Using their mean concentrations, ratios (metabolite/quinidine) of 0.34 and 0.18 can be calculated for the 3-hydroxy and the N-oxide metabolites, respectively.

The cardiac activity of some of these metabolites has been evaluated in different animal models. Drayer and coworkers[48] reported that 3-hydroxy- and 2'-oxo-quinidine were equipotent with quinidine when tested against chloroform- and hypoxia-induced ventricular fibrillation in mice. These same investigators also reported that 2'-oxo-quinidine was equipotent to the parent drug when tested against $BaCl_2$-induced ventricular arrhythmias in rabbits, but that 3-hydroxy quinidine was less potent while appearing to be more toxic.

The disposition characteristics of the metabolites of quinidine have not been reported. Whether their relatively low steady-state plasma concentrations result from disposition factors or are due to the quantitative role of the specific metabolic pathway is not known.

The clinical role of these metabolites remains in question. They are antidysrhythmic and some have potencies similar to that of quinidine. Holford and coworkers[52] concluded that active metabolites are responsible for the greater QTc prolongation seen after quinidine given orally compared with intravenously. However, in most patients, the accumulation of these metabolites is minor, suggesting a minor contribution of these metabolites to the clinical efficacy of quinidine.

## Other Antiarrhythmic Drugs

A recent report has described an active metabolite of propafenone, 5-hydroxy-propafenone.[53] This metabolite was studied in an aconitine-induced arrhythmia model and found to be approximately twice as potent as its parent drug. Whether or not it accumulates in the plasma of patients who are being treated with propafenone remains to be determined.

The metabolism of several other antiarrhythmic drugs remains to be elucidated, and these agents have not been discussed. At least three antiarrhythmic drugs—tocainide, phenytoin and mexiletine—appear to be metabolized primarily to products that are not cardioactive. It is hoped that development of new antiarrhythmic drugs will include evaluation of metabolism and the pharmacology of any resulting metabolites that appear to be potentially active.

## SUMMARY

Most antiarrhythmic drugs are extensively metabolized, and the accumulation of the metabolites of several of these drugs has been documented. In some cases, the steady-state plasma concentrations of metabolites are considerably greater than is the concentration of the parent drug. Several of these metabolites have been evaluated in animal models for antiarrhythmic activity and their potencies have been defined relative to the activity of their parent compound. Evaluations of activity are generally conducted in animal arrhythmia models, and very few metabolites of antiarrhythmic drugs have been evaluated directly in patients. However, from knowledge of antiarrhythmic activity in animals and the degree to which a metabolite accumulates in the plasma of patients, one can make qualitative judgments about its therapeutic role. Such judgments, however, need to be recognized as tenuous. Quantitative judgments require further information regarding the relationship between the parent drug and metabolite when present simultaneously in the myocardium. One must consider whether the effects of the parent drug and metabolite are additive, synergistic, or even antagonistic. The latter case is most possible with drug–metabolite pairs where the metabolite accumulates substantially, but does not have significant antiarrhythmic potency. Other considerations include noncardiac effects of the metabolites. As in the case of the mono-desethyl metabolite of lidocaine, the significance of its accumulation relates more to central nervous system side effects than to direct cardiac actions.

The role of active metabolites also much be considered in regard to differences in the disposition kinetics between the parent drug and metabolite. The most obvious situation where this is important is in designing clinical drug evaluation protocols. As illustrated by the metabolites of encainide and lorcainide, the time course of accumulation and disappearance of the metabolites may be much longer than that of the parent drug. Clinical evaluations at steady state must take into account the time required to achieve steady-state concentrations of the metabolites as well. Similarly, after discontinuation of drug administration, the time required before washout is complete may be totally dependent on the kinetics of the metabolite, and not the parent drug.

Variability in metabolic activity also needs to be considered. It has been shown with procainamide and encainide that genetic factors can influence the rate of production of active metabolites and consequently influence the clinical efficacy of these drugs. Another consideration that deserves attention is the question of drug interactions. It is well recognized that hepatic metabolizing enzymes can be influenced (both inhibited and induced) by drugs. The influence of drug-induced alterations in hepatic function on the clinical efficacy of antiarrhythmic drugs and their active metabolites remains to be elucidated.

Clearly, the metabolites of several antiarrhythmic drugs are clinically important. Determination of the exact role that these metabolites play requires knowledge of their pharmacologic actions, their disposition kinetics, and any interaction that occurs between the metabolite and parent drug. At present, the available knowledge does not support definitive judgments as to the role of metabolites of any antiarrhythmic drugs. However, research is proceeding in this area which promises to provide exciting and useful information that will facilitate the rational evaluation and use of these drugs.

## REFERENCES

1. McMahon, R. E. 1966. Microsomal dealkylation of drugs: Substrate specificity and mechanism. J. Pharm. Sci. **55:** 457–466.
2. Andreasen, F., H. Bjerregaard & P. Gotzsche. 1981. Pharmacokinetics of amiodarone after intravenous and oral administration. Eur. J. Clin. Pharmacol. **19:** 293–299.
3. Riva, E., M. Gerna, R. Latini, P. Giani, A. Volpi & A. Maggioni. 1982. Pharmacokinetics of amiodarone in man. J. Cardiovasc. Pharmacol. **4:** 264–269.
4. Broekhuysen, J., R. Laruel & R. Sion. 1969. Recherches dans la série des benzofurannes: XXXVII. Étude comparée du Transit et du Métabolisme de l'amiodarone

chez diverses espèces animales et chez l'homne. Arch. Int. Pharmacodyn. **177:** 340–359.

5. FLANAGAN, R. J., G. C. A. STOREY, D. W. HOLT & P. B. FARMER. 1982. Identification and measurement of desethylamiodarone in blood specimens from amiodarone-treated patients. J. Pharm. Pharmacol. **34:** 638–643.

6. HARRIS, L., W. J. MCKENNA, E. ROWLAND, G. C. A. STOREY, D. M. KRIKLER & D. W. HOLT. 1981. Plasma amiodarone and desethyl amiodarone levels in chronic oral therapy. Circulation **64** (Suppl. IV): 263.

7. LATINI, R., R. E. KATES, R. REGINATO & A. L. BURLINGAME. 1983. HPLC isolation and FAB-MS identification of di-*N*-desethylamiodarone, a new metabolite of amiodarone in the dog. Biomed. Mass Spect. In press.

8. WELLENS, H. J. J., P. BRUGADA, D. ROX, B. HEDDLE & F. W. BAR. 1982. A comparison of the electrophysical effects of intravenous and oral amiodarone. Am. J. Cardiol. **49:** 1043.

9. KARIM, A. 1975. The pharmacokinetics of Norpace. Angiology **26:** 85–98.

10. RANNEY, R. E., R. R. DEAN, A. KARIN & F. M. RADZIALOWSKI. 1971. Disopyramide phosphate: Pharmacokinetic and pharmacologic relationships of a new antiarrhythmic agent. Arch. Int. Pharmacodyn. **191:** 162–188.

11. AITIO, M. L. 1981. Plasma concentrations and protein binding of disopyramide and mono-*N*-dealkylated disopyramide during chronic oral disopyramide therapy. Br. J. Clin. Pharmacol. **11:** 369–376.

12. GRANT, A. L., R. J. MARSHALL & S. I. ANKEIR. 1978. Some effects of disopyramide and its *N*-dealkylated metabolite on isolated nerve and cardiac muscle. Eur. J. Pharmacol. **49:** 389–394.

13. BAINES, M. W., J. E. DAVIS, D. N. KELLET & P. L. MUNT. 1976. Some pharmacological effects of disopyramide and a metabolite. J. Int. Med. Res. **4** (Suppl. 1): 5–7.

14. KATES, R. E., D. C. HARRISON & R. A. WINKLE. 1982. Metabolite cumulation during long-term oral encainide administration. Clin. Pharmacol. Ther. **31:** 427–432.

15. GOMOLL, A. W., J. E. BYRNE & R. F. MAYOL. 1981. Comparative antiarrhythmic and local anesthetic actions of encainide and its two major metabolites. Pharmacologist **23:** 209.

16. DRESEL, P. E. 1981. Effect of encainide and its two major metabolites on cardiac conduction. Pharmacologist **23:** 209.

17. ELHARRAR, V. & D. P. ZIPES. 1982. Effects of encainide and metabolites (MJ 14030 and MJ 9444) on cainide cardiac Purkinje and ventricular fibers. J. Pharmacol. Exp. Ther. **220:** 440–447.

18. JACKMAN, W. M., E. N. PRYSTOWSKY, R. L. RINKERBERGER, G. V. NACCARELLI, J. J. HEGER & D. P. ZIPES. 1980. Oral encainide increases refractoriness of ventricular, atrium and accessory pathways. Circulation **62** (Suppl. III): III–11.

19. SAMI, M., J. W. MASON, F. PETERS & D. C. HARRISON. 1979. Clinical electrophysiological effects of encainide, a newly developed antiarrhythmic agent. Am. J. Cardiol. **44:** 526–532.

20. CAREY, E. J., H. J. DUFF, D. M. RODEN, R. K. PRIMM, G. R. WILKINSON, T. WANG, J. A. OATES & R. A. WOOSLEY. 1983. Encainide and its metabolites: Comparative effects in ventricular arrhythmia and electrocardiographic intervals. J. Clin. Invest. In press.

21. HOLLUNGER, G. 1960. On the metabolism of lidocaine. I. The biotransformation of lidocaine. Acta Pharmacol. Toxicol. **17:** 365–373.

22. KEENAGHAN, J. B. & R. N. BOYES. 1972. The tissue distribution, metabolism and excretion of lidocaine in rats, guinea pigs, dogs and man. J. Pharmacol. Exp. Ther. **180:** 454–463.

23. NARANG, P. K., W. G. CROUTHAMEL, N. H. CARLINER & M. L. FISHER. 1978. Lidocaine and its active metabolite. Clin. Pharmacol. Ther. **24:** 654–662.

24. NELSON, S. D., W. A. GARLAND, G. D. BRECK & W. F. TRAGER. 1977. Quantification of lidocaine and several metabolites utilizing chemical-ionization mass spectrometry and stable isotope labeling. J. Pharm. Sci. **66:** 1180–1190.

25. COLLINSWORTH, K. A., J. M. STRONG, A. J. ATKINSON, R. A. WINKLE, F. PERLROTH & D. C. HARRISON. 1975. Pharmacokinetics and metabolism of lidocaine in patients with renal failure. Clin. Pharmacol. Ther. **18:** 56–64.

26.  HALKIN, H., P. MEFFIN, K. L. MELMON & M. ROWLAND. 1975. Influence of conges-
     tive heart failure on blood levels of lodocaine and its active monodeethylated metab-
     olite. Clin. Pharmacol. Ther. **17:** 669–676.
27.  STRONG, J. M., M. PARKER & A. J. ATKINSON. 1973. Identification of glycinexylidide
     in patients treated with intravenous lidocaine. Clin. Pharmacol. Ther. **14:** 67–72.
28.  DRAYER, D. E., B. LORENZO, S. WERNS & M. M. REIDENBERG. 1983. Plasma levels,
     protein binding and elimination data of lidocaine and active metabolites in cardiac
     patients of various ages. Clin. Pharmacol. Therap. **34:** 14–22.
29.  BLUMER, J., J. M. STRONG & A. J. ATKINSON. 1973. The convulsant potency of
     lidocaine and its N-dealkylated metabolites. J. Pharmacol. Exp. Ther. **186:** 31–36.
30.  BURNEY, R. G., C. A. DIFAZIO, M. J. PEACH, K. A. PETRIE & M. J. SILVESTER. 1974.
     Antiarrhythmic effects of lidocaine metabolites. Am. Heart J. **88:** 765–769.
31.  FREEDMAN, M. D., J. GAL & C. R. FREED. 1982. Decreased toxicity and equipotent
     antiarrhythmic potency of monoethylglycine xylidide compared to lidocaine. Clin.
     Res. **30:** 87A.
32.  STRONG, J. M., D. E. MAYFIELD, A. J. ATKINSON, B. C. BURRIS, F. RAMON & L. T.
     WEBSTER. 1975. Pharmacological activity, metabolism, and pharmacokinetics of
     glycinexylidide. Clin. Pharmacol. Ther. **11:** 184–194.
33.  MEINERTZ, T., W. KASPER, F. KERSTING, H. JUST, H. BECHTOLD & E. JAHNCHEN.
     1979. Lorcainide. II. Plasma concentration-effect relationship. Clin. Pharmacol.
     Ther. **26:** 196–204.
34.  WINKLE, R. A., D. L. KEEFE, I. RODRIGUEZ & R. E. KATES. 1984. Pharmacodynam-
     ics of the initiation of oral lorcainide therapy. Am. J. Cardiol. **53:** 544–551.
35.  KEEFE, D. L., R. E. KATES, R. A. WINKLE. 1981. Comparative electrophysiology of
     lorcainide and its major metabolite, norlorcainide, in the dog. Circulation **64** (part
     II): IV–127.
36.  ECHT, D. S., R. E. KATES & R. A. WINKLE. 1983. Electrophysiologic effects of
     intravenous lorcainide differ from those of oral lorcainide in ventricular tachycardia
     patients. Circulation **68:** 392–399.
37.  KATES, R. E., D. L. KEEFE & R. A. WINKLE. 1983. Disposition kinetics of lorcainide
     in arrhythmia patients. Clin. Pharmacol. Therap. **33:** 28–34.
38.  REIDENBERG, M. M., D. E. DRAYER, M. LEVY & H. WARNER. 1975. Polymorphic
     acetylation of procainamide in man. Clin. Pharmacol. Ther. **17:** 722–730.
39.  DRAYER, D. E., D. T. LOWENTHAL, R. L. WOOSLEY, A. S. WIES, A. SCHWARTZ &
     M. M. REIDENBERG. 1977. Cumulation of N-acetyl procainamide, an active metabo-
     lite of procainamide, in patients with impaired renal function. Clin. Pharmacol. Ther.
     **22:** 63–69.
40.  JAILLON, P. & R. A. WINKLE. 1975. Electrophysiologic comparative study of pro-
     cainamide and n-acetylprocainamide in anesthetized dogs. Concentration-response
     relationships. Circulation **60:** 1385–1394.
41.  RODEN, D. M., S. B. REELE, S. B. HIGGINS, G. R. WILKINSON, R. E. SMITH, J. A.
     OATES & R. L. WOOSLEY. 1980. Antiarrhythmic efficacy, pharmacokinetics and
     safety of n-acetylprocainamide in human subjects: Comparison with procainamide.
     Am. J. Cardiol. **46:** 463–468.
42.  CONNOLLY, S. J. & R. E. KATES. 1982. Clinical pharmacokinetics of N-acetylpro-
     cainamide. Clin. Pharmacokinetics **7:** 206–220.
43.  KATES, R. E., P. JAILLON, D. S. RUBENSON & R. A. WINKLE. 1980. Intravenous N-
     acetylprocainamide disposition kinetics in coronary artery disease. Clin. Pharmacol.
     Ther. **28:** 52–57.
44.  STEC, G. P., A. J. ATKINSON, M. J. NEVIN, J. P. THENOT, T. I. RUO, T. P. GIBSON,
     P. IVANOVITCH & F. DEL GRECO. 1979. N-acetylprocainamide pharmacokinetics in
     functionally anephric patients before and after pertubation by hemodialysis. Clin.
     Pharmacol. Ther. **26:** 618–628.
45.  REIDENBERG, M. M., M. CAMACHO, J. KLUGER & D. E. DRAYER. 1980. Aging and
     renal clearance of procainamide and n-acetylprocainamide. Clin. Pharmacol. Ther.
     **28:** 732–735.
46.  SCHROEDER, P., N. A. KLITGOARD & E. SIMMONSEN. 1979. Significance of the acety-
     lation phenotype and the therapeutic effect of procainamide. Eur. J. Pharmacol. **15:**
     63–68.

47. CARROLL, F. I., D. SMITH & M. E. WALL. 1974. Carbon-13 magnetic resonance study-structure of the metabolites of orally administered quinidine in humans. J. Med. Chem. **17:** 985–987.
48. DRAYER, D. E., D. T. LOWENTHAL, K. M. RESTIVO, A. SCHWARTZ, C. E. COOK & M. M. REIDENBERG. 1978. Steady-state serum levels of quinidine and active metabolites in cardiac patients with varying degrees of renal function. Clin. Pharmacol. Ther. **24:** 31–39.
49. GUENTERT, T. W., P. E. COATES, R. A. UPTON, D. L. COMBS & S. RIEGELMAN. 1979. Determination of quinidine and its major metabolites by high performance liquid chromatography. J. Chromatogr. **162:** 59–70.
50. HORNING, M. G., A. A. TAYLOR, E. C. HORNING & S. E. BARROW. 1980. Isolation and identification of quinidine metabolites by HPLC. Fed. Proc. **39:** 307.
51. DEWITZ, G., H. R. HA, U. GANZINGER & F. FOLLATH. 1980. Serum konzentration des chinidins und und seiner metabolite nach repetierter dosierung. Schweiz. Med. Wochenschr. **110:** 1706.
52. HOLFORD, N. H. G., P. E. COATES, T. W. GUENTERT, S. RIEGELMAN, & L. B. SHEINER. 1981. The effect of quinidine and its metabolites on the electrocardiogram and systolic time intervals: Concentration-effect relationships. Brit. J. Clin. Pharmacol. **11:** 187–195.
53. PHILIPSBORN, G. V., J. GRIES, & R. KRETZSCHMAR. 1983. Antiarrhythmic and β-sympatholytic effects of the new antiarrhythmic propafenone and its main metabolite 5-hydroxy-propafenone. II World Conference on Clinical Pharmacology and Therapeutics (Abstracts). 105.

# The Role of the Autonomic Central Nervous System in Mediating and Modifying the Action of Cardiac Antiarrhythmic Drugs[a]

AUGUST M. WATANABE AND JOHN C. BAILEY

*Departments of Medicine and Pharmacology, and the*
*Krannert Institute of Cardiology*
*Indiana University School of Medicine*
*Indianapolis, Indiana 46202*

Cardiac function is importantly regulated by the activity of the autonomic nervous system. In general, activation of the sympathetic nervous system results in stimulation of cardiac function, whereas activation of the parasympathetic limb of the autonomic nervous system leads to inhibition of the heart. The nature of the interaction of this dual system in regulating cardiac function is complex. Efferent autonomic nerve activity emanating from vasomotor regulatory centers in the central nervous system (CNS) is influenced by input from higher CNS centers and modulated by afferent nerve traffic originating from baroreceptors.[1] The resulting sympathetic and parasympathetic outflows reflect the complex regulation that occurs at these levels in the CNS.[1] In addition, the two limbs of the autonomic nervous system interact in a complex manner at the level of the nerve terminals and the innervated tissues. At this peripheral level, the interaction between the sympathetic and parasympathetic nervous systems can be subdivided into two major types, prejunctional and postjunctional[2] (FIG. 1). In the prejunctional type of interaction, acetylcholine (ACh) released from parasympathetic terminals can interact with muscarinic receptors on prejunctional sympathetic terminals to inhibit the release of norepinephrine[3] (FIG. 1). Thus, by this mechanism the parasympathetic system can modulate the effects of the sympathetic system. At the postjunctional or tissue level, activation of muscarinic receptors can modulate the tissue response to beta-receptor stimulation[2] (FIG. 1). These types of interactions must be recognized when the cardiac effects of drugs that modify autonomic function are considered.

The role of the autonomic nervous system in mediating and/or modulating the effects of antiarrhythmic drugs will be considered in two sections: (1) interactions occurring in the CNS and (2) interactions occurring at the level of cardiac tissues. This discussion is not meant to be comprehensive in terms of drugs considered, but rather will focus on a few antiarrhythmic drugs which are known to affect the autonomic nervous system and whose mechanisms of action are fairly well characterized, in order to illustrate the point that the effects of certain antiarrhythmic drugs depend importantly on their interaction with the autonomic nervous system.

[a] This work was supported in part by the Herman C. Krannert Fund; by Grants HL18795, HL06308, and HL07182 from the National Heart, Lung and Blood Institute of the National Institutes of Health; and by the American Heart Association, Indiana Affiliate.

The role of the sympathetic nervous system in precipitating and/or maintaining ventricular arrhythmias is well established, both in clinical situations and in animal models for studying arrhythmias.[4-7] In animal models, it has been shown clearly that manipulations that increase efferent sympathetic nerve traffic can be arrhythmogenic.[6,7] In these animal studies, the time course and magnitude of changes in sympathetic traffic correlate well with the development of arrhythmias, thus suggesting strongly a causal relationship between the two. It is therefore not surprising that drugs that decrease efferent sympathetic nerve traffic may be antiarrhythmic as a result of this effect. We will discuss a few examples of such effects of antiarrhythmic drugs and of other drugs, generally not thought of as antiarrhythmic drugs but which decrease efferent nerve traffic.

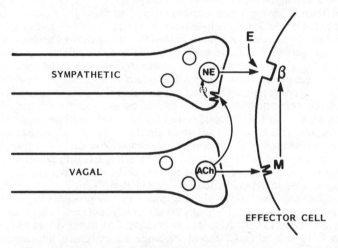

**FIGURE 1.** Diagrammatic representation of sympathetic and vagus nerve terminals and interaction between them. Acetylcholine (ACh) released from vagus nerve endings activates muscarinic receptors (M) on prejunctional sympathetic nerve endings. This results in inhibition of norepinephrine (NE) release. In addition, acetylcholine activates muscarinic receptors on postjunctional effector cells and this activation can modulate the cellular response to beta-receptor activation by catecholamines: E = the circulating catecholamine, epinephrine.

## EFFECTS OF ANTIARRHYTHMIC DRUGS ON EFFERENT SYMPATHETIC NERVE ACTIVITY

Beta-receptor blockers obviously antagonize the cardiac effects of sympathetic stimulation by blocking beta-receptors in cardiac myocytes. In addition, there is evidence from animal studies that beta-receptor blockers that enter the CNS, such as propranolol, can also decrease efferent sympathetic nerve traffic.[8] In anesthetized cats, large doses of ouabain increased directly measured sympathetic nerve activity and produced ventricular tachycardia.[8] Large doses of propranolol administered intravenously normalized the increased sympathetic nerve activity and concomitantly restored the ventricular rhythm to normal sinus rhythm.[8] This drop in nerve activity following propranolol administration occurred in association with a decrease in blood pressure, thus further suggesting that the effects of propranolol were mediated via the CNS.[8] Thus, certain beta-receptor blockers might antagonize arrhythmias dependent on sympathetic activity by decreasing nerve traffic as well as by blocking beta-receptors in the heart.

Diphenylhydantoin is an anticonvulsant drug which also possesses antiarrhythmic activity. Clearly this drug enters the CNS and is capable of altering brain function (that is, anticonvulsant activity). Diphenylhydantoin produces direct effects on cardiac cells.[9–11] In vitro studies with Purkinje fibers showed that this drug shortens action potential duration (APD), decreases automaticity, and increases diastolic membrane potential of partially depolarized fibers.[9] In studies with isolated atrial tissues, diphenylhydantoin has been observed either to enhance[10] or depress[11] membrane responsiveness and conduction. Thus, it seems clear that this agent can produce direct effects on cardiac tissues, and these effects may contribute to the antiarrhythmic activity of this drug.

In addition to having a direct action on cardiac cells, diphenylhydantoin may produce antiarrhythmic effects by modifying sympathetic nerve activity. In anesthetized cats, diphenylhydantoin decreased directly measured activity of cardiac sympathetic nerves.[12] This decrease in nerve activity paralleled reductions in contractile force, blood pressure, and heart rate, supporting the conclusion that the cardiovascular effects of diphenylhydantoin were mediated via reduction in sympathetic nerve activity.[12] In other experiments also done in anesthetized cats, diphenylhydantoin attenuated the increase in cardiac sympathetic nerve activity produced by the cardiac glycoside, deslanoside, and simultaneously converted ventricular tachycardia to normal sinus rhythm.[13] Electrical stimulation of the posterior hypothalamus of cats produced sympathetic nerve hyperactivity and ventricular arrhythmias.[14] Pretreatment of these animals with diphenylhydantoin prevented both the increase in nerve activity and cardiac arrhythmia associated with this increase in sympathetic nerve stimulation.[14]

Lidocaine is an antiarrhythmic drug which clearly produces important direct effects on cardiac tissues. It is equally clear that lidocaine enters the brain and can produce alterations in CNS function, as evidenced by its important and relatively common CNS side effects. Recent evidence suggests that lidocaine's antiarrhythmic activity may depend partially on its ability to decrease efferent sympathetic nerve activity.[15] Cardiac sympathetic nerve activity was directly measured in dogs. Lidocaine given in boluses or by continuous intravenous infusion produced a dose-dependent inhibition of nerve activity.[15] Experiments were performed to exclude an effect of lidocaine on the sympathetic ganglion or nerve terminal. It was concluded that lidocaine can produce a CNS-mediated reduction in sympathetic nerve activity, and it was speculated that this effect might contribute to the antiarrhythmic activity of the drug.[15]

Thus, several antiarrhythmic drugs which are known to have direct effects on cardiac tissues that might explain their antiarrhythmic activities also act in the CNS to reduce efferent sympathetic nerve activity. It is likely that in certain situations, depending on the activity of the sympathetic nervous system and on the dependency of a given arrhythmia on sympathetic tone, the CNS effects of these antiarrhythmic drugs might participate with the direct tissue effects in preventing arrhythmias.

There are other classes of drugs not generally thought of as having antiarrhythmic activity, but which clearly are able to reduce efferent sympathetic nerve activity. Central dopaminergic agonists are in this group. When L-dopa is administered to animals in combination with inhibitors of L-amino acid decarboxylase, the result is a suppression of the cardiovascular system: heart rate, blood pressure, and peripheral vascular resistance fall.[16,17] This occurs without any evidence of impairment of peripheral sympathetic nerve function or of ganglionic transmission. Directly measured postganglionic sympathetic nerve activity demonstrates that these hemodynamic effects of L-dopa are due to reduction in efferent sympathetic nerve traffic[17] (FIG. 2). L-dopa must be converted into dopamine in the CNS for this effect to occur.[16] If CNS as well as extracerebral L-amino acid decarboxylase is inhibited, L-dopa becomes devoid of effects on the cardiovascular system.[16] This centrally mediated inhibition of sympathetic nerve activity produces potent antihypertensive effects in spontaneously hypertensive rats (SHR).[18] L-dopa, given with an extracerebral inhibitor of decarboxylase, lowered directly measured sympathetic nerve activity and, in parallel, reduced heart rate and

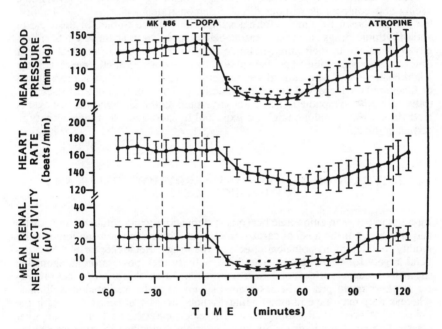

**FIGURE 2.** Effect of L-dopa (30 mg/kg), after MK 486 (10 mg/kg), on mean blood pressure, heart rate and mean renal nerve activity in five anesthetized cats. Drugs were injected over a few seconds to minutes at times indicated. For graphic presentation, mean nerve activity was averaged by measuring the area under the electronically derived curve over a 30-sec period. This value (mean ± S.E.M.), along with blood pressure and heart rate, is plotted at 6-min intervals. *Small asterisks* = p <.05 for difference from control (from reference 17).

blood pressure in these rats.[18] It would be expected that L-dopa, combined with a peripheral decarboxylase inhibitor, would exert antiarrhythmic effects on arrhythmias dependent on increased sympathetic nerve activity.

Indeed, other centrally acting dopaminergic agonists have been shown to possess antiarrhythmic activity in animal models. In chloralose-anesthetized cats intoxicated with deslanoside, the dopamine agonists apomorphine and piribedil prevented the development of ventricular tachycardia and ventricular fibrillation.[19] Apomorphine could produce this effect in much lower doses when given intracerebroventricularly than when administered intravenously, supporting the interpretation that the drug was acting in the CNS.[19] The dopaminergic antagonist haloperidol blocked the antiarrhythmic effect of apomorphine.[19]

Modification of the metabolism of other CNS amine systems also appears to confer antiarrhythmic effects in animal models. The administration of three different central serotonergic agents—melatonin, 5-methoxy-tryptophol, and 6-chloro-2-(1-piperazinyl)-pyrazine (MK-212)—produced significant increases in the vulnerable period for repetitive electrical activity in dogs.[20] The protective effect of MK-212 was blocked by the serotonin antagonist metergoline.[20] It was concluded that an increase in CNS serotonergic activity may inhibit arrhythmogenic efferent sympathetic nerve activity.

Thus, several different classes of drugs, including classical antiarrhythmic agents and compounds without directly demonstrated antiarrhythmic activity, have been shown to inhibit efferent sympathetic nerve traffic. In the case of antiarrhythmic drugs, it seems reasonable to speculate that these CNS effects might contribute to their antiarrhythmic activity. In the case of other classes of drugs, it seems possible that their ability to inhibit sympathetic nerve activity might bestow them with antiarrhythmic activity against arrhythmias precipitated or facilitated by increased sympathetic activity. Thus, drugs known to act centrally to inhibit sympathetic nerve activity, such as the antihypertensive agents methyldopa and clonidine, might be expected to exert antiarrhythmic activity in certain settings.


## INTERACTION BETWEEN ANTIARRHYTHMIC DRUGS AND AUTONOMIC RECEPTORS

Interaction between autonomic nervous system activity and antiarrhythmic drugs can also occur at the level of cardiac tissues and this interaction can importantly modify the electrophysiological effects of the drugs. Beta-receptor blockers depend largely for whatever antiarrhythmic activity they possess on antagonizing the arrhythmogenic effects of beta-receptor stimulation. Accordingly, beta-receptor blockers might protect hearts against sympathetically mediated arrhythmias, whereas they may have minimal antiarrhythmic activity in hearts not under the influence of sympathetic stimulation. The electrophysiological effects of other classical antiarrhythmic drugs are also importantly modified by superimposition of autonomic influences. The effects of two commonly used drugs will be discussed to illustrate these interactions.

The antiarrhythmic drugs quinidine and disopyramide were studied using isolated atria and Purkinje fibers *in vitro* to avoid the influences of nerve activity or circulating neurotransmitters that would be expected in intact animals. Quinidine, disopyramide and procainamide all slowed spontaneous rate of isolated guinea pig right atria[21] (TABLE 1). This expected effect was due to the well-known supressant action of these agents on the automaticity of the sinoatrial node. If, however, quinidine and disopyramide were given to atria that had been pretreated with physostigmine and acetylcholine, spontaneous rate increased.[21] An example of the effect of disopyramide is shown in FIGURE 3. Quinidine and disopyramide sped spontaneous rate by blocking muscarinic cholinergic receptors, thereby antagonizing the rate-slowing effects of acetylcholine (TABLE 1). Procainamide, which has little anticholinergic activity, slowed rate in the presence or absence of muscarinic stimulation[21] (TABLE 1). Thus, in the presence of muscarinic stimulation, the anticholinergic effects of quinidine and disopyramide predominated over

TABLE 1. The Effect of Antiarrhythmic Agents on Rate of Spontaneously Beating Guinea Pig Atria[a]

| Control (n)[b] | Physostigmine (PS) (1 × 10$^{-6}$ M) | PS/Drug | Drug Alone |
|---|---|---|---|
| 223 ± 49 (12) | — | — | 221 ± 57 (atropine, 1 × 10$^{-6}$ M) |
| 264 ± 39 (9) | — | — | 232 ± 32[c] (disopyramide, 7 × 10$^{-6}$ M) |
| 209 ± 39 (9) | — | — | 176 ± 47[c] (disopyramide, 1.4 × 10$^{-5}$ M) |
| 198 ± 34 (7) | — | — | 168 ± 30[c] (quinidine, 1 × 10$^{-5}$ M) |
| 233 ± 75 (12) | — | — | 194 ± 57[c] (quinidine, 2 × 10$^{-5}$ M) |
| 208 ± 69 (5) | — | — | 184 ± 59[c] (procainamide, 2 × 10$^{-5}$ M) |
| 260 ± 43 (6) | 140 ± 28[d] | 216 ± 52[e] (atropine, 1 × 10$^{-6}$ M) | — |
| 236 ± 23 (8) | 101 ± 20[d] | 115 ± 32 (disopyramide, 7 × 10$^{-6}$ M) | — |
| 237 ± 45 (8) | 90 ± 49[d] | 137 ± 53[c] (disopyramide, 1.4 × 10$^{-5}$ M) | — |
| 235 ± 25 (7) | 95 ± 20[d] | 117 ± 17[e] (quinidine, 1 × 10$^{-5}$ M) | — |
| 224 ± 52 (9) | 96 ± 42[d] | 104 ± 47 (quinidine, 2 × 10$^{-5}$ M) | — |
| 243 ± 54 (6) | 113 ± 17[d] | 103 ± 24 (procainamide, 2 × 10$^{-5}$ M) | — |

[a] Values are mean ± S.D. depolarizations per minute.
[b] Number of guinea pig right atria studied.
[c] Slowed compared to control after 5 min of drug exposure, p < 0.01.
[d] Slowed compared to control after 15 min of drug exposure, p < 0.005.
[e] Accelerated compared to rate observed at 15 min of PS, p < 0.05.

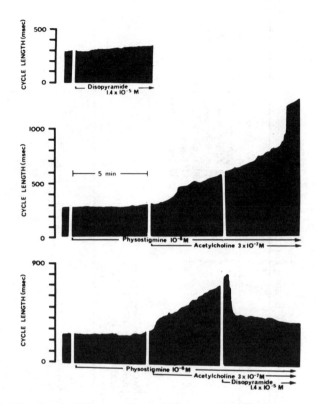

**FIGURE 3.** Directionally different effects of disopyramide on cycle length of spontaneously depolarizing guinea pig right atrial preparations, depending on the level of muscarinic cholinergic receptor stimulation. *Top panel:* Disopyramide slows the rate of spontaneous depolarization in control state. *Middle panel:* Superfusion of physostigmine plus acetylcholine markedly increases spontaneous cycle length. *Lower panel:* During muscarinic cholinergic stimulation with physostigmine and acetylcholine, disopyramide causes acceleration of spontaneous rate, an effect opposite to that observed in top panel. In each panel the initial portion of the record represents the last minute of a stable 20-min control period prior to drug treatment.

the direct automaticity-suppressing effects, and spontaneous rate increased instead of falling. The effects of quinidine and disopyramide on spontaneously beating guinea pig right atria were thus qualitatively different depending on the nature of the ambient autonomic tone.

The effects of quinidine and disopyramide on properties of isolated canine cardiac Purkinje fibers are also modified by autonomic activity. Drugs were administered to Purkinje fibers *in vitro,* and isoproterenol and/or acetylcholine were added to simulate autonomic tone. The electrophysiological property measured in these studies was action potential duration (APD). First, the effects of autonomic agonists on APD of isolated Purkinje fibers paced at a constant rate will be described. Stimulation of beta-adrenergic receptors with isoproterenol shortened

APD[22] (FIG. 4). This APD shortening was reversed by the administration of ace-tylcholine[22] (FIG. 4). The muscarinic reversal of the APD-shortening effect of beta agonists is an electrophysiological manifestation of the well-known and exten-sively studied postjunctional sympathetic-parasympathetic antagonism.[1] Atro-pine added to Purkinje fibers exposed to both isoproterenol and acetylcholine shortens APD because of its reversal of the effects of acetylcholine[22] (FIG. 4).

When disopyramide and quinidine were given alone to isolated Purkinje fibers, APD was prolonged.[21] An example of the effect of disopyramide is shown in FIGURE 5. However, when these drugs were given during simultaneous activation of beta and muscarinic receptors, APD was shortened, because of the anticholin-ergic effects of these drugs[21] (FIG. 6). As shown in FIGURE 6, isoproterenol alone shortened APD. The addition of acetylcholine prolonged APD because of the antiadrenergic effect of the choline ester. Because of their anticholinergic effects, disopyramide or quinidine administered during beta-adrenergic and muscarinic stimulation shortened APD[21] (FIG. 6; TABLE 2). This effect resembled that of atropine. Thus, during simultaneous stimulation of beta-adrenergic and mus-carinic receptors, the anticholinergic effects of disopyramide and quinidine pre-dominated over the direct membrane effects, and APD was shortened (TABLE 2). Procainamide, which has little anticholinergic activity, prolonged APD in the presence or absence of autonomic receptor stimulation (TABLE 2).

To verify that in these *in vitro* studies disopyramide and quinidine were pro-ducing their effects by interacting with muscarinic receptors, two types of bio-chemical studies were done.[23] First, cyclic GMP levels were measured in guinea pig atria. Acetylcholine stimulated cyclic GMP levels as expected (FIG. 7). Atro-pine and disopyramide both inhibited acetylcholine stimulation of cyclic GMP

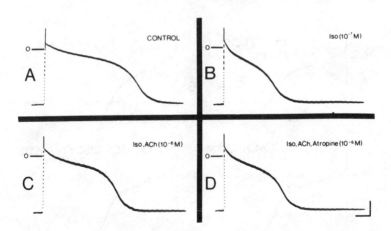

**FIGURE 4.** Effect of acetylcholine on action potential shortening produced by isopro-terenol. (**A**) Control action potential from a canine cardiac Purkinje fiber. (**B**) Isoproterenol ($10^{-7}$ M) elicits action potential duration shortening. (**C**) Addition of acetylcholine ($10^{-6}$ M) partially reverses the action potential duration shortening produced by isoproterenol. (**D**) Addition of atropine ($10^{-6}$ M) blocks the effect of acetylcholine, and action potential dura-tion returns toward that seen in (**B**). Calibrations: *horizontal bar* = 50 msec; *vertical bar* = 25 mV.

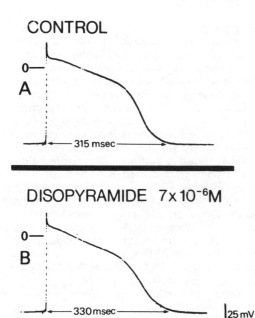

**FIGURE 5.** Effect of disopyramide on action potential duration. (**A**) Control action potential from a canine cardiac Purkinje fiber. (**B**) Disopyramide (7 × 10⁻⁶ M) prolongs action potential duration.

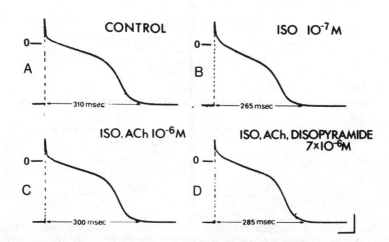

**FIGURE 6.** Effect of disopyramide on action potential duration during simultaneous adrenergic-muscarinic cholinergic receptor stimulation. (**A**) Control canine cardiac Purkinje fiber action potential. (**B**) Isoproterenol (10⁻⁷ M) shortens action potential duration. (**C**) Addition of acetylcholine (10⁻⁶ M) antagonizes action potential duration shortening effects of isoproterenol. (**C**) Addition of disopyramide (7 × 10⁻⁶ M) partially reverses the effects of acetylcholine, causing shortening of action potential duration. Calibrations as in FIGURE 4.

**TABLE 2.** The Effect of Antiarrhythmic Agents on Action Potential Duration of Canine Cardiac Purkinje Fibers[a]

| Control (n)[b] | Isoproterenol (ISO) ($10^{-7}$ M) | ISO/Acetylcholine (ACh) ($3 \times 10^{-7}$ M) | ISO/ACh Drug | Drug Alone |
|---|---|---|---|---|
| 367 ± 49 (5) | — | — | — | 369 ± 51 (atropine, $1 \times 10^{-6}$ M) |
| 343 ± 16 (5) | — | — | — | 348 ± 12 (disopyramide, $1 \times 10^{-6}$ M) |
| 313 ± 40 (5) | — | — | — | 334 ± 41[c] (disopyramide, $7 \times 10^{-6}$ M) |
| 351 ± 27 (9) | — | — | — | 367 ± 29[c] (disopyramide, $1.4 \times 10^{-5}$ M) |
| 373 ± 27 (6) | — | — | — | 378 ± 22 (quinidine, $1 \times 10^{-6}$ M) |
| 331 ± 42 (9) | — | — | — | 359 ± 40[c] (quinidine, $1 \times 10^{-5}$ M) |
| 323 ± 46 (7) | — | — | — | 365 ± 51[c] (quinidine, $2 \times 10^{-5}$ M) |
| 368 ± 25 (7) | — | — | — | 384 ± 35[c] (procainamide, $2 \times 10^{-5}$ M) |
| 340 ± 43 (12) | 269 ± 30[d] | 293 ± 28[e] | 280 ± 34[f] (atropine, $1 \times 10^{-6}$ M) | — |
| 383 ± 30 (8) | 323 ± 33[d] | 356 ± 32[e] | 343 ± 25[f] (disopyramide, $1 \times 10^{-6}$ M) | — |
| 324 ± 52 (9) | 265 ± 27[d] | 297 ± 30[e] | 289 ± 25 (disopyramide, $7 \times 10^{-6}$ M) | — |
| 350 ± 18 (8) | 284 ± 20[d] | 315 ± 15[e] | 320 ± 17 (disopyramide, $1.4 \times 10^{-5}$ M) | — |
| 354 ± 31 (6) | 293 ± 20[d] | 313 ± 15[e] | 313 ± 18 (quinidine, $1 \times 10^{-6}$ M) | — |
| 338 ± 19 (6) | 253 ± 18[d] | 275 ± 16[e] | 274 ± 18 (quinidine, $1 \times 10^{-5}$ M) | — |
| 337 ± 32 (5) | 259 ± 18[d] | 281 ± 37[e] | 269 ± 36[f] (quinidine, $2 \times 10^{-5}$ M) | — |
| 327 ± 49 (5) | 208 ± 33[d] | 248 ± 31[e] | 266 ± 37[g] (procainamide, $2 \times 10^{-5}$ M) | — |

[a] Values are mean ± S.D. of total action potential duration in msec.
[b] Number of Purkinje fibers studied.
[c] Prolonged from control after 5 min of drug alone, $p < 0.01$.
[d] Shortened from control after 5 min of ISO, $p < 0.001$.
[e] Prolonged from ISO after 5 min of ISO plus ACh, $p < 0.05$.
[f] Shortened from ISO/ACh after 5 min of ISO/ACh plus drug, $p < 0.05$.
[g] Prolonged from ISO/ACh after 5 min. of ISO/ACh plus drug, $p < 0.05$.

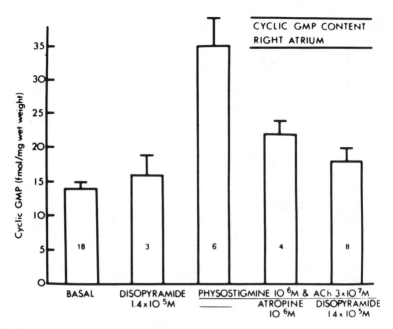

**FIGURE 7.** Antagonism of physostigmine-induced increases in cyclic GMP levels in guinea pig right atria by muscarinic antagonists. Disopyramide alone had no effect on cyclic GMP levels. Physostigmine significantly elevated cyclic GMP levels. Atropine and disopyramide both antagonized the elevation in tissue cyclic GMP produced by physostigmine. Values are means ±S.E.M. Numbers in bars signify $n$.

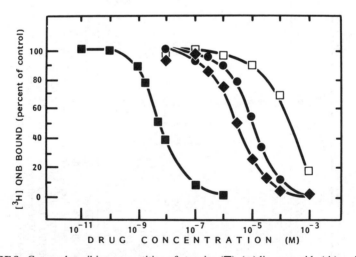

**FIGURE 8.** Curves describing competition of atropine (■), (±)disopyramide (♦), quinidine (●), and procainamide (□) with [³H]QNB for binding to muscarinic receptors in guinea pig right atrium. Each point is the mean of values obtained from triplicate determinations in three separate experiments with S.E. ≤ 5%. [³H]QNB concentration was approximately 80 pM. Control [³H]QNB binding in the separate experiments (fmol/mg protein, expressed as a mean ±S.E.) was: atropine 42.4 ± 3.2; (±)disopyramide 41.0 ± 1.9; quinidine 48.1 ± 1.4; procainamide 43.4 ± 1.4. Derived inhibition constants ($K_i$) were: atropine $1.2 \times 10^{-9}$ M; (±)disopyramide $8.5 \times 10^{-7}$ M; quinidine $2.8 \times 10^{-6}$ M; procainamide $5.6 \times 10^{-5}$ M. (From Mirro *et al.*[23] Reproduced by permission.)

levels, verifying that both drugs produced anticholinergic effects by blocking muscarinic receptors (FIG. 7). In addition, direct radioligand binding studies were performed utilizing [$^3$H]quinuclidinyl benzilate (QNB) to label muscarinic receptors. Disopyramide and quinidine both effectively competed with [$^3$H]QNB for binding to muscarinic receptors, albeit less potently than atropine (FIG. 8).[23] Procainamide was virtually without activity except at nonpharmacologic concentrations.[23]

Thus, drugs might produce antiarrhythmic effects specifically because they interact with autonomic receptors (for example, beta blockers in the setting of high sympathetic tone) or, as illustrated in the examples, the electrophysiological effects of antiarrhythmic drugs might be importantly modified because of their interaction with autonomic receptors. The nature of this modification will depend on the level and type of autonomic nerve activity.

## SUMMARY

The autonomic nervous system, particularly the sympathetic nervous system, plays an important role in initiating or perpetuating cardiac arrhythmias in various animal models and presumably also in man. The parasympathetic and sympathetic nervous systems interact in a complex manner in regulating the electrophysiologic properties of cardiac tissues. To the extent that a given arrhythmia is influenced by autonomic tone, the alteration in autonomic tone produced by an antiarrhythmic drug will modify the effects of the antiarrhythmic drug. Several antiarrhythmic drugs that are known to have direct electrophysiologic effects on cardiac tissues also reduce efferent sympathetic nerve activity by acting in the CNS. This centrally mediated effect on sympathetic activity likely plays an important role in the antiarrhythmic effects of these drugs. Other antiarrhythmic drugs interact directly with autonomic receptors on cardiac tissues in addition to producing their direct electrophysiological effects. The electrophysiologic effects of such antiarrhythmic drugs that interact with autonomic receptors are qualitatively modified by the magnitude and nature of the prevailing autonomic tone. These interactions between the autonomic nervous system and antiarrhythmic drugs must be kept in mind when the mechanism of action of these drugs is considered.

## REFERENCES

1. LEVY, M. N. & P. J. MARTIN. 1979. Neural control of the heart. *In* Handbook of Physiology, Section 2, The Cardiovascular System. R. M. Berne, Ed.: 581–620. American Physiological Society. Bethesda, MD.
2. WATANABE, A. M. 1983. Cholinergic agonists and antagonists. *In* Cardiac Therapy. M. R. Rosen & B. F. Hoffman, Eds.: 95–144. Martinus Nijhoff. Amsterdam.
3. MUSCHOLL, E. 1980. Peripheral muscarinic control of norepinephrine release in the cardiovascular system. Am. J. Physiol. **239:** H713–720.
4. ZIPES, D. P., J. B. MARTINS, R. RUFFY, E. N. PRYSTOWSKY, V. ELHARRAR & R. F. GILMOUR, JR. 1981. Roles of autonomic innervation in the genesis of ventricular arrhythmias. *In* Disturbances in Neurogenic Control of the Circulation.: 225–250. American Physiological Society. Bethesda, MD.
5. LOWN, B. 1979. Sudden cardiac death: The major challenge confronting contemporary cardiology. Am. J. Cardiol. **43:** 313–328.
6. VERRIER, R. L. 1980. Neural factors and ventricular electrical instability. *In* Sudden Death. Martinus Nijhoff. Amsterdam.

7. MARTINS, J. B. & D. P. ZIPES. 1980. Effects of sympathetic and vagal nerves on recovery properties of the endocardium and epicardium of the canine left ventricle. Circ. Res. **46:** 100–110.
8. GILLIS, R. A. 1979. Cardiac sympathetic nerve activity: Changes induced by ouabain and propranolol. Science **166:** 508–510.
9. BIGGER, J. T., JR., A. L. BASSETT & B. F. HOFFMAN. 1968. Electrophysiological effects of diphenylhydantoin on canine Purkinje fibers. Circ. Res. **22:** 221–236.
10. STRAUSS, H. C., J. T. BIGGER, JR., A. L. BASSETT & B. F. HOFFMAN. 1968. Actions of diphenylhydantoin on the electrical properties of isolated rabbit and canine atria. Circ. Res. **23:** 463–477.
11. JENSEN, R. A. & B. G. KATZUNG. 1970. Electrophysiological actions of diphenylhydantoin on rabbit atria. Circ. Res. **26:** 17–27.
12. GILLIS, R. A., J. R. McCLELLAN, T. S. SAUER & F. G. STANDAERT. 1971. Depression of cardiac sympathetic nerve activity by diphenylhydantoin. J. Pharmacol. Exp. Ther. **173**(3): 599–610.
13. EVANS, D. E. & R. A. GILLIS. 1975. Effect of ouabain and its interaction with diphenylhydantoin on cardiac arrhythmias induced by hypothalamic stimulation. J. Pharmacol. Exp. Ther. **195**(3): 577–586.
14. EVANS, D. E. & R. A. GILLIS. 1974. Effect of diphenylhydantoin and lidocaine on cardiac arrhythmias induced by hypothalamic stimulation. J. Pharmacol. Exp. Ther. **191**(3): 506–517.
15. MILLER, B. D., M. D. THAMES & A. L. MARK. 1983. Inhibition of cardiac sympathetic nerve activity during intravenous administration of lidocaine. J. Clin. Invest. **71:** 1247–1253.
16. WATANABE, A. M., L. C. PARKS & I. J. KOPIN. 1971. Modification of the cardiovascular effects of L-dopa by decarboxylase inhibitors. J. Clin. Invest. **50:** 1322–1328.
17. WATANABE, A. M., W. V. JUDY & P. V. CARDON. 1974. Effect of L-dopa on blood pressure and sympathetic nerve activity after decarboxylase inhibition in cats. J. Pharmacol. Exp. Ther. **188:** 107–113.
18. JUDY, W. V., A. M. WATANABE, D. P. HENRY, H. R. BESCH, JR., W. R. MURPHY & G. M. HOCKEL. 1976. Sympathetic nerve activity: Role in regulation of blood pressure in the spontaneously hypertensive rat. Circ. Res. **38:** II-21–II-29.
19. HELKE, C. J. & R. A. GILLIS. 1978. Centrally mediated protective effects of dopamine agonists on digitalis-induced ventricular arrhythmias. J. Pharmacol. Exp. Ther. **207**(2): 263–270.
20. BLATT, C. M., S. H. RABINOWITZ & B. LOWN. 1979. Central serotonergic agents raise the repetitive extrasystole threshold of the vulnerable period of the canine ventricular myocardium. Circ. Res. **44:** 723–730.
21. MIRRO, M. J., A. M. WATANABE & J. C. BAILEY. 1980. Electrophysiological effects of disopyramide and quinidine on guinea pig atria and canine cardiac Purkinje fibers: Dependence on underlying cholinergic tone. Circ. Res. **46:** 660–668.
22. BAILEY, J. C., A. M. WATANABE, H. R. BESCH, JR. & D. A. LATHROP. 1979. Acetylcholine antagonism of the electrophysiological effects of isoproterenol on canine cardiac Purkinje fibers. Circ. Res. **44:** 378–383.
23. MIRRO, M. J., A. S. MANALAN, J. C. BAILEY & A. M. WATANABE. 1980. Anticholinergic effects of disopyramide and quinidine on guinea pig myocardium. Mediation by direct muscarinic receptor blockade. Circ. Res. **47:** 855–865.

# Clinical Trials in the Evaluation of Antiarrhythmic Drugs: Design, Drugs, and Double-Blind Considerations[a]

ARTHUR J. MOSS

*Heart Research Follow-up Program*
*University of Rochester*
*School of Medicine and Dentistry*
*Rochester, New York 14642*

As of October 1983 only five generic drugs (quinidine, procainamide, lidocaine, disopyramide, and verapamil) have been approved by the Food and Drug Administration (FDA) as primary antiarrhythmic agents. Although beta blockers have some antiarrhythmic properties, these drugs exert their effects through antiadrenergic actions and thus should be considered secondary antiarrhythmic agents. It is well recognized by the pharmaceutical industry, clinical pharmacologists, cardiologists, and primary care physicians that an enormous number of patients are troubled with annoying palpitations and a smaller number with potentially life-threatening arrhythmias. Furthermore, the existing oral antiarrhythmic agents have limited efficacy and a high incidence of adverse side effects. Presently, the ideal antiarrhythmic drug suitable for chronic usage does not exist. Thus, the challenge exists for developing and scientifically substantiating the safety and efficacy of new antiarrhythmic agents. At the present time at least ten antiarrhythmic agents are undergoing active clinical testing in the United States; these are amiodarone, aprindine, encainide, ethmozin, flecainide, imipramine, lorcainide, mexiletine, propafenone, and tocainide. How should clinical trials with these agents be carried out, and what are the pitfalls in drug testing that are unique to this class of agents?

## FDA PHASES OF CLINICAL DRUG RESEARCH

The FDA has established general guidelines in the investigative evaluation of new drugs including antiarrhythmic agents. Phase I studies are the earliest studies in humans and usually involve single-dose trials in a small number of healthy volunteers. The primary aim of these studies is to establish drug pharmacokinetics and to identify any major side effects. The studies are usually carried out by a clinical pharmacologist and are characterized by multiple measurements on a few patients. The statistical design is straightforward and the study is usually not blinded.

Phase II studies are the preliminary efficacy investigations, and in the case of antiarrhythmic agents are designed to evaluate the suppression, control, or termi-

[a] This work was supported in part by Grant HL22982 from the National Institutes of Health.

nation of cardiac arrhythmias. The patients are highly selected for manifestations of a specific arrhythmia, and the drug's fundamental effectiveness is evaluated in restricted circumstances. Dose-ranging studies are the first step, and subsequent investigations usually include evaluation of the dose–response effect of the drug on pertinent electrophysiologic and hemodynamic parameters. Common subjective and biochemical side effects are uncovered during Phase II studies. The trials are usually conducted by a clinical pharmacologist with special interest in cardiac arrhythmias or by an investigative cardiologist with an involvement in the pharmacologic control of arrhythmias. The individual studies generally involve fewer than 50 patients, are often single-blinded, and frequently use a crossover design to increase the power (minimize the type II error) in view of the small sample size. For the most part these studies are carried out at a single center for a relatively short follow-up period.

Phase III trials are the definitive studies to evaluate drug efficacy in a large representative population with a spectrum of arrhythmia manifestations, but above some arbitrary cutoff point. The number of patients studied requires a multicenter approach. Statistical design and analysis may be quite complex and sophisticated statistical input is essential. The principal investigator is usually an investigative cardiologist. The trials almost always utilize a randomized, double-blind, placebo or comparison drug controlled approach. The anticipated sample size is determined in advance and is predicated on the magnitude of the anticipated effect and the type I (false positive) and type II (false negative) error rates one is willing to accept relative to the cost of the study. If the study is carefully carried out, safety (with the exception of rare adverse effects) can also be evaluated.

## STATISTICAL CONSIDERATIONS IN PHASE III TRIALS

The reader is referred to standard texts for detailed considerations concerning trial design and analysis.[1] What follows is an attempt to highlight certain basic principles.

The fundamental purpose of a randomized, double-blind, placebo-controlled trial is to minimize chance (type I and type II errors) as a likely explanation of the results. Furthermore, one is trying to eliminate systematic bias by a randomization procedure in drug assignment, by randomizing within each center in multicenter studies and through analysis of the data on an intention-to-treat basis. The object is to insure that the two clinical groups (active drug and placebo) are similar and that the observed findings are not the result of differences in the baseline characteristics of the two groups.

In determining the sample size to be studied, it is important to have accurate figures on the anticipated event rate in the placebo-treated patients who realistically will be enrolled in the study. Once the event rate is known, the sample size can be computed from the percent reduction in the event rate anticipated with the drug, the alpha and beta error rates acceptable to the investigators, and adjustments necessitated by anticipated "drop-in" and "drop-out" rates.[2] Furthermore, the sample size usually has to be expanded as a result of frequent "peeks" at the data during the course of the study for safety monitoring. Each "peek" costs the study power which can only be compensated for by an augmented sample size.[3]

Two sample-size problems are frequently encountered in most clinical trials. The number of patients who will meet the enrollment criteria is almost always less than predicted. "Lasagna's law" teaches us that the incidence of the disease under study will drastically decrease once the study begins.[4] A corollary of this law is that the disease incidence will not return to its previous level until the completion of the study. Secondly, the event rate in the placebo-treated patients is almost always lower than the prestudy rates on which the sample size was calculated. There are many possible reasons for this, but major ones relate to excessively stringent enrollment criteria that exclude appropriate patients. The net result is a refined population with the purest-of-the-pure sample that has a disturbingly low event rate.

In the interpretation of the data, it is important to differentiate between the statistical significance (p value) of the results, the strength of the association (odds ratio, relative risk) between drug administration and arrhythmia suppression, and the clinical significance of the findings. The latter refers to the magnitude of the effect in terms of the gradient or percent reduction in the manifest arrhythmia and necessitates the inclusion of a 90–95% confidence interval to be clinically meaningful.

Intervention trials usually involve a rolling enrollment and a common stopping date. Patients are exposed to the drug from the date of enrollment until either the end-point event (death or the specified arrhythmia), the date the study last had contact with the patient if he/she was lost to follow-up (censored), or the stopping date—whichever comes first. Thus, the trial time (the time for which the patient was at risk) is variable. Exact dates when patients experienced the defined event or were last seen must be determined. Data collected in this way lend themselves to life-table (survivorship) methods of analysis. This approach requires calculation of the proportion of a group of patients not experiencing the event at sequential times after randomization, with due allowance for censoring. The fundamental computation utilizes the concept of probabilities. The likelihood of not having an event for $x$ days from randomization is the probability of not experiencing the event for $(x - 1)$ days multiplied by the chance of not experiencing the event on day $x$ after living $(x - 1)$ days. This multiplication of probabilities is all that underlies the calculation of "life-table" survival curves of the Kaplan-Meier type.[5] Sophisticated Cox-type life-table methods permit the evaluation of the independent contribution of selected variables to the survivorship model. This technique utilizes regression analysis, and the model assumes proportional relationships for the instantaneous rates of death (hazard rate) between two or more subgroups, that is, a proportional hazards model.[6]

In the evaluation of drug efficacy using survival data, a comparison of life-table event rates in the two treatment groups is carried out. In such analyses information is utilized from all patients who are exposed to the drug. Peto et al. have pointed out erroneous methods in the analysis of survival data which are inefficient, misleading, or actually wrong[7]: (1) It is invalid to compare survival graphs at one point in time, thereby ignoring their structure elsewhere. (2) A simple count of the numbers with an event in each group is inefficient and it wastes valuable information about when each event occurred. (3) Analysis of survival should begin with the date of randomization rather than the date treatment was initiated. (4) If no overall significant treatment effect exists between the two groups being compared (active drug versus placebo), then it is invalid to seek out differences between various subgroups of the two populations since observed differences are more likely to be due to chance than would be intuitively expected. (5) Studies that calculate p values after excluding protocol deviants or any other category of withdrawn patients should be mistrusted, that is, studies should be analyzed on the basis of the intention-to-treat principle.

## ENDPOINTS IN ANTIARRHYTHMIC TRIALS

A variety of endpoints (dependent variable) may be used in antiarrhythmic drug trials. When the trial involves ventricular arrhythmias, short-term studies usually involve evaluation of the efficacy of suppressing inducible repetitive ventricular arrhythmias. In susceptible patients, the repetitive rhythms frequently can be induced by programmed electrical stimulation. Drug efficacy and safety can then be evaluated by a change in the ease of inducibility following treatment. Studies of this type require multiple tests since time-dependent variations in cardiac electrophysiologic measurements may occur. Furthermore, inducibility may be quite variable at different endocardial sites.

A second endpoint that is frequently utilized in antiarrhythmic drug trials is the suppression of spontaneously occurring repetitive ventricular arrhythmias. The patients must be preselected for having a high likelihood of manifesting this arrhythmia over a specified time before entering the trial. Similarly, one can evaluate the efficacy of suppressing the frequency of ventricular ectopic activity, and once again, proper preselection of patients is required. Patients with low ectopic activity are unlikely to contribute much information to the drug trial and should be excluded.

The interest in suppressing ventricular arrhythmias reflects the hypothesis that patients with frequent or complex ventricular ectopy, which complicates existing cardiac disease, are at high risk of sudden cardiac death and that suppression of this ectopy with an antiarrhythmic agent will diminish this risk. Thus, the ultimate antiarrhythmic drug trial should evaluate drug efficacy in terms of reduction in cardiac death, and more specifically, a reduction in arrhythmia-related sudden cardiac death.

## PROBLEMS IN THE EVALUATION OF ANTIARRHYTHMIC DRUGS

Several problems exist in the evaluation of antiarrhythmic drugs that have contributed to the slow progress in this field. There is large variability in ectopic beat frequency and complexity from one day to the next. Thus, prolonged periods of Holter monitoring are required to properly evaluate arrhythmia suppression in any clinical trial. At the present time we do not know the clinical significance of "rare events" such as one salvo of 3 or 4 repetitive ventricular ectopic beats over 24 hours of Holter monitoring on the mechanism of cardiac death months to years later. Several studies have shown a strong association between repetitive runs and subsequent death, but the relationship to sudden cardiac death is less clear-cut.

Several investigative groups have recently shown that drug efficacy in suppressing inducible (programmed electrical stimulation) ventricular arrhythmias is associated with improved survival in a select subset of very high-risk patients. Unfortunately, we do not know if such information is applicable to lower-risk patients. Thus, it may be dangerous to extrapolate findings from a specific high-risk group to the much larger population at risk.

Measurement of antiarrhythmic drug levels is important in the evaluation of efficacy studies whether they utilize ectopic beat counts or cardiac death as the endpoint. The problem is compounded by drug metabolites which may be more potent or active than the parent compound and by the effects of drug interactions. Furthermore, there seems to be a poor understanding of the relationship between the therapeutic drug level required for arrhythmia suppression and that required for elevating the threshold for fibrillation. In this regard, we frequently carry out triple-blind antiarrhythmic drug trials. Not only are the patients and the physicians blind to active versus placebo medication, but we as investigators are also blind to the drugs' ability to raise the fibrillation threshold.

## REFERENCES

1. FLEISS, J. L. 1981. Statistical Methods for Rates and Proportions, 2nd ed.: 138–143. Wiley. New York, NY.
2. HALPERIN, M., E. ROGOT, J. GURIAN & F. EDERER. 1968. Sample sizes for medical trials with special reference to long-term therapy. J. Chron. Dis. 21: 13–24.
3. O'BRIEN, P. C. & T. R. FLEMING. 1979. A multiple testing procedure for clinical trials. Biometrics Res. 35: 549–556.
4. GORRINGE, J. A. L. 1970. Initial preparations for clinical trials. In Principles and Practice of Clinical Trials. E. L. Harris & J. D. Fitzgerald, Eds.: 41–46. Livingston. Edinburgh.
5. KAPLAN, E. L. & P. MEIER. 1958. Non-parametic estimation from incomplete observation. J. Am. Stat. Assoc. Res. 53: 457–481.
6. COX, D. R. 1972. Regression Models and Life-Tables. J. Royal Stat. Soc. [B] Res. 34: 187–200.
7. PETO, R., M. D. PIKE, P. ARMITAGE, N. E. BRESLOW, D. R. COX, S. V. HOWARD, N. MANTEL, K. MCPHERSON, J. PETO & P. G. SMITH. 1977. Design and analysis of randomized clinical trials requiring prolonged observation of each patient. Br. J. Cancer Res. 35: 1–39.

# Technological Status and Problems of Ambulatory Electrocardiographic Monitoring

ROGER A. WINKLE,[a] INEZ RODRIGUEZ, AND
DEBORAH A. BRAGG-REMSCHEL

*Cardiology Division*
*Stanford University Medical Center*
*Stanford, California 94305*

A precise technological evaluation of all ambulatory electrocardiographic monitoring equipment would be extremely difficult. Considerable information is needed which generally greatly exceeds that available to any individual user or evaluating group. In many instances the precise details of system operation or algorithm function are proprietary information. Furthermore, even having detailed specifications about the mechanical and electrical function of a system does not permit one to evaluate the device's functional capabilities and accuracy in arrhythmia analysis. These types of evaluation are only possible through extensive use of a system. Few investigators have had the opportunity to evaluate in detail more than one or two systems and papers in this area are either nonexistent or have been published in noncritically peer-reviewed journals. This review, therefore, must of necessity deal largely only in general terms and will stress concepts important to clinical research and patient care.

## AMBULATORY ELECTROCARDIOGRAMS FOR ARRHYTHMIA EVALUATION

### Continuously Recording Ambulatory ECG Systems

*Equipment*

Most systems designed to continuously record ambulatory ECG data consist of small battery-operated recording devices and larger playback or scanning units on which the recorded data are subsequently analyzed. The recording units are small and easily worn by most older children or adult patients. Their size occasionally limits recording capability in young children. Most systems are AM, but there are a few FM recorders in use. Virtually all systems currently in use record two bipolar ECG channels. They contain an event marker, which makes an electronic signal either by overwriting data on one of the two channels or by recording a signal on a separate portion of the tape. These recording systems have the major advantage of recording all ECG data for subsequent evaluation. The playback scanning units are generally large and based either in a hospital or physician's office. They may either make a printout of the entire ECG signal for 24 hours in a

---

[a] To whom correspondence should be addressed.

miniature ECG format or permit a preliminary ECG analysis in varying detail and give isolated rhythm strips. The arrhythmia analysis may be carried out by relatively inexpensive analog circuits, the use of one or more microprocessors or mini- or mainframe computer systems. These playback units often provide trend plots of heart rate versus time and ventricular arrhythmia frequency versus time. Frequently they are fitted with automatic alarms to identify periods of excessive bradycardia, tachycardia or long R-R intervals. ECG data are printed out either as direct analog signals from the magnetic tape or as reconstructed signals from digitized analog data. These systems all require technician-operator intervention. As a general rule, the more accurate the arrhythmia analysis, the greater the degree of operator intervention required.

## Arrhythmia Detection Accuracy

Arrhythmia detection accuracy must be considered in two ways. First one must consider how a system functions on a group of preselected tapes such as a standardized data base, and second, one must have some knowledge of a system's performance on each individual tape being scanned. Many system developers and manufacturers provide data on the accuracy of performance in a selected group of tapes. Of necessity, initial evaluations are often done by the persons developing, building, or selling the system. For many custom systems it is difficult to have independent outside evaluations. The accuracy of each system depends on many factors other than the arrhythmia identification algorithms; these factors include the quality of the tapes recorded, the skills and persistence of individual technicians, and the types of arrhythmias being recorded. For these reasons it is important that each commercially available system be evaluated on site during a trial period before purchase. During this trial period the potential user can perform his or her own independent evaluation of a system's arrhythmia detection accuracy on a previously evaluated set of representative tapes from that center. Most evaluations of systems for arrhythmia detection accuracy have a major emphasis only on the detection and quantification of ventricular arrhythmias. Evaluation of these systems' ability to detect second- or third-degree AV block, significant bradyarrhythmias, atrial fibrillation, or paroxysms of supraventricular tachycardia are either nonexistent or are made on the basis of a small number of tapes with these arrhythmias.

It is insufficient to rely strictly on a prior evaluation of a system for considering the accuracy of arrhythmia diagnosis. Some measure of a system's performance must be available for each tape. This may range from as simple a process as having the technician who scans the tape indicate whether or not the data were clean and the automated analysis system providing a reasonably representative picture of events actually on the tape or having a more formal quantitative assessment of false-positive and false-negative detections of arrhythmia events. Since the latter type of analysis requires a considerable amount of counting by hand and technician time, the former approach is preferable for most clinical settings.

## Esophageal Recording

One of the limitations of standard surface electrocardiographic monitoring, especially when only two channels are available, is the difficulty in distinguishing P waves. While this is generally not a problem during sinus rhythm, it does

present difficulties during various narrow and wide QRS complex tachyarrhythmias. Arzbaecher[1] has developed a small bipolar electrode which is placed in
a gelatin capsule and swallowed easily by the patient. This electrode is connected
to the body surface by a small pair of connecting wires. The signal is preprocessed
to filter out respiratory artifact and can then be recorded simultaneously with the
surface ECG leads. This technique is best carried out with recorders able to
record more than two channels so that both surface leads may be preserved. At
the present time, however, most systems can only play back two channels at a
time. If multichannel recording is not available, the esophageal recording may be
made on the second channel of a standard two-channel recorder. These esophageal recordings are generally well tolerated by patients, although occasionally
younger patients may regurgitate the electrode. They provide high-quality atrial
complexes which are equal to or larger than the ventricular QRS complexes.
They are useful for differentiating various types of supraventricular tachycardias
as well as for diagnosing ventricular tachycardia when atrioventricular dissociation is present.

## Suitability for Clinical and Research Purposes

There is considerable disparity between the most frequent clinical indication
for performing ambulatory ECG monitoring and the most frequent research application. The most frequent clinical application is for the evaluation of a symptomatic patient to determine whether or not arrhythmias are the cause of the patient's symptoms. In this situation clinicians may be searching carefully for a
variety of supraventricular tachyarrhythmias as well as any one of several bradyarrhythmias. Almost any of the types of continuously recording systems are
suitable for this clinical use. The most widely utilized research indication for
ambulatory ECG monitoring is for quantitative assessment of ventricular arrhythmias, either for prognostic stratification studies in patients with diseases such as
coronary heart disease or to document the antiarrhythmic activity of antiarrhythmic agents. In such studies the accuracy of quantitation of ventricular arrhythmias is considerably more important than it is for the routine clinical use of
ambulatory ECG recordings. For these reasons systems that may be suitable for
clinical use may not be adequate for research purposes. The major cause for this
discrepancy is that pharmaceutical companies and investigators have paid little
attention to evaluating patients' symptomatic improvement, while researchers
have failed to prove that reduction in highly quantitated but asymptomatic ventricular arrhythmias influences subsequent morbidity or mortality. For the present
time, continuous ambulatory ECG systems should probably remain the "gold
standard" for evaluation of most symptomatic patients and certainly for all research patients, and should not be replaced by real-time systems (see below). The
reason for this is that all ECG data will be available for subsequent review either
at the time the patient's symptoms occur or in order to validate the accuracy of
arrhythmias detection.

## S-T SEGMENT ANALYSIS

### Standard Ambulatory ECG

#### Fidelity of Recording Equipment

Although early reports question the ability of ambulatory ECG equipment to
faithfully record and reproduce S-T segment shifts because of the inadequate low-

frequency response of the equipment,[2] most recent manufacturers' claims suggest that they meet the American Heart Association standards. These standards for electrocardiographic equipment require that the 3-dB cutoff point be less than 0.05 Hz or greater than 100 Hz and that the frequency–response curve be essentially flat (±6%) between 0.14 and 50 Hz. It is important to note that most manufacturers report that their recorders meet AHA standard, but do not comment on the frequency response of the entire recorder-playback system. In addition, there are no AHA standards for phase shift and, in fact, it is difficult to appreciate fully the impact of phase shift on ECG quality. (Phase shift is the shifting of one frequency in time relative to another.) Since each ECG signal can be thought of as being made of the sum of a number of frequencies, with S-T segment shifts being relatively low-frequency information and QRS complexes being high-frequency information, one can think of phase shift of lower frequencies as being the equivalent of shifting the S-T segment relative to the QRS complex.

In order to analyze in greater detail the technical qualities of recording-playback equipment for S-T segment analysis, we obtained equipment from several manufacturers of ambulatory ECG devices.[3,4] These included two recorders of each manufacturer and one standard calibrated playback unit. In order to plot

**TABLE 1.** Frequency Response Characteristics[a]

|  | Low-Frequency Cutoff (−3dB) | High-Frequency Cutoff (−3dB) | Linearity |
|---|---|---|---|
| AHA | 0.05 | 100 | ±6% (.14–50 Hz) |
| Advance Med | 0.07 | 18 | Nonlinear |
| American Optical | 0.11 | 19 | Nonlinear |
| Avionics | 0.09 | 27 | Nonlinear |
| CardioBeeper | 0.22 | 18 | 0.4–7 Hz |
| Hittman | 0.15 | 25 | Nonlinear |
| ICR | 0.06 | 18 | Nonlinear |
| Oxford AM | 0.16 | 22 | Nonlinear |
| Oxford FM | 0.05 | 41 | 0.2–10 Hz |

[a] From Bragg-Remschel *et al.*[3] Reprinted by permission.

frequency–response curves, we provided standard signal generator inputs using a sinewave ranging from 0.05 to 100 Hz. We found that virtually no manufacturer met AHA standards in terms of the low- or high-frequency cutoff, and, potentially more importantly, that the systems were extremely nonlinear, generally showing marked peaks (indicating data amplification) at approximately .1 Hz (TABLE 1). Although these were inherent problems in the equipment, it was more difficult to demonstrate that they made any clinical difference in ECG signal. In order to evaluate this we played standardized ECG signals into each recorder-playback system with flat-line S-T depression ranging from 1 to 10 mm. Almost all systems provided a clinically useful replication of this ECG signal. Only one manufacturer had results that were clearly unacceptable, with a near doubling of the amount of S-T segment depression at each level.

In addition, we found a significant phase shift for each system (TABLE 2), but once again the clinical importance of this was not determinable.

Thus, although no ambulatory ECG monitor system clearly met AHA standards, it was not possible to prove from our study that in most instances this made a great deal of difference. Most systems provided at least a qualitatively acceptable reproduction of the S-T segment and could have been utilized to diagnose important shifts of the S-T segment. Clinical or research use of these devices with attempts to measure subtle (1 mm) shifts or to determine precisely whether S-T segment shifts are exactly flat-line or up-sloping might be difficult given the technical limitations we noted. In particular, inadequate low-frequency response can cause a flat-line depression to appear to be slightly up-sloping.

### Clinical and Research Applications

It has been well documented that some patients with ischemic heart disease have a large number of episodes of S-T depression.[5,6] Only approximately 20% of these episodes are associated with angina and they generally occur without significant changes from the patient's normal heart rate during everyday activities. Other studies have indicated that the diagnosis of coronary artery disease may be made using ambulatory ECG recordings.[7,8] Despite these reports there has been little widespread clinical use of these recordings for these purposes. Lead systems are not well standardized and only two channels of ECG data are available for

**TABLE 2.** Phase Distortion at Selected Frequencies[a]

|  | 0.05 Hz | 0.1 Hz | 0.5 Hz |
|---|---|---|---|
| American Optical | 65° | 35° | 10° |
| Avionics | 135° | 75° | 20° |
| Hittman | 150° | 90° | 20° |
| ICR | 120° | 50° | 0° |
| Oxford AM | 150° | 90° | 15° |
| Oxford FM | 60° | 32° | 8° |

[a] Bragg-Remschel et al.[3] Reprinted by permission.

analysis. Ischemia involving areas of the heart other than those for which the patient was initially connected might go undetected. Although depression of the 80-msec point has been used as the gold standard, it is possible that other parameters such as S-T segment slope, S-T segment area, or other variables might be important. Although there is accumulating evidence to suggest that these silent S-T segment depressions do in fact represent ischemia,[9] it is not clear that they do so necessarily in all patients. While it is possible to record and quantitate S-T segment shifts in patients undergoing antiangina drug trials, the precise clinical relevance of these measurements remains unclear. The benefit to the patient of reducing the amount of silent ischemia also remains uncertain.

Clinicians have been appropriately slow in adopting ambulatory ECG recordings as a method for diagnosing ischemia. It is clear in the everyday practice of medicine that exercise treadmill tests and coronary arteriography are the primary means for diagnosing coronary artery disease. Ambulatory ECG recordings have achieved use primarily in the subset of patients with suspected Prinzmetal's angina. Even in this condition, patients experiencing frequent episodes of pain are most frequently hospitalized and the disease documented by 12-lead electrocardiography performed during attacks of pain or by ergonovine provocation of coronary arterial spasm during coronary arteriography.

## REAL-TIME AMBULATORY ECG SYSTEMS

### *Equipment*

These devices evaluate one, two, or three channels of ECG data. These systems, rather than recording all of the ECG data for later analysis, analyze the ECG by a microprocessor-based set of algorithms as it is made. These devices have ECG storage memory for as few as 16 brief two-channel ECG strips to as many as several hours of ECG data that can be stored on a magnetic tape. The majority of data are stored as number of events rather than the actual ECG. Thus, the number of runs of ventricular tachycardia and their length may be stored rather than the ECG from all runs. The primary reason for this method of storage is the limited memory available. The major limitation of these recorders is that not all of the ECG is recorded and it is therefore not available for subsequent analysis. The major advantage is that since ECG analysis is completed at the time the recording is completed, scanning time is brief and can be done by a technician not extremely knowledgeable in arrhythmia diagnosis.

### *Accuracy of Arrhythmia Evaluation*

These devices can be evaluated carefully against known standard libraries of ECG tapes. Most reports done to date have been performed by the manufacturers or builders of the equipment and none has been reported in great detail in the scientific literature. Since all of the ECG data are not available, it becomes almost impossible to make a detailed evaluation of the accuracy of arrhythmia analysis in a given individual patient. These devices label ECG strips with the automated microprocessor arrhythmia diagnosis and, despite our limited experience in evaluating these real-time systems, the errors made by the microprocessor in calling slight areas of artifact or normal ECG as episodes of tachycardia or bradycardia, for example, leave us with less than perfect confidence that the trend plots they report with numbers of events of each type of arrhythmia are accurate (FIG. 1).

### *Clinical and Research Uses*

Real-time systems have considerable appeal to the practicing cardiologist. They are often less expensive than more complicated continuous tape systems, for while the recorders are somewhat more expensive, the playback systems are less so. The major appeal to the clinician is the automated analysis, which requires little technician interaction. Nonetheless, it is recognized at most centers at which ambulatory ECG analysis is frequently done that strong technician interaction and editing of data are at the heart of accurate arrhythmia evaluation and clinically relevant ECG diagnosis. Therefore clinicians must be wary of systems that do not permit subsequent analysis of all of the actual ECG, but that rely heavily on trend plots and data that can never be verified. Their use is to be strongly discouraged for research purposes. If and when such systems can combine real-time analysis with recording of the entire 24 hours of ECG data, they may then become useful for clinical and research purposes.

## TRANSTELEPHONIC ECG MONITORING

### *Equipment*

One major problem with continuous or real-time ambulatory ECG recordings is that they are generally of a finite, usually 24-hour, duration. Many patients with

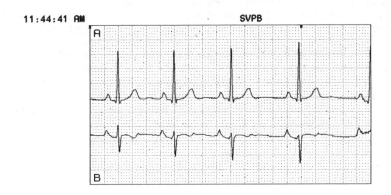

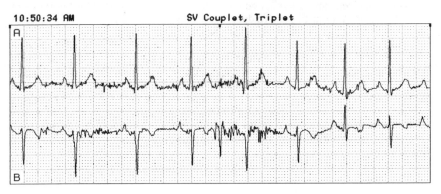

**FIGURE 1.** Mislabeling of rhythm strips by a real-time ECG system. In such systems a number of events are stored in order to later construct a trend plot of number of events over time. Only a limited number of ECG examples are stored. (*Top*) rhythm strip with a slight sinus arrhythmia which the real-time system has incorrectly diagnosed as being a supraventricular premature beat (SVPB). (*Bottom*) sinus rhythm with a minor amount of baseline artifact. In this case the real-time system has incorrectly diagnosed the presence of supraventricular (SV) couplets or triplets. Such errors are not a problem when all data are available for retrieval and subsequent validation. They represent a more serious problem in real-time systems with limited memory, where most episodes cannot actually be recalled for verification.

serious and/or symptomatic arrhythmias may experience these only every few days or even less frequently. For such patients, a negative 24-hour monitoring period is not of clinical value unless the patient experienced typical symptoms during that time. The past few years has seen a marked increase in the use of transtelephonic ECG monitoring. This employs small FM transmitting devices which send the ECG over telephone lines to a receiving station which transforms the signal into a standard ECG rhythm strip. As originally conceived, these devices were carried by the patient and when a symptomatic arrhythmia episode occurred, the patient immediately went to a telephone and placed the electrodes of the device on the precordium or in the axillae and transmitted a real-time ECG signal. Because of the difficulty in getting to telephones and the brief duration of many symptomatic arrhythmias, these devices have recently been modified to include memories containing 20 to 40 seconds of ECG. Thus the ECG can be recorded and transmitted at a later time. These devices have the drawback of not recording the arrhythmia onset. In addition, at times, P waves are difficult to see in the single-channel output and in some patients, especially elderly patients with tremor or anxiety at the time of symptoms, the tracings may have some artifact. Recent devices require the patient to wear electrodes continuously attached to the body. When the symptoms occur, the patient activates the recorder with a memory loop so as to catch the ECG 10 to 20 seconds before the precise moment symptoms were perceived.

### *Clinical Value*

These transtelephonic ECG recordings have markedly improved the clinical usefulness of ambulatory ECG monitoring for the practicing physician. It is possible to exclude or include the diagnosis of an arrhythmia in any patient who has symptoms suggestive of arrhythmia occurring with a frequency of once weekly or more and whose symptoms last for several seconds or longer. These devices, especially those not requiring permanent electrode fixation, are well received by the patients. Specially modified units have a better frequency response for recording S-T segment shifts. In general, to achieve the best fidelity for S-T segment recordings, gel electrodes should be utilized. In addition, the leads in which potential ischemia might be occurring should be known ahead of time so as to optimize lead placement for the single-channel recordings. One major advantage of these devices is their low price, which enables patients with serious arrhythmias to purchase the device and transmit the ECG recording of arrhythmias when symptoms occur.

### CONCLUSIONS

Ambulatory ECG equipment has improved markedly over the past decade, both in terms of the types of recorders/transmitters available as well as the technical quality of these devices. A large body of information and experience about their uses and limitations has accumulated. The recent introduction of real-time analysis systems raises major questions about the accuracy of arrhythmia analysis since for the first time all data are not available for subsequent review and verification. More effort should be placed on independent review of systems with publication in peer review scientific journals.

### REFERENCES

1. ARZBAECHER, R. 1978. A pill electrode for the study of cardiac arrhythmia. Med. Instrum. **12:** 227–281.

2. HINKEL, L. E., JR., J. MEYER, M. STEVENS & S. T. CARVER. 1967. Tape recordings of the ECG of active men. Limitations and advantages of the Holter-Avionics instruments. Circulation 36: 752–765.
3. BRAGG-REMSCHEL, D. A., C. M. ANDERSON & R. A. WINKLE. 1982. Frequency response characteristics of ambulatory ECG monitoring systems and their implications for ST segment analysis. Am. Heart J. 103: 20–31.
4. BRAGG-REMSCHEL, D. A., C. M. ANDERSON & R. A. WINKLE. 1981. New methods to evaluate the frequency response and ST segment reproducibility of ambulatory ECG systems. Comput. Cardiol. 91–96.
5. ALLEN, R. D., L. S. GETTES & M. D. AVINGTON. 1976. Painless ST-segment depression in patients with angina pectoris. Chest 69: 467–473.
6. SCHANG, S. J., JR. & C. J. PEPINE. 1977. Transient asymptomatic S-T segment depression during daily activity. Am. J. Cardiol. 39: 396–402.
7. STERN, S., D. TZIVONI & Z. STERN. 1975. Diagnostic accuracy of ambulatory ECG monitoring in ischemic heart disease. Circulation 52: 1045–1049.
8. STERN, S. & D. TZIVONI. 1974. Early detection of silent ischaemic heart disease by 24-hour electrocardiographic monitoring of active subjects. Br. Heart J. 36: 481–486.
9. CHIERCHIA, S., M. LAZZARI, B. FREEDMAN, C. BRUNELLI & A. MASERI. 1983. J. Am. Coll. Cardiol. 1(3): 924–930.

# Computer Recognition of Cardiac Arrhythmias and Statistical Approaches to Arrhythmia Analysis

JOEL MORGANROTH[a]

*Likoff Cardiovascular Institute*
*Hahnemann University*
*Philadelphia, Pennsylvania 19102*

## INTRODUCTION

Long-term ambulatory (Holter) electrocardiographic monitoring has provided important insights into the mechanisms and potential means to prevent sudden cardiac death. In patients fortuitously wearing a Holter monitor at the time of sudden cardiac death it was demonstrated that the most common mechanism of sudden death was a ventricular tachyarrhythmia that degenerated into ventricular fibrillation.[1] Left ventricular dysfunction and electrical instability are the two primary markers in identifying the high-risk patient[2-4] and it is hoped that the correction of ventricular arrhythmias will be an important means of primary prevention of sudden death.

Before 1978, only arbitrary criteria existed to define whether or not a therapeutic approach was successful in correcting electrical cardiac instability.[5] The fact that ventricular arrhythmias have a marked spontaneous variability in frequency from hour to hour or day to day allows different approaches to be used to define antiarrhythmic drug efficacy. All of these approaches are statistically based and allow one to be certain that it is the drug therapy (antiarrhythmic agents, for example) rather than spontaneous variability alone that is responsible for the observed changes in arrhythmia frequency.

The purpose of this article is to detail the various definitions of antiarrhythmic drug efficacy using sophisticated statistical approaches that have evolved since 1978 and then to define briefly the different methods available for recording and analyzing long-term ambulatory ECG monitoring data.

## SPONTANEOUS VARIABILITY OF VENTRICULAR ECTOPY

In 1978, Winkle and coworkers[6] studied 20 hospitalized patients undergoing evaluation of new antiarrhythmic drug therapy. Eleven half-hour Holter monitoring recordings were analyzed from a 5.5-hour monitoring session for each person. The initial half-hour was considered the control, and subsequent half-hour periods were compared to that control frequency. Statistical evaluation was made using the Wilcoxin rank sum nonparametric statistical technique.

[a] Address for correspondence: Joel Morganroth, M.D., Director, Sudden Death Prevention Program, Hahnemann University Hospital, 230 N. Broad Street, Philadelphia, Pennsylvania 19102.

A large spontaneous variation in the frequency of ventricular ectopy was identified: Variations ranged from a 99% decline to a 1100% increase in frequency. During the first 3 hours after the initial half-hour control period, in 14 of 20 (70%) of the patients a 50% or greater reduction in ventricular ectopic frequency was demonstrated, thus eliminating the prior arbitrary definition of a 50% reduction in ventricular ectopic frequency as a definition of therapeutic drug efficacy. Using limited Holter monitoring data, these investigators concluded that only by requiring complete ectopic suppression during a single half-hour period or more than 90% suppression for 2–3 consecutive half-hour periods would therapeutic drug efficacy seem to be present.

In 1978, we[7] reported our investigation of the degree of spontaneous variability present in ventricular ectopy frequency in 15 hospitalized patients prior to evaluation with a new antiarrhythmic agent. These patients had to meet the requirement of having at least 30 ventricular premature complexes (VPCs) per hour per day during placebo monitoring for 3 days, and they also had to demonstrate the presence of stable underlying cardiac conditions and medications. Before entry to the hospital, all patients had antiarrhythmic therapy discontinued for at least 7 days, and 3 consecutive 24-hour periods of ambulatory monitoring data were used during controlled conditions on placebo therapy for this analysis. Five of these patients were selected at random to undergo a repeat 72-hour ambulatory monitoring recording session approximately 3 months apart.

The statistical analysis technique used in this study was analysis of variance.[7] This technique allows for isolation of the contribution of each of many components of an observed variation of a complex model. This model was, therefore, used to define the sources of variability between subjects and within a subject. To define the extent of spontaneous variability in ectopic frequency a pure model II four-factor nested analysis of variance was used and spontaneous variability "between patients", "between days" within patients, "between 8-hour periods" within days, and "between hours" within 8-hour periods were analyzed. Analysis of variance calculations were made by the least-squares regression technique since not all subjects had complete 24-hour recordings because of technical problems in monitoring techniques at that time. Therefore, we did not study the possible model assuming that the dose "period" and "hour" were fixed effects. Since these variance components are additive, the total variation in hourly ectopic frequency for all patients was determined by the formula: $S^2$ (total) = $S^2$ (between patients) + $S^2$ (between days) + $S^2$ (between periods) + $S^2$ (between hours), where S = the standard deviation for each of the respective variances. This equation underlies the four-factor nested analysis of variance principle, and estimates of the variance components were pooled for all patients. Since five patients were studied at a subsequent time, the variance calculations were redetermined from a five-factor nested analysis by adding the source "between 3-day periods in the same patients." In this statistical approach, all frequencies of ventricular ectopy were transformed to the natural logarithm using the formula: ln (VPC + 1) to insure that the statistical assumptions of normal distribution and homogeneous variance would be closely satisfied. The number "1" was added to each ectopic frequency value since some hours had zero arrhythmia frequency. The variance ($V$) of the daily average arrhythmia frequency was calculated using the formula:

$$V(\text{average}) = S^2(\text{``between days''})$$

$$+ \frac{S^2(\text{``between periods''})}{P} + \frac{S^2(\text{``between hours''})}{PH}$$

where $P$ is the number of 8-hour periods sampled and where $H$ is the number of hours per period. The 95% confidence limit for the difference between any control period when compared to a test period in which an intervention was being evaluated was calculated by the formula:

$$D = 2\sqrt{\text{average variance} \left(\frac{1}{C} + \frac{1}{T}\right)},$$

where $C$ is the number of days in the control period and $T$ the number of days in the test period. The percentage reduction from control during the test period was calculated by the formula:

$D = \ln(\text{test}) - \ln(\text{control})$,

$$\text{which equals } \ln \frac{\text{test}}{\text{control}},$$

$$\text{therefore, } e^D = \frac{\text{test}}{\text{control}}.$$

The percent change =

$$100 \times \frac{\text{test}}{\text{control}} - 1, \text{ which therefore} = 100(e^D - 1).$$

Sensitivity analysis was also conducted to determine the effect of the dose-period variance component on the results demonstrating the minimal percent reduction in ventricular ectopic frequency required to demonstrate an effect attributable to the intervention itself rather than to spontaneous variability. These reduction guidelines would change little even in the unlikely event that the dose-period variance component was zero. For example, if the $S^2$ (periods) = zero, then the percent reduction for 3 control days and 7 test days would change from minus 58.4% to only minus 52.4% for VPCs.

In addition, the data from this study[7] were subjected to a determination of variation using the formula:

$$\text{Coefficient of variation} = \frac{(\text{S.D. of the mean 72-hr VPC frequency}) \times 100}{\text{mean hour VPC frequency}}$$

This analysis revealed quite clearly that the more frequent the control ectopic frequency, the less the degree of spontaneous variability and the less the percent reduction required for the definition of therapeutic efficacy (TABLE 1).

In a subsequent analysis of an additional 20 patients we evaluated[8] the spontaneous variability of beats of ventricular couplets and ventricular tachycardia. These patients had to meet the same entrance criteria as in the previous study.[7]

TABLE 2 details the sources of variation as seen in these studies and defines that the major source of variation in ectopic frequency variability is "between patients." Within individual patients the source of variance "between hours" contributed approximately one-half of the variance as the "between 8-hour periods" and "between days" values, in which each contributed approximately 25%. TABLE 3 details the suggested guidelines using various lengths of ambulatory ECG monitoring recording for control and treatment periods which can be used to define therapeutic efficacy using the statistical approach.

**TABLE 1.** Variance (%) from Each Source

| | Ventricular Ectopy ($n = 15$) | Ventricular Couplets ($n = 22$) | Ventricular Tachycardia ($n = 14$) |
|---|---|---|---|
| Pooled data | | | |
| Between patients | 66 | 64.5 | 46.2 |
| Between days | 8 | 4.3 | 6.4 |
| Between 8-hour periods | 10 | 8.4 | 9.4 |
| Between hours | 16 | 22.8 | 38.0 |
| Total | 100 | 100 | 100 |
| Data from individual patients | | | |
| Between days | 23 | 12.1 | 12.1 |
| Between 8-hour periods | 29 | 23.7 | 17.3 |
| Between hours | 48 | 64.2 | 70.6 |
| Total | 100 | 100 | 100 |
| Between three-day monitoring periods | 37 | | |
| Between patients | 35 | | |
| Between days | 7 | | |
| Between 8-hour periods | 8 | | |
| Between hours | 13 | | |
| Total | 100 | | |

NOTE: Data adapted from References 7 and 8.

**TABLE 2.** Mean Frequency of Ventricular Premature Complexes (VPCs)[a]

| Mean Frequency of VPCs/hr/24 hrs | Coefficient of Variation (%) |
|---|---|
| <100 | 59 |
| 100–200 | 66 |
| 200–1000 | 35 |
| >1000 | 13 |

[a] Adapted from Morganroth et al.[7]

**TABLE 3.** Guidelines to Define Therapeutic Efficacy Using Holter Monitoring[a]

| Length of Monitoring | Number of Periods | | Minimal Percent Reduction Required | | |
|---|---|---|---|---|---|
| | Control | Test | VPCs[b] | Couplets[c] | VTACH[d] |
| 8 hours | 1 | 1 | −90.3 | −85.7 | −75.9 |
| 24 hours | 1 | 1 | −83.4 | −75.3 | −64.8 |
| 24 hours | 3 | 3 | −64.6 | −55.4 | −45.3 |
| 24 hours | 7 | 7 | −49.3 | −41.1 | −32.6 |
| 24 hours | 14 | 14 | −38.2 | −31.2 | −24.4 |

[a] Adapted from Morganroth et al.[7]
[b] Ventricular premature complexes.
[c] Ventricular couplets.
[d] Ventricular tachycardia.

In these studies[7,8] there was no evidence that a decrease in ectopic frequency during sleep was other than a trend and not directly attributable to the decrease in heart rate seen with sleep. In fact, no statistically significant correlation between VPC frequency and complex arrhythmia frequency was noted nor was there a correlation between the frequency of complex arrhythmias and underlying heart rate.

In 1980, Sami et al.[9] evaluated a statistical model based on the linear regression analysis technique to establish the degree of spontaneous variability in 21 patients with coronary artery disease with chronic VPCs. These patients had to have only 6 VPCs per hour to enter the study. Antiarrhythmic drugs were discontinued for at least 7 days before entry. Since this was an outpatient study, data were obtained on an initial 24-hour ambulatory Holter monitor, and then patients were given a placebo and a second 24-hour recording was obtained 2 weeks later. The comparison of these two single 24-hour monitoring periods was the basis for their analysis. VPC frequency was again transformed to logarithm using VPC + 1 for reasons similar to those used in our earlier study.[7] Linear regression analysis was used to describe the relationship between ventricular ectopic frequency between the two ambulatory monitoring periods. The slope and intercept of the linear regression curves were estimated and confidence intervals were computed for the expected placebo response given a specific baseline ectopic frequency level. Ninety-five and 99% confidence lines representing a "one-tailed" lower confidence interval for individual data points were determined, and the sensitivity threshold was defined as that point at which the 95 or 99% confidence line crossed the baseline ventricular ectopic frequency line. Baseline frequencies below the sensitivity threshold could not be used to evaluate antiarrhythmic drug efficacy. The minimal percent reduction required using these guidelines in patients with a baseline of ventricular ectopic frequency of $\geq$ 30/hr was 65%. This study suggested that patients with as few as 2.2 VPCs per hour could be tested for antiarrhythmic drug efficacy and would require at least a 90–100% reduction to establish drug efficacy at the 95% confidence level. This study differs from the ones reported above and such differences may be attributable to (1) the facts that patients utilized in this study had only one cardiac disease (coronary artery disease) and that only the total ventricular ectopic frequency for the entire 24-hour period was used rather than an analysis of variations within the 24-hour day, (2) the effects of hospitalization versus ambulatory states and (3) the differences in statistical design.

Shapiro et al.[10] studied 162 untreated patients with three 24-hour Holter monitoring recordings and 8 untreated patients with two 24-hour recordings for a total of 170 patients. These recordings were obtained within a 14-day period in which at least 30 VPCs per hour on average were required for entry into the study. This study compared the analysis of the sources of variability by the nested analysis of variance technique[7,8] as well as the linear regression model.[9] There was a very close agreement between the linear regression and one-tailed nested analysis of variance methods. Seventy-three to 84% reduction was determined to be required using these data of Shapiro et al.[10] on linear regression. This is in contrast to the data from Sami et al.,[9] which required only a 65% reduction. This discrepancy was probably accounted for by the observation that the correlation between days in Shapiro's data[10] was not as high as that obtained in Sami's original report.[9] Differences reflect also the heterogeneity of diagnoses in the Shapiro data compared with those of Sami's data. Both analysis of variance and linear regression technique required similar percent reductions when performed on a "one-tail" basis. While linear regression is easier to apply, this method does not use all of the information available in the database and the advantage of the nested analysis of variance approach is that it accommodates a variable number of days' data, utilizing more information in the database and therefore possibly yielding a better estimate of percent reduction required to eliminate spontaneous variation.

In summary, while the various approaches to define the input or spontaneous variability of VPCs have used different statistical techniques and assumptions, these experiments clearly show that the role of spontaneous variability of ventricular ectopic beats is important in defining guidelines to determine therapeutic efficacy using ambulatory monitoring. Before a well-controlled clinical trial is undertaken to determine whether sudden cardiac death can be prevented, we recommend that a minimum of a 75% reduction for VPCs be required when a single 24-hour ambulatory monitoring period is compared with another. It must be recognized, however, that such a reduction may not necessarily prevent sudden cardiac death, but will define only therapeutic or drug efficacy, eliminating spontaneous variability as the cause for an observed reduction in ectopic frequency. Consideration must be given to details of long-term sudden death trials before a definition of efficacy based on biological rather than statistical observations is possible. It is inherent in this analysis that proper consideration be given to the quality of ambulatory ECG monitoring recordings and to analysis systems. Different approaches to such recording and analysis will be reviewed later in this paper.

## RECOMMENDATIONS FOR CONDUCT OF CLINICAL ANTIARRHYTHMIC DRUG TRIALS

In view of the fact that there is a high degree of spontaneous variability in ventricular ectopic frequency, individual patient data in which the percentage of patients demonstrating a response to an antiarrhythmic drug is compared with that of a placebo should be the basis for reporting drug efficacy data. This is in contradistinction to the averaging of VPC frequency using all patient data obtained on control and on drug therapy. Since most studies utilize patient populations with (1) a great deal of heterogeneity both in the underlying clinical state and in concomitant medication and (2) more than a 100-fold variation in frequency of VPCs, pooling of ventricular ectopic data from all patients in a study to compare mean changes on drug compared to placebo will mask proarrhythmic effects or seriously compromise the usefulness of the results to predict therapeutic efficacy. After considering the impact of spontaneous variability, we have recommended that patients be considered candidates for chronic antiarrhythmic drug testing protocols when they have at least 30 VPCs per hour per 24 hours during the baseline placebo control period. While it has been shown[4] that after a myocardial infarction patients have an increased risk of sudden death with as few as 10 VPCs per hour per day, such patients will have a higher degree of spontaneous variability and require a greater than 90% reduction in VPCs to define therapeutic drug efficacy. By use of such efficacy guidelines, patients can be entered into trials with only $\geq 10$ VPCs per hr with the recognition that the degree of spontaneous variability will be higher. It is obviously essential that subjects with chronic ventricular arrhythmias undergo a placebo-controlled period to define the baseline frequency of ventricular ectopy so that an estimate of the degree of spontaneous variability can be made. This placebo period should extend for at least a 5–7-day interval after at least a 5–7-day period of cessation of prior antiarrhythmic agents. When digitalis, beta blockers, or calcium channel blockers are not used for arrhythmia control, they can be continued concomitantly as long as their dosage is not changed throughout the study and no serious adverse drug interactions are expected.

Whether crossover or parallel design trials are instituted, one should expect to see at least a 50% return of ventricular ectopy to the baseline control period during the interim or final placebo period. We particularly believe that the crossover design is more powerful and thus useful, for it requires fewer numbers of patients and is less costly, and the potential for any bias in a carryover effect from one period to another in the crossover design can be eliminated by using the objective endpoint provided by ambulatory Holter monitoring data.

Because of spontaneous variability, initial antiarrhythmic drug studies should be of a relatively short duration (less than 14 days), and at least a minimum of two 24-hour ambulatory Holter recordings should be obtained during the placebo baseline control period. This will define the degree of spontaneous variability and characterize the baseline. Dose-titration periods can be conducted with changes every 7 days using one or preferably two 24-hour monitoring sessions at each dose level. Long-term studies should include a reintroduction of placebo at least every 6 months to evaluate the continuing presence of ventricular arrhythmias and the necessity for continued therapy. We often observe that variability may be high enough so that a sufficient return (compared to the baseline) of ventricular ectopy frequency during a final placebo period in short-term studies or during the reintroduction of placebo in long-term studies is not observed. Ambulatory ECG monitoring in long-term efficacy and tolerance studies is usually done at 1, 3, 6, 9, and 12 months. It is important to remember in the general evaluation of antiarrhythmic drug therapy that interaction studies with digoxin and coumadin are needed. Trials with new agents are also necessary in patients with marked left ventricular dysfunction, during acute ischemia (such as in the early phases of myocardial infarction), and in other special settings.

## LONG-TERM AMBULATORY ECG RECORDERS AND ANALYSIS SYSTEMS

In 1961, Norman J. Holter, D.Sc.,[11] developed a miniaturized battery-operated recording device which enabled long-term, continuous recording of cardiac rhythm for up to 10 hours. It was not until the mid to late 1960s that the first playback scanners became commercially available; these systems were completely analog in nature and did not have the ability to automatically detect ventricular arrhythmias. These units were typically slow in operation (30–60 × real time) and required the constant interpretation and interaction of an analyst to detect the ventricular ectopy. The Avionics Model 650 electrocardioscanner, which was able to analyze single-channel ECG data, was the prototype instrument. It was not until several years later that analog hardwired ventricular arrhythmia detecting devices were introduced and integrated into these playback scanners to enhance analysis of ECG waveforms. These newer instruments resulted in a marked increase in accuracy of VPC detection and documentation, but they were deficient in adaptability for one patient to the next and thus suffered from a lack of precision (accuracy). Reproducibility of data analysis was also difficult since the operator or analyst was still required to perform an intricate activity in the first-pass wave-shape discrimination. Technician fatigue and inter-technician variability in determining arrhythmia reduction continued to be a problem. It has only been within the last 5 to 7 years that advances in both recorder and playback techniques have allowed for a rapid dissemination of accurate ambulatory monitoring.[12] At present there are at least 30 manufacturers of instruments for ambulatory monitoring and analysis, and at least a 15–20% growth rate yearly is projected for the number of procedures to be performed. It has been estimated that the total amount of money spent on Holter monitoring in the United States in 1980 was 55 million dollars and in 1984 more than 120 million dollars; this amount is expected to increase to more than 200 million dollars by 1987. New advances in analysis techniques and in different methods have not only markedly expanded the potential for Holter monitoring, but have also introduced a degree of confusion as to the most preferable system.

## AMBULATORY ECG RECORDING DEVICES

Ambulatory ECG data may be recorded in three different modes: continuous, intermittent (patient- or time-activated), and real-time analytical. Because the continuous and real-time analytical recording devices have become so sophisticated, intermittent recorders have become less important.

Continuous recorders share such common features as recording direct analog signals only, providing at least the potential for two or more recording channels for physiologic data, and providing at least 24 hours of continuous recording using a magnetic media (cassette or reel-to-reel tape). The ECG signal is detected from the input into the recorder, which consists of a dual bipolar precordial lead system. In addition to having an external ground, negative electrodes are used to complement each exploratory electrode. A three-lead system eliminates both the ground wire and one of the negative poles and is not recommended since a single electrode dislodgement will result in no ECG signal input into the recorder on either channel. Factors that account for poor quality of recording include partial disconnection of the lead system, severe skin irritation, use of inferior materials, or poor construction. These cause the baseline to wander and artifact to occur, which confuses ECG analysis.

The most common type of magnetic recording device used in continuous recorders is the cassette. The cassette recorders are lighter than reel-to-reel counterparts, less obtrusive for patient use, and more convenient for the technician to use. Reel-to-reel recorders, however, have a better signal-to-noise ratio, dynamic range, and a more consistent speed stability with less wow and flutter. Fewer recording failures are encountered with reel-to-reel recorders than are found with cassette recorders. Reel-to-reel recorders employ a ¼-inch tape of either chromium dioxide or ferric oxide with a thickness of 4–5 mil. They use wide two-track recording heads, and frequently three-phase motors. Most cassette recorders, however, use ⅛-inch tape of ferric oxide which is only 2–3 mil in thickness. Narrower four-track recording heads and less stable motor/transmission configurations are used. We therefore believe that for research reel-to-reel devices are still the method of choice and should include an internal millivolt calibration system.

Most recorders currently available in the United States use amplitude modulation (AM) as the method of recording. The potential of using frequency modulation (FM), which will provide an ultra-wide frequency response, is under investigation. At present it is unclear whether FM recording will be a major advantage in the context of ambulatory ECG monitoring. All currently available AM records display frequency response characteristics from .05–100 Hz (−3 dB), which are more than sufficient for recording without distortion even the slowest of the S-T T-wave patterns. Cassette recorders seem to be perfectly suitable for the clinical ambulatory outpatient setting since they are smaller, self-contained, and less expensive. Other recorders are available, such as the ICR 7200 and the Marquette 8500, which are "slow-speed" recorders (1 mm/sec) as opposed to the more conventional 2 mm/sec used by other recorders. This slower speed allows for the use of a C-60 cassettes, which are less costly than the C-120 cassette. However, there is a greater inherent tendency towards wow and flutter and, therefore, distorted ECG patterns are more common with the slower recorders.

The second type of recorder is the real-time analyzer, in which the body of the recorder contains a microprocessor which actually analyzes the ECG data at input in the Holter monitor as it is taking place in real time. The recorder stores those patterns selected as abnormal by the microcomputer and thus does not require the immediate attention of a technician or physician. These recorders do have dual-channel recording capabilities lasting up to 24 hours. They can be symptom-activated and use disposable batteries, and they have internal millivolt calibrations and a real-time clock display. These devices weigh 50–100% more than do the continuous recording devices. The major disadvantage is that these recorders cost up to five times more than a continuous recorder. However, the playback system for these real-time analyzers is considerably less expensive. The primary limitation of this system is lack of storage of real data for reanalysis and lack of demonstrable accuracy and reproducibility compared to those of the well-standardized continuous recording techniques, especially for infrequent complex VPCs.

## ANALYSIS SYSTEMS FOR AMBULATORY HOLTER MONITORING RECORDERS

Although recorders tend to be fairly uniform in design and performance features, Holter monitoring tape analysis systems differ greatly with respect to their hardware, their method of detecting QRS complexes, and their general cost and other specifications.[13] The recent marked improvement in computer technology and the availability of powerful byte processors has allowed for very sophisticated digital analysis systems to be developed. We would anticipate that further improvements in storage density for basic memory chips and more powerful logic chips will translate into faster, more accurate cost-effective analysis systems. We believe that the hardware-based analog tape scanners, which have been the basic analyzers for the past 15 years, have become almost entirely outmoded within the last few years because of advances in computer technology. The analog-type of arrhythmia analyzer will cease to be used in the future as these newly improved computer analyzers become more widely available to the marketplace.

New analytical models have evolved including (1) high-speed data reduction processors (accelerated semiautomatic analysis), (2) manual systems for the complete display of continuous Holter recording, and (3) real-time analyzers. The lack of precise guidelines and standardization of Holter analysis equipment has resulted in this wide diversity of analysis models. The recent availability of standardized Holter tapes to determine the quality of various systems will help in the proper selection process; however, these standard database tapes were developed for the validation of real-time coronary care unit monitoring systems rather than for high-speed Holter monitoring tape playback systems, and therefore limitation in this regard is present.

The first group of analyzers are those that have an accelerated analysis by processor/technician interface using a semiautomatic mode of processing. The most powerful subset in this group of systems employs a 16-byte microcomputer as the central processing unit buffered with a disk-drive which provides flexibility in analysis. There are those systems that are entirely digital, but that lack the flexibility afforded by a fixed based system. The rigid-disk-based systems are the most advanced analysis systems available and their detection algorithms are complex and adaptive for VPC detection. All of the systems use a patient's normal QRS pattern as the reference to compare new test beats against beats for potential aberration. The systems offer a 16-byte resolution, thus enabling a more accurate QRS representative to be constructed, resulting in better template-matching with feature extraction and correlation techniques. The unfiltered analog ECG signal from the cassette or reel-to-reel recorder is filtered for frequency and/or voltage artifacts and the QRS complexes are identified by the software-controlled systems during the first pass. During this first pass, analog-to-digital conversion occurs and the data are stored on a hard disk. During the second pass the digital QRS data are analyzed in core memory automatically by the VPC-detection algorithms using featured extraction and correlation techniques, and initial strip documentation is generated. Editing of numerical and selected wave-shaped data by an analyst occurs prior to generation of the final report. The recent availability of dual-lead, simultaneous analysis (such as that provided by United Medical Corporation's CT240 system) may be an important advance in detecting and eliminating artifact, which is the commonest concern in these analysis systems. These systems can process data at speeds up to 240 times real time. Some analysis systems (Marquette's Model 8000, for example) complete the entire analysis without user interface. If this is proven to be quantitatively accurate, the need for much technician interface will decline. These new advances will require further evaluation.

The analysis systems that do not use a disk-based digital process system are the semiautomated processing systems and these may be looked at as being halfway between the old conventional analog approach and the microcomputer-based systems discussed earlier. These systems execute but one function and are programmed for any computer function that the user desires. These systems do not analyze dual leads simultaneously and they have limited graphic capabilities. Their advantage is, of course, that their price is less than that of the disk-based systems. In the traditional analog tape-processing system (such as Oxford's Medilog II) the wave-shape analysis and discrimination of VPC presence occurs in hardware only. This analysis is performed using voltage–time variations as recorded on magnetic tape. These systems are inexpensive and easy to operate, but the accuracy of the data may be limited.

Another method of analyzing Holter monitoring tapes employs the manual approach, in which the entire ECG information (all 24 hours) is displayed on the screen and may be printed photographically. Since this is a manual and fatiguing method of counting and defining ventricular ectopic frequency, we believe it to be a most imprecise method of analysis. This system may be useful, however, for gross qualitative analysis of a 24-hour ambulatory monitoring record. Its use for accurate quantitation in both clinical and research tapes has not yet been established.

Real-time analytical recorder and analysis devices are digitally based systems that detect arrhythmias automatically during the recording process. Since wave-shape analysis occurs in real time instead of at high speed, many computer instructions can be executed, allowing for a more sophisticated algorithm. These systems may be completely solid-state without moving parts, and incorporate a 64K-byte memory which may execute the programs and analyze the ECG in real time. Dual-channel ECG signals may be digitalized at 250 points/sec and a 16–32-beat template may be formed to analyze each complex for shape and area change. These systems theoretically have great power, but until they are proven to be accurate, and reproducible, they are limited in terms of their potential research and clinical capabilities. Real-time analyzers provide no provision for recall of particular segments of the 24-hour period for verification of results, and the ability to distinguish artifact from true VPCs has not been clearly demonstrated. Such determinations often require the knowledge of a skilled technician working with the analysis device.

## SUMMARY

The recognition of marked spontaneous variability in the frequency of ventricular ectopy has required the analysis of various statistical approaches to define appropriate guidelines for determining that a therapeutic agent, rather than spontaneous variability alone, is the cause of an observed reduction in VPC frequency. Analysis of variance or linear regression techniques have been applied to ambulatory ECG data obtained on different patient population groups. When similar patient groups are studied with comparable assumptions, then either of these statistical techniques provides similar guidelines to detect spontaneous variation as the cause of ventricular ectopic reduction. A 75% minimal reduction in VPC frequency should be required when comparing one 24-hour ambulatory monitoring period with another. The impact of spontaneous variability of ventricular ectopy on clinical trial designs is discussed, as is the categorization of various ambulatory ECG monitoring recorders and analysis systems.

## REFERENCES

1. PANIDIS, I. & J. MORGANROTH. 1982. Holter monitoring during sudden cardiac death: Clues to its etiology and prevention. Circulation 66: II–25.
2. MOSS, A. J. 1980. Clinical significance of ventricular arrhythmias in patients with and without coronary artery disease. Prog. Cardiovas. Dis. 23: 33.
3. MORGANROTH, J., E. N. MOORE, et al., Eds. 1981. The Evaluation of New Antiarrhythmic Drugs. Martinus Nijhoff. The Hague.
4. BIGGER, J. T., F. M. WELD & L. M. ROLNITSKY. 1981. Prevalence, characteristics and significance of ventricular tachycardia (three or more complexes) detected with ambulatory electrocardiographic recording in the late hospital phase of acute myocardial infarction. Am. J. Cardiol. 48: 815.
5. HARRISON, D. C., J. W. FITZGERALD & R. A. WINKLE. 1976. Ambulatory electrocardiography for diagnosis and treatment of cardiac arrhythmias. N. Engl. J. Med. 294: 373.
6. WINKLE, R. A. 1978. Arrhythmia drug effect mimicked by spontaneous variability of ventricular ectopy. Circulation 57: 1116.
7. MORGANROTH, J., E. L. MICHELSON, L. N. HOROWITZ, M. E. JOSEPHSON, A. S. PEARLMAN & W. B. DUNKMAN. 1978. Limitations of routine long-term ambulatory electrocardiographic monitoring to assess ventricular ectopic frequency. Circulation 58: 408.

8. MICHELSON, E. L. & J. MORGANROTH. 1980. Spontaneous variability of complex ventricular arrhythmias detected by long-term electrocardiography recordings. Circulation **61:** 690.
9. SAMI, M., H. KRAMEMER, D. C. HARRISON, N. HOUSTON, C. SHIMASAKI & R. F. DEBUSK. 1980. A new method of evaluating antiarrhythmic drug efficacy. Circulation **62:** 1172.
10. SHAPIRO, W., W. B. CANADA, G. LEE, A. N. DEMARIA, R. I. LOW, D. T. MASON & A. LADDU. 1982. Comparison of two methods of analyzing frequency of ventricular arrhythmias. Am. Heart J. **4:** 874–875.
11. SOKAL, R. R. & F. J. ROHLF. 1969. Biometry.: 253–298. W. H. Freeman. San Francisco, CA.
12. WEGSCHEIDER, K., D. ANDRESEN, E. R. LEITNER & R. SCHROEDER. 1982. A new method for evaluating antiarrhythmic drug efficacy in the individual patient using 24 hour ECG recordings. Circulation **66:** II–1486.
13. BRAGG-REMSCHELD, D. A. & R. A. WINKLE. 1983. Ambulatory monitoring of electrocardiograms: Current technology of recording and analysis. Physiologist **26:** 39.

# Therapeutic Drug Monitoring Techniques: An Overview

C. E. PIPPENGER[a]

*Section of Applied Clinical Pharmacology*
*Department of Biochemistry*
*Cleveland Clinic Foundation*
*Cleveland, Ohio 44106*

It has been clearly established that routine therapeutic drug monitoring (TDM) is invaluable to both patient and clinician, since it helps to ensure the best possible patient care. Historically, the measurement of serum drug concentrations was one of the functions of the clinical pharmacology laboratory, but the increasing demand for such measurements to be performed routinely exceeded the capacity of many laboratories, and necessitated the establishment of special sections within many clinical chemistry laboratories for processing large numbers of patient specimens. Over the last decade, the demand for TDM has increased geometrically to the point where therapeutic drug monitoring has evolved into a new scientific discipline.[1,2]

Physicians have had a longstanding interest in establishing why a fixed drug dosage is therapeutically effective in some individuals, but not in others. For years appropriate dosage regimens of drugs were established only by an empirical trial-and-error approach. Modern analytic techniques have provided an alternative, the ability to correlate serum or plasma drug concentrations, and, by inference, tissue concentrations, with the observed clinical effect of a given agent, and this has provided new insights into therapeutics. Today, utilizing new analytical techniques, we have begun to understand the interrelationships between drug dose and pharmacologic effect. We know that the desired pharmacologic effect is achieved only after a specific plasma drug concentration is achieved and that there is an optimal plasma concentration range for successful drug therapy. Above this optimal range, patients can be expected to experience undesirable drug side effects. Below the optimal concentration range, patients may fail to achieve the desired relief from the disease or symptom for which they are receiving therapy. Rapid advances in clinical pharmacology over the past decade are directly attributable to TDM; the availability of TDM, in turn, is directly related to the rapid advancement in technology associated with the quantitation of drug compounds.[1-5]

Clinicians should be aware of the various methods that can be utilized to quantitate drug concentrations in biological fluids. The purpose of this article is to provide a brief overview of these techniques. Detailed descriptions of the analytical techniques utilized to quantitate antiarrhythmic drug concentrations are available in Drayer's excellent reviews.

Historically, therapeutic drug monitoring has been associated with clinical laboratory medicine since World War II, when the search for antimalarial com-

---

[a] Address for correspondence: C. E. Pippenger, Ph.D., Department of Biochemistry, Cleveland Clinic Foundation, 9500 Euclid Avenue, Cleveland, Ohio 44106.

pounds resulted in improved analytic instrumentation and techniques for drug quantitation and new insights into the relationship between drug concentration and therapeutic effectiveness. The first studies correlating plasma drug concentrations with their therapeutic efficacy were published in the late 1950s and early 1960s.

Not until the late 1960s did TDM become widespread.[6-10] Gas-liquid chromatography (GLC) represented a major breakthrough because it provided a method of rapidly separating and quantitating individual drugs within a given class. Gas-liquid chromatographic techniques were further refined and improved so that by the early 1970s GLC analysis of various therapeutically monitored agents was performed routinely in many clinical chemistry laboratories. One of the major disadvantages of GLC had been the complexity of the instrumentation, which necessitated a highly trained and skilled analyst. More recent advances in the development of the nitrogen-phosphorus detector and capillary columns have increased the sensitivity of the instruments to such an extent that drug analyses can be performed routinely on micro volumes of plasma.

The development of radioimmunoassay (RIA) techniques permitted quantitation of drug concentrations in microvolumes of serum. Unfortuantely the complexity of the technique as well as the lack of radioimmunoassays for a wide variety of drugs prevented its widespread adaption for routine drug monitoring. Making TDM available to all laboratories and physicians required simple technology that could be performed by a technician without special training or instrumentation. This was achieved with the development of the homogeneous enzyme multiple immunoassay technique (EMIT), which is capable of performing assays on less than 40 $\mu$l of serum. The major advantages of the system are its microcapability and accuracy, and rapidity and ease of operation of the assays. More recently substrate-labeled fluorescent immunoassays (SLFIA) and fluorescence polarization immunoassays (FPIA) for the rapid quantitation of drugs have become available.

A large number of drugs exist for which antibodies are not available, but which must be therapeutically monitored. The most promising and practical method of monitoring these agents is by high-pressure liquid chromatography (HPLC). Within the last 10 years the development of HPLC has provided laboratories with a system having many of the same advantages as the homogeneous enzyme immunoassay system: it is capable of processing microsamples (100 $\mu$l), it is rapid and specific, and the instrumentation is relatively simple. In addition, HPLC can be adapted to simultaneously quantitate a large variety of drugs as well as their metabolites. High-pressure liquid chromatography permits simultaneous drug analysis and is a valuable tool for establishing correlations between drug and drug metabolite concentrations in biological fluids.

As with any new laboratory discipline, TDM is not a panacea that will solve all problems associated with drug therapy. There are, however, specific clinical applications for which information derived from TDM has clinical utility, just as there are situations where TDM will probably serve no useful purpose in management of a given patient.

Therapeutic drug monitoring is most applicable when the drug in question has a narrow therapeutic range, is administered chronically, has potentially toxic side effects if overdosed, and has minimal therapeutic effects if underdosed, as previously described.[6-7] Therapeutic drug monitoring can be utilized for the following reasons.

1. *Recognition of noncompliance.* Many patients, in particular those who have chronic disease requiring therapy over a prolonged period of time, tend not to

take their medications as prescribed. Moreover, patients with a chronic disease that does not necessarily cause pain or other unusual discomfort (for example, the epilepsies, asthma, or hypertension) may easily neglect to take their medicine. The end result of such noncompliance is an exacerbation of the existing disorder at some time in the future. Studies have clearly demonstrated that noncompliance is a major factor in treatment failures.

2. *Compensation for individual variations in drug utilization patterns.* In any population of individuals, a drug dosage based solely on body weight results in a fixed steady-state serum concentration. If the plasma concentrations following a specific dosage are analyzed in a large patient population, the distribution of drug levels will be gaussian. The vast majority of patients will have levels within the range expected from a dosage calculated on the basis of a given body weight and age. But patients who are genetically either "fast" or "slow" drug metabolizers will have levels at the extreme ends of the curve. Fast drug metabolizers require significantly higher doses to achieve the same plasma concentrations and consequently the desired therapeutic effect. Slow drug metabolizers become intoxicated and experience side effects from standard therapeutic doses of the drugs, and therefore, can be maintained at optimal drug concentrations on dosages well below the standard regimen.

3. *Compensation for altered drug utilization associated with various disease states.* Patients on long-term drug therapy may become acutely ill and need additional therapeutic agents. Drug interactions may then cause these patients to respond in an unexpected manner to a fixed dosage of some adjunctive therapy. Acute or chronic uremia can dramatically decrease the elimination of a drug that is primarily dependent on urinary excretion, and renal failure can alter the protein-binding characteristics of many drugs to albumin. In both situations the ratio of free to total drug may increase to the point where free drug concentrations are high enough to produce a clinically evident drug response, although the total serum drug concentrations are within optimal therapeutic range.

Hepatic disease can extensively alter a given therapeutic response by impairing a patient's ability to metabolize drugs. Most drugs depend on liver detoxification for conversion to water-soluble products, which are easily eliminated from the body. Thus, a precipitous rise in parent drug concentrations can occur as the unmetabolized drug, which normally would have been eliminated from the system, accumulates.

4. *Adjustment of therapeutic drug regimens to compensate for changing physiologic states.* Normal alterations in physiologic state also change drug utilization patterns. Therapeutic drug monitoring is crucial to successful adjustment of dosage regimen in pregnancy, puberty, and old age.

Recent studies have shown that decreased drug absorption during pregnancy is associated with a decrease in serum phenytoin concentration and exacerbation of seizures in epileptic gravidas. The use of therapeutic drug monitoring from the onset of pregnancy, with appropriate dosage regulation to maintain therapeutic drug concentrations, significantly decreases the number of seizures that occur, thus decreasing potential harm to the fetus.[11]

The normal process of maturation involves a large number of physiologic changes that can dramatically alter drug utilization. Children utilize drugs at a faster rate than adults, and therefore require almost twice as much drug on a body weight basis as an adult to achieve the same therapeutic drug concentration. As a child enters puberty, drug utilization rapidly changes, to the extent that by early pubescence the conversion to adult patterns is complete. These changes usually occur between the ages of 10 and 13, appearing earlier in girls than in boys.

Therapeutic drug monitoring must be carried out carefully for any drug administered chronically to early pubescent children. Failure to adjust the child's therapeutic regimen to compensate for the associated physiologic changes may result in exposure to unnecessary and prolonged drug toxicity, with its attendant sequelae.[12,13]

As the maturation process continues and the efficiency of normal physiologic functions decreases, so does the ability to bind drugs to plasma protein. Geriatric patients often exhibit reduced rates of drug elimination, thereby requiring reduced drug dosages. Geriatric patients may have total drug plasma concentrations within the optimal therapeutic range, but elevated free drug concentrations that can produce adverse side effects. The clinical signs of drug intoxication in the elderly often present clinically as lethargy and confusion, and therapeutic drug monitoring provides a means of distinguishing drug-induced confusion from organic deterioration.

5. *Identification of the baseline concentrations associated with an optimal therapeutic regimen.* After the patient has undergone a strenuous workup to define an appropriate therapeutic regimen, the physician can establish a baseline drug concentration at which the patient responds well. Should the patient return in the future in an uncontrolled state, the physician can rapidly document whether the patient has been compliant, or whether a new disease state has altered the pharmacologic response to the drug.

A physician utilizing drug concentrations as well as the clinical pathologist or chemist providing routine monitoring services must understand the principles and techniques of clinical pharmacology as applied to patient care. Such an understanding enables the physician to more effectively interpret drug concentration data encountered in various clinical situations and to optimize a specific patient's therapeutic regimen.

## ANALYTICAL METHODS

### Gas-Liquid Chromatography

For gas-liquid chromatography (GLC) the analyte is first extracted from an appropriate biological fluid into an organic solvent. The extracted material is either injected directly into the gas chromatograph, "derivatized" prior to injection to enhance its chromatography or derivatized directly on the GLC column at an elevated temperature (usually 200–350°C), where it is volatilized. The "carrier gas" (nitrogen, helium or argon) then carries the sample through the column in the gas chromatograph, which contains a "stationary phase" that is an inert solid-support of diatomaceous earth coated with a nonvolatile liquid polymer. In the case of capillary GLC the stationary phase is coated directly on the column walls. The interaction between the analyte and the stationary phase results in the separation of the analyte from other components present in the specimen. After passing through the column, the gas containing the separated components is passed through a detector which quantitates the compounds eluted from the column. GLC detectors available include flame ionization, electron capture, nitrogen-phosphorus (NP), and mass spectrometers. Flame ionization and NP detectors are most commonly utilized for routine drug analysis. The major factors regulating separation of analytes by gas chromatography are the amount of stationary phase and the column temperature. An internal standard which is similar in structure to the analyte is added in known concentrations to the specimen prior to analysis. The relative peak heights of the analyte and internal standard, or the area under these peaks, is utilized to quantitate the analyte concentrations. After sample preparation, the actual GLC analysis usually requires from 5–35 minutes of instrument time per specimen.

Nonpolar drugs, which are stable at elevated temperatures, are most applicable to GLC analysis, whereas more polar drugs usually require chemical derivatization prior to analysis. Gas-Liquid Chromatography (particularly capillary GLC) remains a valuable tool for screening specimens submitted for toxicological analysis as well as routine drug monitoring.

### Liquid Chromatography

The principles of liquid chromatography (LC) are similar to those of GLC except that the carrier phase in LC is a liquid (the "mobile phase," which usually consists of acetonitrile or methanol mixed with an aqueous buffer) and the chromatography is usually performed at ambient temperature. This prevents the destruction of heat-labile compounds, thus possessing a distinct advantage over GLC methods, where analyte may be destroyed at high temperature. The technique of utilizing high pressure to force the liquid through the column is referred to as HPLC (high-pressure or high-performance LC). The pressures necessary for HPLC range from 200–1000 psi. Since the analyte is eluted from the LC column in a liquid solvent, the commonly used detectors for LC analyses are flow cell detectors utilizing either ultraviolet absorbance, fluorescence, electrochemical detection, or refractive index.

Compared with immunoassay techniques, the chromatography methods (GLC and LC) have distinct differences. Both GLC and LC methods can often quantitate both drugs and their metabolites in a single analysis, whereas immunoassays usually quantitate only the parent compound. A major advantage of chromatographic methods lies in the ability to develop and adapt assays for new analytes quickly without the time restrictions imposed by the development of specific antibodies for immunoassays. It is to be noted, however, that chromatographic methods may be subject to interferences from unidentified contaminants, such as other drugs or normal physiological constituents present in individual patient specimens. Although the cost of reagents for GLC and LC are less per test than the immunoassay reagents, this advantage is offset by the need for more expensive instrumentation and dedicated technologists. The major disadvantage of GLC and HPLC is that the sample throughput is significantly less per unit of time (even with the use of automated systems) than sample throughput with immunoassay techniques.

## IMMUNOASSAY METHODS

### Radioimmunoassay

Radioimmunoassay (RIA) is based upon utilization of an antibody as the specific binding agent. The key characteristics for antibodies used in RIA (or any immunoassay) are specificity and high affinity. These characteristics, combined with instrumentation to detect radiolabels with extreme sensitivity, allow the routine quantitation of analytes at nanogram or picogram concentrations. Since it is possible to develop antibodies with specificity towards a wide variety of analytes (such as drugs, hormones, and proteins), RIA is a versatile technology.

In RIA, the analyte (A) present in a sample in an unknown concentration is allowed to compete with a constant amount of radiolabeled ($^{57}$Co, $^3$H, and $^{125}$I, for example) analyte (A-$^3$H) for a limited number of antibody-binding sites (Ab).

$$\underset{\text{``free''}}{\text{A + Ab + A-}^3\text{H}} \leftrightarrow \underset{\text{``bound''}}{(\text{Ab}:\text{A}) + (\text{Ab}:\text{A-}^3\text{H})}$$

At equilibrium, both the labeled and unlabeled analyte exist either bound to the antibody or "free" (not bound to the antibody). Since the binding is competitive, the amount of labeled analyte bound to the antibody is inversely proportional to the amount of unlabeled analyte. Analyte concentrations in a serum sample can be determined after separation of the bound and free fractions, and by comparing the amount of radioactivity in either fraction with that obtained from analyte standards. The separation step is essential since antibody binding has no effect on radioactive decay, and thus it is impossible to determine the distribution of label between the bound and free forms without separation of the two forms. There are a number of modifications of the above RIA procedure; however, they all require a separation step. All immunoassays which require a separation step are usually referred to as heterogeneous. Digoxin and digitoxin are the most commonly monitored drugs by RIA because of their presence in low nanogram concentrations. Most radioimmunoassays utilized in therapeutic drug monitoring employ $^{125}$I labels and thus require gamma counters. Since RIA procedures are heterogeneous it is difficult to completely automate the assays.

RIA offers the advantage of sensitivity and low cost per test. Its major disadvantages include the inconvenience associated with radiolabels, such as short shelf-lives of the radiolabeled reagents, the licensing requirements, disposal, and record keeping.

### Enzyme Immunoassay

The enzyme multiple immunoassay technique (EMIT) and the enzyme-linked immunosorbent assay (ELISA) are the two predominant forms of enzyme immunoassay technique utilized in therapeutic drug monitoring.

The ELISA technique is a heterogenous assay similar to the RIA methods. The major distinction is the use of an enzyme as the label in ELISA instead of a radioisotope. The separated bound or free phase must be treated with a substrate for the labeling enzyme in the ELISA technique. As the enzyme converts the substrate to its product, a spectrophotometric change is monitored and converted to analyte concentration. ELISA assays for digoxin and theophylline, and various endogenous compounds are currently available.

In the EMIT method, pioneered as the first homogeneous immunoassay by the Syva Company (Palo Alto, CA), an analyte (A) and a known amount of a specially prepared conjugate, which is composed of the analyte covalently linked to an enzyme (usually glucose phosphate dehydrogenase [G6PD] or lysozyme) (A-E), compete for a limited number of binding sites on an antibody (Ab). The amount of enzyme-labeled analyte bound to the antibody is inversely proportional to the amount of unlabeled analyte:

$$\underset{\text{free}}{\text{A + Ab + A-E}} \leftrightarrow \underset{\text{bound}}{(\text{Ab}:\text{A}) + (\text{Ab}:\text{A-E})}$$

Since EMIT is a homogeneous assay, that is, the bound and free antibody are not separated during analysis, the amount of enzyme activity elicited by the bound and free forms of the conjugate must be substantially different, so that they may be easily distinguished from one another. When antibody binds to the analyte-enzyme conjugate, the antibody either sterically prevents access of substrate to the active site of the enzyme or causes a conformational change in the enzyme which alters its activity. Therefore, the activities of the bound forms of the conjugate are modulated and are easily distinguished from those of the free forms.

With competitive binding, the level of free A-E present at equilibrium is directly proportional to the level of analyte in the specimen. Since the bound and free forms of the conjugate have different degrees of enzyme activity, the assay is by definition homogeneous and there is no separation step there prior to adding substrate and determining the analyte concentration spectrophotometrically.

The basic instruments used in conjunction with EMIT assays are a pipettor and a spectrophotometer. The EMIT procedure is readily adaptable to other instruments including the DuPont automatic clinical analyzer (ACA), Abbott VP, and centrifugal analyzers including the Cobas-Bio and IL Multistat. The conversion of NAD to NADPH to the final reaction in the EMIT procedure can also be read fluorometrically. Thus the Advance fluorometer system, introduced by Syva, will perform routine EMIT assays. The EMIT assays are convenient to perform, rapid, cost-effective, and provide a broad range of assays which can be performed in a semiautomated or completely automated mode.

### Fluorescent Immunoassays

The substrate labeled fluorescent immunoassay (SLFIA) is a homogenous assay developed by the Ames Division of Miles Laboratories (Elkhart, IN). The analyte is covalently attached to a fluorogenic enzyme substrate, galactosylumbelliferone. The substrate-labeled drug (—F—D) is not fluorescent until it reacts with the enzyme, $\beta$-galactosidase, to produce a fluorescent product (—F—D). When the substrate-labeled analyte is bound to an analyte specific antibody, it is inactive as a substrate for the enzyme. The free label produces fluorescence in SLIFA while the antibody-bound label does not. In a competitive binding reaction, substrate-labeled analyte and analyte from the sample compete for a limited number of binding sites. When $\beta$-galactosidase is added, the fluorescence produced is proportional to the analyte concentration in the specimen.

Since the free and antibody-bound forms of the label possess different activities, SLIFA requires no separation steps and is homogeneous. SLIFA assays can be performed manually, in a semiautomated or fully automated mode (utilizing the Ames/Gilford OPTIMATE or the Abbott VP). These systems offer the same advantages as EMIT.

The fluorescence polarization immunoasay (FPIA) is a homogeneous assay developed by Abbott Diagnostics (North Chicago, IL). The analyte is covalently attached to a fluorophore derived from fluorescein. The fluorophore-labeled analyte conjugate, when excited by polarized light, produces a polarized fluorescence emission. The degree of polarization of a fluorescent solution is correlated to the fluorophore's rotational Brownian movement. Fluorescence polarization is sensitive to changes in the fluorophore's molecular size. The fluorophore-analyte is relatively small and has a very rapid rotational Brownian movement, which results in fluorescence that is substantially depolarized. When the fluorophore-analyte conjugate binds to the analyte-specific antibody, the complex has a much greater mass. Thus, the fluorophore-analyte bound to antibody has a decreased Brownian rotational motion which is manifested by an increased fluorescence polarization. In competitive binding assays the ratio of free and antibody-bound analyte conjugate is governed by the level of analyte in the specimen. In the FPIA competitive binding, as the specimen concentration of analyte increases, the amount of antibody-bound analyte decreases, resulting in a decreased level of fluorescence polarization compared to that observed in the absence of analyte.

The FPIA requires, of course, an instrument capable of determining the polarization of fluorescence. An automated instrument capable of performing therapeutic drug assays, the Abbott TDX®, which is capable of determining fluorescence polarization, is currently available. This system offers a high degree of automation and all of the advantages of the EMIT system.

### Nephelometric Inhibition Immunoassay

Small analytes can be covalently linked to large molecules such as proteins to produce a protein conjugate which possesses several analyte antigenic determinants. In the presence of an antianalyte antibody, crosslinking between the analyte determinants on the protein will occur. The development of these large complexes can be followed by determining changes in the light-scattering properties of the solution.

The analyte-protein conjugate may be used as a label in competitive binding assays. The analyte present in the specimen competes with the conjugate-label for antibody binding sites. As the analyte concentration increases, the amount of antibody available for crosslinking the conjugate-label decreases, and thus the light-scattering ability of the solution is decreased. There is a concentration-dependent inverse relationship between light scattering and analyte concentration. The application of nephelometric inhibition immunoassays to therapeutic drug monitoring has been developed by Beckman Instruments (Fullerton CA), utilizing their Immunochemistry System (ICS) with both semiautomated and automated instruments.

### Apoenzyme Reactive Immunoassay

Recently a major technological breakthrough in analytical technology was achieved by the Ames Company with the introduction of their Apoenzyme Reactive Immunoassay System (ARIS). ARIS is the first example of dry-phase immunology. The antibody and enzyme necessary for the immunoassay are impregnated on paper strips. The patient's serum is added directly to the strip, and the antibody-drug interaction takes place followed by a peroxidase reaction to produce a blue color. The color produced is proportional to the drug concentration. Quantitative analysis is achieved by measuring the reflectance of light from the strip in a reflectometer (Ames Seralyzer®).

At the present time, theophylline can be quantitatively determined with the ARIS with the same accuracy and precision as that achieved by the methods described above. The clear advantage of the system is its rapid, accurate quantitation. The instrument is portable and simple to operate. Thus drug concentrations can be easily measured at the patient's bedside.

Over the past five years our understanding of the interrelationships between drug dosage, drug concentrations in biological tissues, and the observed clinical response have become crystallized.

The concept of dry-phase immunochemistry represents a major step forward because it allows bedside and/or acute care monitoring.

We can anticipate that within the near future routine monitoring of cardioactive drugs will be able to be carried out in the intensive care unit, at the patient's bedside, and in the physician's office. On the basis of our current knowledge of applied clinical pharmacokinetics and the availability of accurate and specific technologies for monitoring drug concentrations, physicians everywhere should be utilizing therapeutic drug monitoring as a guide to individualizing patient therapy today.

[NOTE: The material contained in this review has been compiled from previous publications by the author as well as from other sources.]

## REFERENCES

1. AVERY, G. S., Ed. 1980. Drug Treatment: Principles and Practice of Clinical Pharmacology and Therapeutics, 2nd ed. ADIS. Sydney, Australia.
2. MELMON, K. L. & H. I. MORELLI, Ed. 1978. Clinical Pharmacology: Basic Principles in Therapeutics, 2nd ed. Macmillan. New York, NY.
3. GILMAN, A. G., L. S. GOODMAN & A. GILMAN. 1980. The Pharmacological Basis of Therapeutics, 6th ed. Macmillan. New York, NY.
4. PIPPENGER, C. E. 1979. Therapeutic drug monitoring: An overview. Ther. Drug Monit. 1: 3–9.
5. MUNGALL, D. R., Ed. 1983. Applied Clinical Pharmacokinetics. Raven Press. New York, NY.
6. DRAYER, D. E. 1981. Antidysrhythmics: Analytical techniques. In Therapeutic Drug Monitoring. A. Richens & V. Marks, Eds.: 393–403. Churchill Livingstone. New York, NY.
7. DRAYER, D. E. 1982. Methods for the analysis of antiarrhythmic drugs in serum. In Applied Therapeutic Drug Monitoring. I. Fundamentals. T. P. Moyer & R. L. Boeckx, Eds.: 167–172. American Association for Clinical Chemistry. Washington, DC.

# Monitoring of Antiarrhythmic Drug Levels: Values and Pitfalls

JOEL KUPERSMITH[a]

*Departments of Medicine and Pharmacology*
*Mount Sinai School of Medicine of the*
*City University of New York*
*New York, New York 10029*

The clinical use of drug level monitoring has been considered by some to be a *sine qua non* of scientific medicine. This technique brings to bear a unique type of expertise, that of the pharmacologist, in more precisely evaluating therapeusis. However, as with any new laboratory test or technique, problems arise in interpretation and use. This review will be concerned with the benefits and pitfalls in interpreting serum levels of antiarrhythmic drugs.

## VALUE OF SERUM LEVEL DETERMINATION

There are no controlled-perspective studies on the value of drug level determinations for antiarrhythmic agents; such studies are a difficult but not impossible task. One study on digoxin by the Boston Collaborative Drug Surveillance Program showed a lower incidence of toxicity at a hospital where serum levels of the drug were determined than at one where the test was not performed.[1] In a more recent study, assays of digoxin and phenytoin were performed several months apart. More levels were found in the therapeutic range in the second assay indicating that the attending physician had used the test to modify the digoxin dose.[2] However, even though more extensive and conclusive studies have not been done, it is clear that drug level monitoring has value in the management of patients.[3–5]

The value of drug monitoring mainly relates to the fact that all drugs have significant individual variations pharmacokinetically. Therefore, knowledge of a dose of a particular drug does not necessarily predict how much is actually being delivered to the individual patient.

Some of the important reasons for variations are as follows:

1. Variation of absorption may occur because of the concurrent administration of food, antacids, or complexing agents or there may be an intrinsic variation in bioavailability (a particular problem in the case of digoxin[6]).

2. Problems related to high hepatic extraction ratio and consequent extensive first-pass heptic metabolism may also exist.[7,8] Drugs with high hepatic extraction ratios have important variations in both bioavailability (increased by food, exercise, and other drugs) and elimination (influenced by cardiac output and interacting drugs). These effects are all unpredictable in degree. Antiarrhythmic drugs with a high hepatic extraction ratio include lidocaine, verapamil, and propranolol. Lorcainide has a special problem—it exhibits extensive first-pass metabolism, but

[a] Address for correspondence: Joel Kupersmith, M.D., Mount Sinai Medical Center, One Gustave L. Levy Place, New York, New York 10029.

also has saturable hepatic enzymes. This leads to a particular problem in estimating the amount of hepatic drug passage during the loading phase (when hepatic enzymes are in the process of becoming saturated) as well as during steady state.[9]

3. Hepatic elimination overall is subject to individual variation by virtue of drug interactions (which may induce or interfere with enzymes) or hepatic disease.

4. Renal elimination may vary among patients, in part because of renal failure[10] (where it may for many reasons vary unpredictably), but also in relation to the acidity of urine. Where pK of a drug is close to the range of urinary pH, drug elimination can vary in relation to urinary pH.[11] Mexiletine, for example, displays increased elimination in acidic urine (though the practical importance of this is questionable because of the large proportion of nonrenal clearance of mexiletine).

5. Michaelis–Menten (also called "zero order") kinetics may lead to great individual variation. Here the enzymes that metabolize the drug become saturated at a certain drug dose, above which elimination is much slower. Among antiarrhythmic drugs, phenytoin exhibits Michaelis–Menten kinetics. At doses above 300 mg/day of phenytoin there is a disproportionate and highly variable increase in serum level.[12] Lidocaine exhibits a related phenomenon: after 24 hours, lidocaine levels tend to increase even though the dose remains constant. It is postulated that accumulation of a metabolite of lidocaine that interferes with the enzymes responsible for eliminating the parent compound causes this effect.[13]

6. Variation in patient compliance is another (obvious) factor that influences the amount of drug received and serum level studies are especially valuable in detecting this. In the case of antiarrhythmic drugs, this may be a particular problem, since the drugs are used in many situations in which pain or other symptoms are infrequent or absent. Because there are few symptoms to constantly remind the patient of disease, compliance is lessened. In our own study of this problem, in a typical medical center clinic, we found an appallingly low rate of compliance in 100 consecutive patients given local anesthetic agents (quinidine, procainamide and disopyramide) for ventricular premature beats. Many patients were not taking the drug at all (zero level) or taking amounts much lower than expected, resulting in lower than expected serum levels.[58]

Although the aforementioned variables are to some extent predictable, what is important about them in relation to serum levels is that they lead to individual variability in amount of drug effectively delivered. Proper determination of drug levels is a way to compensate for these problems and as such offers an important step beyond dose in individually titrating the amount of drug offered to the patient.[5]

## SERUM LEVELS OF ANTIARRHYTHMIC DRUGS

Antiarrhythmic drugs have certain properties that make them particularly suitable for the determination of their levels in serum. On the basis of clinical studies, each drug (at least each local anesthetic drug) has a proposed therapeutic window. As we will see later, there are flaws in the concept of an overall therapeutic window for any drug, but at least an important step has been taken in an orderly manner for the study of these drugs. This has not been done for many other categories of agents.

Secondly, the relationship between drug and receptor is a reasonably simple one. The receptor is the $Na^+$, $K^+$, or $Ca^{2+}$ channel of the cell sarcolemmal membrane and this is in fairly close contact with the serum. Local anesthetic drugs reach the receptor by local diffusion (not active transport) and interchange rapidly. There is no evidence or reason to think that local anesthetic agents cause changes in the number of channels (that is, up- or down-regulation). Thus it may be expected that drug levels will have a reasonably close relationship to activity both in degree and in timing.

On the other hand, there are also reliable drug pharmacodynamic variables to follow in patients receiving antiarrhythmic drugs. Most agents have predictable, measurable effects on the electrocardiogram (for example, prolongation of QRS or Q-T interval in the case of most local anesthetics and decreased heart rate for beta blockers). These can be as easily monitored as drug levels to assess the effects and the possibility of toxicity. For assessment of arrhythmias, apart from electrophysiologic studies, which are performed acutely, one uses ambulatory monitoring and, less reliably, exercise tests.

While it is true that determinations of serum levels of antiarrhythmic drugs are most useful, it is also true that there are many pitfalls in interpreting these levels. The basic assumption one makes is that the relationship between drug level and drug effect is definite and very predictable. Unfortunately, many factors confound this relationship and thus limit the usefulness of the test, at least in its broadest application. Problems arise in many areas, including those associated with the relationship between serum level and dynamic effect, interaction with receptors, and so forth. Some of these problems occur with all drugs, while others are specific to antiarrhythmic agents.

## ACCURACY OF TEST

As with any laboratory test there are problems of measurement inaccuracy. Under highly controlled research laboratory conditions, blood is drawn and drug level measured very carefully. However, when the test moves from the research laboratory to widespread general use, greater inaccuracy is apt to occur. While the extent of the problem may not be great, there is at least some disturbing information in the literature. Measurement differences of a dummy sample of phenytoin, for example, were found to be great among various laboratories in the United States and abroad.[14]

One curious technical problem that has arisen in the case of lidocaine is a "rubber-stopper effect." A chemical (Tris-2-butoxyethyl phosphate) found in rubber stoppers of many Vacutainers displaces lidocaine from its plasma protein binding sites, causes more partition into red blood cells, and thus increases the free fraction.[15] This must be taken into account when drawing blood for serum laboratory levels.

## LOADING PHASE

Problems of interpretation related to kinetics during the loading phase are well known to clinical pharmacologists. During the loading phase, before peripheral tissues are saturated, drug levels are a particularly inaccurate representation of dynamics. Levels are changing very rapidly (from minute to minute) in both peripheral tissues and in blood. In addition, active metabolites are much less prominent, both at this time and in early steady state (that is, it takes longer for active metabolites to reach steady state).

Interpretive problems related to the loading phase may arise, for example, in electrophysiologic drug testing. Here, testing may be performed after single intravenous injections of drug, when the patient is not in the "steady state." Serum levels at this juncture are not comparable or applicable to those in chronic phases of drug administration. There is general awareness of this problem, however, and the important drug testing is made when a patient is on oral therapy in early steady state (although even at this time the lesser role of active metabolites should be considered).

## PROTEIN BINDING

All drugs are bound in varying degrees to serum proteins. In general, acidic drugs (negative radicals) are bound largely to albumin, while basic drugs (positive radicals, and including all local anesthetics, beta blockers, and calcium channel blockers) are bound in large proportion to alpha-1 acid glycoprotein lipoprotein.[16] The bound form of the drug is, of course, inactive and the free form, active. When there are changes in binding protein (let us say elevation), a predictable sequence of events occurs: increased binding protein, increased binding ratios, increased concentrations of bound drug, the same concentration of free drug, and ultimately higher serum levels—but, in fact, a falsely elevated serum level because the free (active) form is unchanged. When binding proteins diminish, the converse occurs.

Variations in drug-binding proteins occur in several clinical settings. Alpha-1 acid glycoprotein, which carries lidocaine and propranolol among other drugs, is an acute-phase reactant. It increases in concentration during acute illness, most notably acute myocardial infarction. Lidocaine is, of course, commonly administered during this condition. Over the first few days of myocardial infarction, alpha-1 acid glycoprotein level progressively rises. In patients receiving lidocaine, this increase causes a progressive "false" elevation of total lidocaine due to an increase in bound drug, while free drug remains the same.[17] This is a most important confounding factor in interpreting serum lidocaine levels during acute myocardial infarction. In fact, it may have caused errors in some of the important research studies on the drug before it was recognized.

A number of diseases such as hepatic disease, nephrosis, or malignancy cause a serum albumin decline. These diseases would cause a contrary effect—a falsely low serum level. In addition, uremia seems to cause an increase in percent of unbound drug, most notably in the case of phenytoin, and this change would also lead to a falsely low drug level.

Disopyramide presents a specific problem since its binding varies with the drug level. As the disopyramide level increases, the binding protein becomes saturated so that a progressively higher proportion of the drug becomes unbound.[18] The therapeutic range of disopyramide is approximately 2–7 mg/liter. Disopyramide protein saturation occurs at 3 to 6 mg/liter. When serum concentration increases from 1 to 6 mg/liter, protein binding increases from 17.4 to 40%. When drug level increases from 2–4 mg/liter (right in the middle of the therapeutic range), the free drug increases four-fold. Because these numbers vary from patient to patient, it is very difficult to estimate the free and active drug concentration on the basis of a report of total drug level. A similar though less marked phenomenon occurs with lidocaine. Binding of quinidine also seems to vary greatly among patients.

TABLE 1. Protein Binding of Antiarrhythmic Drugs[a]

| Drug | Percent Bound |
|------|---------------|
| Aprindine | 90 |
| Disopyramide | 40–90[b] |
| Diltiazem | 70 |
| Lidocaine | 25–50[b] |
| Lorcainide | 70–80 |
| Nifedipine | 90 |
| Phenytoin | 93 |
| Procainamide | 15–20 |
| Quinidine | 60–90 |
| Tocainide | 50 |
| Verapamil | 90 |

[a] From Kates.[57]
[b] Concentration-dependent binding.

Plasma protein displacement by concurrently administered drugs has been a much discussed phenomenon related to serum levels. However, these interactions appear to be far more complex (involving multiple binding sites, binding related to changes in pharmacokinetics, and so forth) and perhaps less important than first appreciated.[19] Without considering the complexities, such a drug interaction is thought to proceed as follows. In a patient in steady state on a highly protein-bound drug (A), addition of another highly protein-bound and therefore displacing drug (B) causes an immediate jump in the level of free drug (A), which then declines to the original baseline level in a few days. During this time there might be a transient enhancement of the effects of (A) on the body. A gradual decline in bound drug (A) also occurs so that in the new steady state there is a falsely low total serum level—low bound (A), and the same level of free (A). For many reasons (for example, multiple binding sites—eight in the case of albumin) this is an oversimplified view, and particularly in the case of antiarrhythmic drugs the importance of this type of drug interaction is unclear.[19,20]

Another interaction worthy of note is the fact that free fatty acids, where increased in acute myocardial infarction, tend to displace drugs from their binding sites.

TABLE 1 shows the percent protein binding of various antiarrhythmic drugs and thus gives an indication of the relative likelihood of erroneous interpretations due to alterations in binding. Of course, one may get around binding-related problems by assaying the amount of free as well as total drug. This is technically feasible but not yet in clinical use except in the case of phenytoin at some centers.[21] Such an assay would do much to improve the validity and usefulness of drug level determinations.

## PHARMACODYNAMIC FACTORS

The relationship between drug levels and drug effect can be influenced by a large number of humoral, ionic and other factors which influence pharmacodynamics. For example, serum $K^+$ strongly influences the action of digoxin and the local anesthetics. High serum $K^+$ potentiates the depressant effects of local anesthetics on the $Na^+$ channel and thus on cardiac conduction, and it may therefore potentiate toxic or therapeutic effects of these drugs. Low $K^+$ does the converse, although it may potentiate blocking effects on the $K^+$ channel. Low $K^+$ also predictably potentiates certain adverse effects of digoxin preparations. Magnesium, $Ca^{2+}$, pH, and hypoxia have important effects on all categories of antiarrhythmic drugs. Among hormonal effects, thyroid hormone obviously interferes with digitalis-induced slowing of the rate of atrial fibrillation and, insofar as it may potentiate ischemia, can interfere with any antiarrhythmic drug. Regarding drug interactions, dynamic (as distinguished from kinetic) interactions may also be important—$K^+$ depletion with diuretics, arrhythmogenic and chronotropic effects of beta agonists, and so on. The list of such dynamic interactions is endless and each may importantly confound the relationship between drug level and effect.

## ACTIVE METABOLITES

Many antiarrhythmic drugs have been active metabolites (see TABLE 2). Metabolites are often not routinely measured, but even when they are, many questions remain. For an active metabolite to play an important role in the pharmacology of a drug besides exhibiting (in this case) antiarrhythmic and electrophysiologic properties, it must have potency close to (or greater than) that of the parent compound; it must be present in concentrations at which it has activity, and it must have a half-life of some duration (many active metabolites are very polar and are eliminated rather quickly).

The clinical role of many of the active metabolites listed in TABLE 2 is unfortunately not yet clear. 3-OH-quinidine, for example, is present in relatively low concentrations in blood and therefore usually of relatively little significance.[22] Procainamide and its metabolite N-acetyl procainamide (NAPA) have been the most studied.

TABLE 2. Active Metabolites of Antiarrhythmic Drugs[a]

| Drug | Metabolite | Relative Potency | Relative Plasma Concentration[b] |
|------|-----------|------------------|----------------------------------|
| Aprindine | Desethylaprindine | 1[c] | 0.2 |
| Disopyramide | Mono-N-dealkylated disopyramide | <0.5[d] | — |
| Encainide | O-dimethyl encainide 3-methoxy-O-dimethyl encainide | — | 1–4 |
| Lidocaine | Monoethylglycinexylidide | 0.83[e] | 0.5–2 |
|  | Glycinexylidide | 0.1[e] | 0.1–1 |
| Lorcainide | Norlorcainide | <1[f] | 0.5–4 |
| Procainamide | N-acetylprocainamide | <1[g] | 0.5–2.5 |
| Quinidine | 3-hydroxyquinidine | 1[h] | 0.2–0.8 |
| Verapamil | Norverapamil | 0.25[i] | 1 |

  [a] From Kates.[57]
  [b] Chronic dosing.
  [c] Tested with ouabain-induced arrhythmias in dogs.
  [d] Tested with acute infarcted dog model.
  [e] Tested with ouabain-induced arrhythmias in guinea pig atrial model.
  [f] Tested in patients with premature ventricular contractions.
  [g] Electrophysiologic studies in dogs.
  [h] Tested with chloroform-induced ventricular fibrillation in mice.
  [i] Tested in conscious dogs.

Procainamide is eliminated by the kidney, and is also converted to a variable degree to a metabolite, NAPA. This metabolite is also primarily eliminated by the kidney (with a tiny amount metabolized back to procainamide).[23] NAPA has electrophysiologic and antiarrhythmic properties in concentrations at which it is present in blood.[24-26] It also has a longer half-life than the parent compound (6–7 versus 3.5 hr).[24,25]

Acetylation of procainamide to NAPA is variable and depends on a genetic trait. "Fast acetylators" convert a high proportion of procainamide to NAPA; "slow acetylators" a much lower proportion.[27] (This is a general enzymatic trait and influences the conversion of all drugs that are acetylated such as hydralazine and isoniazid). One consequence of the acetylation of procainamide concerns a particular toxic effect. Fast acetylators have a much lower incidence of procainamide-induced lupus erythematosus, since the parent compound, but not NAPA, is involved in this disorder.[28]

Since NAPA is generated in highly variable amounts and is active, assay of the procainamide level alone is an inadequate test. For this reason, assays of NAPA have become routine and various arithmetic ways to consider the relative effect of parent compound and metabolite have been advanced to enable evaluation of overall antiarrhythmic versus toxic effects. However, there are problems with this sort of evaluation. First, NAPA has different kinetics than procainamide (such as lower clearance and longer elimination half-life), so that the metabolite and parent compound are present in plasma in constantly varying amounts; an assay at any particular time may thus reflect only a momentary ratio of the two. Second, and more important, procainamide and NAPA are not equivalent compounds. While there is some dispute over whether the two compounds have a similar antiarrhythmic spectrum, there is no doubt that they have much different basic electrophysiologic properties. NAPA has a much lesser effect on action potential upstroke (considerably less depression of membrane responsiveness, rate of rise of the action potential and conduction velocity), much less or no effect on automaticity, and a much greater effect in prolonging action potential duration.[26] It is possible in many instances that NAPA does not contribute to the antiarrhythmic effects of procainamide, but only to its electrical toxicity, especially by virtue of its propensity to cause marked prolongation of action potential duration.[26] Overall, it is clear that no formula of adding the levels of parent compound and metabolite will suffice as an estimate of overall drug efficacy or likelihood of toxicity, and in my view the approach to this problem is still in doubt.

It should be noted that active metabolites tend to be in much higher concentrations and of much greater importance in renal failure (because they are generally generated in the liver and eliminated by the kidney).

Encainide also has active metabolites (O-dimethyl and 3 methoxy-O-dimethyl encainide) that appear to play a primary, although probably not exclusive, role in encainide's antiarrhythmic effects and toxicity.[29-31] These metabolites are present in high levels in blood.[29] Obviously, because encainide has two (and possibly more) active metabolites, in addition to its own activity,[29,30-32] encainide levels are most difficult to interpret.

## THERAPEUTIC WINDOW

Virtually every antiarrhythmic drug has a proposed therapeutic window (TABLE 3). Usually this is obtained in studies on control of ventricular premature beats, at times during acute myocardial infarction. Unfortunately, criteria for establishing the upper and lower limits of the therapeutic range are by no means standard. The method is usually as follows: In a study in which the drug is given for control of arrhythmias, the particular drug levels at which there is antiarrhythmic control and the levels at which there are toxic effects are listed. The numbers are then pooled to arrive at the "minimum effective" and "toxic" concentrations. Regarding the latter, at times there is an overlap between levels that are needed in some patients for control of arrhythmia and levels at which toxicity occurs in others (this is true for aprindine, for example). In other instances the upper therapeutic limit represents the level at which (acute) toxicity has occurred in any patient (for example, with procainamide). The results of such a study, which is usually performed in a modest number of patients, are then applied to large numbers of patients to whom the drug is ultimately administered.

Unfortunately, no standardized method is used to determine the therapeutic range and, in any case, it would be difficult to do. It would not be judicious, for example, to administer graded increments of drug to the point of toxicity in each of a large number of patients. For certain drugs there may in any event be a necessary overlap in toxicity and therapeusis at the upper level of the therapeutic

**TABLE 3.** Therapeutic Plasma Concentrations[a]

| Drug | Therapeutic Range ($\mu$g/ml) |
|---|---|
| Aprindine | 1–2 |
| Disopyramide | 3–6 |
| Lidocaine | 1.4–6 |
| Mexiletine | 0.75–2 |
| Phenytoin | 10–18 |
| Procainamide | 4–8 |
| Quinidine | 2–5 |
| Tocainide | 6–15 |

[a] From Kates.[57]

window. It should also be noted that in some instances therapeutic range has been promulgated in studies in which there has been little or no indication of how such dosages were determined.

There is also another important concern related to therapeutic window of antiarrhythmic drugs. The promulgated therapeutic window is generally made on the basis of studies of drug action against one specific type of arrhythmia. Unfortunately, the assumption that the therapeutic window is the same for every type of arrhythmia is not valid. The textbook-listed therapeutic windows of most antiarrhythmic drugs were determined by drug-induced reduction in the frequency of the ventricular premature beats,[33-35] although some were determined more broadly.[37] An entirely different drug level may be necessary to control ventricular tachycardia. For example, in the case of procainamide, some studies in the past showed that much higher levels of procainamide were required to control ventricular tachycardia[38] than had been needed for control of ventricular premature beats.[35] More recently, Myerburg found that the average drug level for reduction of VPCs was higher than that for control of ventricular tachycardia.[39] (Incidentally, an important corollary here is that there are problems with using reduction of ventricular premature beat frequency as an index of control of more severe arrhythmias.)

The therapeutic range of a drug may thus be different for each arrhythmia. The range may also vary for the same type of arrhythmia in a different situation. For example, a lower level of drug may be necessary to reduce the frequency of ventricular premature beats during acute myocardial infarction than in the chronic state.[35-39] In fact, variabilities may be such that the concept of an overall therapeutic range for an antiarrhythmic drug is an oversimplification and can be considered only an approximation.

One value of studies in which therapeutic ranges are determined seems to be that they indicate the levels at which an "acute" type of adverse effect is likely— for example, neurologic toxicity in the case of lidocaine, mexiletine, or tocainide and electrocardiographic toxicity in the case of quinidine-like drugs. On the other hand, certain more "chronically" occurring adverse effects (such as procainamide-induced lupus erythematosis), although dose-related, have not been precisely related to serum levels.

## RECEPTORS

Antiarrhythmic properties of a drug are based mainly on electrophysiologic actions within the heart. A number of considerations concerning the nature of drug interaction with its cardiac receptor are important in understanding clinical variability and alteration of the relationship between drug level and effect. The receptor for local anesthetic drugs is the cell sarcolemmal membrane on its inside surface. Movement to the receptor is by passive diffusion, but with one complexity. As has been shown in the case of lidocaine, the nonionic form of drug moves into the cell (nonionic moieties in general move through membranes better), but the ionic form is that which blocks the $Na^+$ channel.[40] It has also been shown (most clearly for tetrodotoxin, a local anesthetic neurologic and cardiac toxin)[41] that relatively few drug molecules are required to block the $Na^+$ channel. Many local anesthetic drugs also influence the $K^+$ channel, inhibition of which causes prolongation of action potential duration. The site of action of $Ca^{2+}$ channel blockers is also the sarcolemmal membrane, but details of binding of these drugs are less well established than for the local anesthetics. Verapamil appears to exert its effect on the inside of the membrane calcium channel, nifedipine (which does not have antiarrhythmic properties) on the outside.[42] Obviously, beta-adrenergic blocking agents have a different sort of receptor.

The nature of the receptor for membrane-active antiarrhythmic drugs has certain implications. First, this receptor appears to have a closer and more immediate relationship to the blood than to the cytoplasm of cardiac cells, where it is perhaps complexly bound. Therefore, tissue drug levels, even if they were obtainable, should have much less value than blood levels. The cytoplasm's only role may be that of a reservoir of drug after blood levels have declined.

Second, one might expect a very close temporal relationship between drug level and electrophysiologic effect. This is generally true (perhaps more so with antiarrhythmic agents than for other types of drugs), but with qualifications. In tissue bath studies on antiarrhythmic drugs, there is always a lag time (usually 15–30 minutes) between washout of drug and reversal of membrane effect. A long washout time suggests partly reversible enzyme inhibition. However, even with a strictly membrane-blocking effect, drug slowly released from cardiac cytoplasmic sites could play a role even after the blood levels have declined. Another variable is that the nature and timing of channel blockade may be different for each channel. For example, the procainamide or quinidine interaction with the $Na^+$ channel (responsible ultimately for prolongation of QRS duration) may have different kinetics than that for the $K^+$ channel (responsible ultimately for prolongation of Q-T interval).

Limited data are available on these points. One example: procainamide's effect in prolonging Q-T interval has been temporally compared with its effect on blood level. The curve of Q-T prolongation had characteristics of a compartment that was intermediate between the central and the peripheral—slower than the central, but faster than the peripheral. Decay of change in Q-T was slower than decay of procainamide level.[43]

Another point worthy of note is that central nervous system properties of several antiarrhythmic drugs, the local anesthetics, as well as beta-adrenergic blocking agents, are thought to play a role in their cardiac effects. Movement in and out of the central nervous system may have a totally different time course than in the cardiac sarcolemmal membrane, which would also serve to confound the temporal relationship between drug level and effect.

In general, slight temporal differences between drug level and effect would not have many practical consequences. Even large differences may not diminish the value of drug levels as long as they are taken into account.

## ISCHEMIA

A number of factors may influence the interaction of drug with its receptor site on the cell membrane; these include pH, local levels of $K^+$, and local blood flow. The presence of acute ischemia and infarction provide one setting in which many of these factors may play a role in altering the drug's blood level/effect relationship. We have been particularly interested in drug effects in ischemia since this circumstance may point out issues that are important in other situations.[44] FIGURE 1 shows previously published data on the electrophysiologic effects of lidocaine on the infarcted heart compared with levels of lidocaine in the blood and indicates that: (1) Lidocaine slows conduction in the ischemic but not in the normal zones. (2) The temporal relationship between blood level and effect on conduction is very close. (3) Lidocaine prolongs the effective refractory period (which was determined on the epicardial surface of the heart) in the infarcted zone only. (4) The temporal relationship between blood level and effect on refractory period is much different than that for conduction.

The following aspects could be important to a drug's distinctive effects in ischemia and infarction: (1) Local $K^+$ levels are increased, which may potentiate local anesthetic effects in the ischemic zone[45] (our postulate for lidocaine). (2) pH in the infarcted zone is acidic, which may also enhance lidocaine's effect on the ischemic zone. Lidocaine $pK_a$ is close to physiologic pH, and a move downward in pH causes a shift to the ionized form of lidocaine, which is the active form (once it crosses the sarcolemmal membrane, which may be defective in ischemia); experimental evidence[46] supports this. (3) Metabolites generated during ischemia may influence drug action. (4) Cell structural alteration may influence drug action. (5) Hemodynamic alteration may influence drug electrophysiologic effects. (6) Because of coronary artery obstruction, perfusion of drug into the infarcted zone may be diminished.

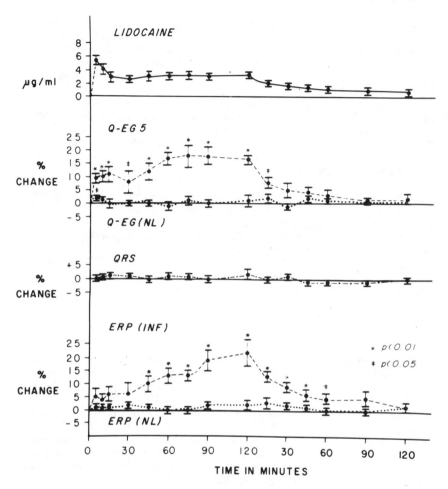

**FIGURE 1.** Effect of lidocaine on conduction intervals from the onset of the QRS to the major deflection of locally recorded electrogram (Q-EG) and effective refractory periods (ERP) in the infarcted and normal zones of the heart and on QRS duration. The *broken lines* indicate determinations made in the infarcted zone and the *dotted lines* indicate those made in the normal zone. The **top curve** shows the serum lidocaine concentration in $\mu$m/ml ± S.E. during and after the lidocaine infusion; the lidocaine infusion was discontinued at 120 minutes. The **second curve** (Q-EG-5) shows the changes in the Q-EG-5 interval determined by means of one of the pairs of electrodes on the intramyocardial electrode in the infarcted zone, during and after the lidocaine infusion; the **third curve** {Q-EG(NL)} shows the changes in the Q-EG interval in the normal zone; the **fourth curve** (QRS) shows the changes in QRS duration; the **fifth curve** [ERP(INF)] shows the changes in the effective refractory period in the infarcted zone; and the **bottom curve** [ERP(NL)] shows the changes in the effective refractory period in the normal zone. Each point on these curves represents the mean percent change ± S.E. from control values determined before lidocaine was administered. The asterisks indicate $p < 0.01$ and the double daggers indicate $p < 0.05$. See the text for further discussion. (From Kupersmith *et al.*[44] Reprinted by permission.)

Temporal differences between effects on conduction and refractory period in infarction are of interest. Our interpretation of the data in FIGURE 1 was as follows: Conduction was primarily influenced by effects on Purkinje fibers, which are close to the left ventricular cavity and therefore would receive lidocaine very quickly in spite of diminished coronary flow. Effective refractory period, on the other hand, was determined on the epicardial surface and it would take longer for tissue levels to build up there.[44] Subsequently, however, we found that lidocaine levels in the ischemic subepicardium were, in any case, almost that in normal tissue (vide infra).[47] Lidocaine's effect on effective refractory period may be influenced differently by the local factors in ischemia than is its effect on conduction.[48]

Regarding the diminished coronary blood flow, it might be expected to severely restrict the amount of drug reaching infarcted tissue; however, this does not appear to be the case. For lidocaine, we found a reduction of blood flow to 46% and 17% in the ischemic subepicardium and subendocardium, respectively. Local lidocaine levels were reduced to a lesser degree than blood flow, i.e., only to 91% and 58% of normal zone in these regions[49] (In the case of procainamide, when coronary blood flows were reduced to less than 10% of control values, local procainamide fell only to 42% of the control.[50])

The infarcted zone can be considered a separate and delayed compartment (with its own special temporal and biochemical reactivity). Drugs distributed to it might be quite variable both among different drugs and among different patients (depending on the number of vessels involved, the presence of collaterals, and so forth). Thus, the relationship of drug level to pharmacodynamic effect would also be variable.

As can be seen from the example of lidocaine, many factors could influence both the temporal and biochemical reactivity of the ischemic zone to drugs and thus the relationship between serum level and effect. Ischemia and infarction are, of course, important states in their own right and one of the important reasons for treatment of arrhythmias. However, some of these issues may also be important in other situations, particularly in states of chronic fibrosis, where drug delivery and other local factors may play a role.

## DRUG INTERACTIONS

One pharmacokinetic drug interaction which is of interest in relation to the drug level/effect relationship is digoxin–quinidine.[50,51] It has been found that when quinidine was administered to patients already receiving digoxin, the serum level of digoxin increased. Subsequent work has shown that the reasons for this include: release of digoxin from receptors,[52] diminished renal and nonrenal clearance of digoxin,[53] and diminished volume of distribution of digoxin.[53] While it would seem that any interaction that raises serum levels would foster toxicity, this is not necessarily the case. The elevated drug levels resulting from the interaction would foster toxicity, but the release from receptors would tend to reverse this. There have, in fact, been very few instances of documented digoxin toxicity attributable to the digoxin–quinidine interaction. It is even possible (although admittedly less likely) that in an occasional instance the interaction would result in less functional digoxin effect because of the release from receptors of the drug (at the very least it probably increases the level of serum digoxin required for a given effect).

## DRUGS AND THE ELDERLY

Pharmacology of drugs in the elderly has recently been the subject of greater and well-deserved attention. The elderly utilize drugs in different ways. There are kinetic differences: for example, quinidine has diminished hepatic clearance in the elderly. Other biologic changes that occur in elderly persons may alter the drug level/effect relationship. These include altered receptor number, affinity (for beta-adrenergic blocking agents, for example), and cellular responsiveness. These changes have been previously delineated for certain drugs, but not for the local anesthetics. Clearly, certain types of altered responsiveness displayed by the elderly to antiarrhythmic drugs are due to one or more of these factors: for example, central nervous system toxicity of lidocaine and other antiarrhythmic agents is greater in relation to plasma concentration in the elderly.[54] Thus, although it is important to determine drug levels in the elderly because of altered pharmacokinetics, it must also be recognized that the meaning of the test may be different in this group of patients.

## WHEN TO USE SERUM LEVEL DETERMINATIONS

In the clinical use of serum level determinations the first point to remember is that therapeutic ranges are not exact, but rather are only rough guidelines (for reasons indicated earlier). In addition, antiarrhythmic drugs generally have target-organ ("effect") and toxicity variables that are accessible to determination. For example, local anesthetic drugs affect the QRS and Q-T interval and beta blockers affect the pulse; neurologic toxicity is relatively easily assessed for mexiletine and tocainide, and so on. Antiarrhythmic effects are determined initially by electrophysiologic studies or repeated ambulatory monitoring studies (or, to a lesser extent, exercise tests, since the results of these are not reproducible except in children).[55]

In view of these aspects and of those enumerated previously, it would appear that best use of blood level studies of antiarrhythmic drugs is as follows: Initially determine the level of drug that is therapeutic for each individual patient either by electrophysiologic studies or by 24–72-hour monitoring. Then aim for this level in chronic therapy (we should remember, of course, some of the potential problems that may intermittently confound the blood level/effect relationship, such as changes in serum $K^+$). In this way, one "individualizes" therapeutic blood levels, i.e., one determines the therapeutic blood level in each and every case and works from there. This is a much more useful way to approach the problem than to aim for a literature-established therapeutic range that may or may not apply for that particular patient. Blood level determinations can be used to assess compliance, changes in kinetics due to drug interactions, abnormalities that may develop in organs of metabolism or elimination, and so forth. Since blood level determinations are not expensive, this is a cost-effective approach.

Arrhythmia still has to be assessed intermittently by ambulatory monitoring and evidence of toxicity must be checked in part by routine electrocardiography (for QRS duration and Q-T interval) and by other methods as well. However, drug level monitoring is a cost-effective test which can be done frequently (at best, Holter monitoring is not cost-effective and there are many problems in evaluating Holter recordings as well).

Even in certain instances where end-organ effect is obvious, such as the use of digoxin to control the ventricular rate in atrial fibrillation, drug level determinations may not seem useful, but they still have important purposes. For example, if a patient on a maintenance dose of digoxin develops an unexpected increase in ventricular response rate, determining the level of drug in the blood and comparing it with previous levels at which rate control was good will help to show whether the rate increase is due to a lack of compliance or change in bioavailability (lower blood level) versus a change in dynamic factors (similar blood level). Thus, the test can save both time and money.

During the loading phase, drug level information is less useful, except in one instance—when a less-than-expected effect occurs with a given dose of drug. Again, however, one must remember the caveats noted earlier.

When drugs are used for prophylaxis (of sudden death, for example) without a clear arrhythmia endpoint, there is a problem in selecting dosage. No therapeutic range for prevention of sudden death has been established nor is it at all clear whether local anesthetic drugs do in fact prevent sudden death. Diminution in the number of ventricular premature beats on ambulatory monitoring has been used as an endpoint in this situation. While the value of such monitoring in this situation is unclear, it seems the best of the alternatives for the present. One study has suggested that maintenance of previously established "therapeutic" levels of antiarrhythmic drugs, regardless of effect on ventricular premature beats, may prevent sudden death, but these data were highly preliminary and thus far unconfirmed.[56]

## REFERENCES

1. DUHME, D. W., D. J. GREENBLATT & J. KOCH-WESER. 1974. Reduction of digoxin toxicity associated with measurement of serum levels. Ann. Int. Med. 80: 516–519.
2. BERGMAN, U., A. RANE, F. SJÖQVIST & B. E. WILHOLM. 1981. Digoxin and phenytoin analyses as part of consultation in clinical pharmacology: A study on the use of drugs. Therapeutic Drug Monitoring 3: 259–269.
3. LATINI, R., M. BONATI & G. TOGNONI. 1980. Clinical role of blood levels. Therapeutic Drug Monitoring 2: 3–9.
4. KOCH-WESER, J. 1972. Serum drug concentrations as therapeutic guides. N. Engl. J. Med. 287: 227–231.
5. KOCH-WESER, J. 1981. Serum drug concentrations in clinical perspective. Therapeutic Drug Monitoring 3: 3–16.
6. LINDENBAUM, J., M. H. MELLOW, M. O. BLACKSTONE & V. P. BUTLER, JR. 1971. Variation in biologic availability of digoxin from four preparations. N. Engl. J. Med. 285: 1344–1347.
7. WILLIAMS, R. L. & R. D. MAMELOK. 1980. Hepatic disease and drug pharmacokinetics. Clin. Pharmacokinetics 5: 528–547.
8. GIBALDI, M., R. N. BOYES & S. FELDMAN. 1971. Influence of first-pass effect on availability of drugs on oral administration. J. Pharm. Sci. 60: 1338–1340.
9. JUST, H. & T. MAINERTZ. 1979. Lorcainide. I. Saturable presystemic elimination. Clin. Pharmacol. Ther. 26: 187–197.
10. REIDENBERG, M. M. 1977. The biotransformation of drugs in renal failure. Am. J. Med. 62: 482–485.
11. PRESCOTT, L. F., A. POTTAGE & J. A. CLEMENTS. 1977. Absorption, distribution and elimination of mexiletine. Postgrad. Med. J. 53 (Suppl. 1): 50–60.
12. HOUGHTON, G. W. & A. RICHENS. 1974. Rate of elimination of tracer doses of phenytoin at different steady-state serum phenytoin concentration in epileptic patients. Br. J. Clin. Pharmacol. 1: 155–161.

13. LE LORIER, V., D. GRENON, Y. LATORER, G. CAILLE, G. DUMONT, A. BROSSEAU & A. SOLIGNAC. 1977. Pharmokinetics of lidocaine after prolonged intravenous infusion in uncomplicated myocardial infarction. Ann. Int. Med. **87:** 700–710.

14. PIPPENGER, C. E., J. K. PERRY, B. G. WHITE, D. D. DALY & R. BUDDINGTON. 1976. Interlaboratory variability in determination of plasma antiepileptic drug concentrations. Arch. Neurol. **33:** 351–355.

15. STARGEL, W. W., C. R. ROE, P. A. ROUTLEDGE & D. G. SHAND. 1979. Importance of blood collection tubes in plasma lidocaine determination. Clin. Chem. **25:** 617–619.

16. PIAFSKY, K. M. 1980. Disease-induced changes in the plasma binding of basic drugs. Clin. Pharmacokinetics **5:** 246–262.

17. ROUTLEDGE, P. A., W. W. STARGEL, G. S. WAGNER & D. G. SHAND. 1980. Increased alpha-1 acid glycoprotein and lidocaine disposition in myocardial infarction. Ann. Int. Med. **93:** 70–74.

18. MEFFIN, P. J., E. W. ROBERT, R. A. WINKLE, S. HARAPAT, F. A. PETERS & D. C. HARRISON. 1979. Role of concentration-dependent plasma protein binding in disopyramide disposition. J. Pharmacokinetics Biopharm. **7:** 29–39.

19. SELLERS, E. M. 1979. Plasma protein displacement interactions are rarely of clinical significance. Pharmacology **18:** 225–227.

20. ROWLAND, M. 1980. Plasma protein binding and therapeutic drug monitoring. Therapeutic Drug Monitoring **2:** 29–37.

21. BOOKER, H. E. & B. DARCEY. 1973. Serum concentrations of free diphenylhydantoin and their relationship to clinical intoxication. Epilepsia **14:** 177–184.

22. DRAYER, D. E., D. T. LOWENTHAL, K. M. RECTIVO, A. SCHWARTZ, C. E. COOK & M. M. REIDENBERG. 1978. Steady state serum levels of quinidine and active metabolites in cardiac patients with varying degrees of renal function. Clin. Pharmacol. Ther. **24:** 31–39.

23. STEC, G. P., T. I. RUO, J. P. THENOT, A. J. ATKINSON, JR., Y. MORITA & J. J. L. LERTORA. 1980. Kinetics of N-acetylprocainamide deacetylation. Clin. Pharmacol. Ther. **28:** 659–666.

24. RODEN, D. M., D. B. REELE, S. B. HIGGINS, G. R. WILKINSON, R. F. SMITH, J. A. OATES & R. L. WOOSLEY. 1980. Antiarrhythmic efficacy, pharmacokinetics and safety of N-acetylprocainamide in human subjects: Comparison with procainamide. Am. J. Cardiol. **46:** 463–468.

25. WOONG-KU, L., J. M. STRONG, R. F. KEHOE, J. S. DUTHCER & A. J. ATKINSON, JR. 1975. Antiarrhythmic efficacy of N-acetylprocainamide in patients with premature ventricular contractions. Clin. Pharmacol. Ther. **19:** 508–514.

26. DANGMAN, K. H. & B. F. HOFFMAN. 1981. In vivo and in vitro antiarrhythmic and arrhythmogenic effects of N-acetylprocainamide. J. Pharmacol. Exp. Ther. **217:** 851–861.

27. REIDENBERG, M. M., P. E. DRAYER, M. LEVY & H. WARNER. 1975. Polymorphic acetylation of procainamide in man. Clin. Pharmacol. Ther. **17:** 722–730.

28. WOOSLEY, R. L., D. E. DRAYER, M. M. REIDENBERG, A. S. NIER, K. CARR & J. A. OATES. 1978. Effect of acetylator phenotype on the rate at which procainamide induces antinuclear antibodies and the lupus syndrome. N. Engl. J. Med. **298:** 1157–1159.

29. RODEN, D. M., S. B. REELE, S. B. HIGGINS, R. F. MAYOL, R. E. GAMMANS, J. A. OATES & R. L. WOOSLEY. 1980. Total suppression of ventricular arrhythmias by encainide: Pharmacokinetic and electrocardiographic characteristics. N. Engl. J. Med. **302:** 877–882.

30. HARRISON, D. C., R. WINKLE, M. SAMI, & J. MASON. 1980. Encainide: A new and potent antiarrhythmic agent. Am. Heart J. **100:** 1046–1054.

31. RO, J., J. GILLON & J. KUPERSMITH. 1981. Electrophysiologic effects of encainide following coronary artery occlusion in dogs. J. Cardiovasc. Pharmacol. **3:** 532–540.

32. CARMELIET, E. 1979. Electrophysiological effects of encainide on isolated cardiac muscle and Purkinje fibers and on the Langendorff-perfused guinea-pig heart. Eur. J. Pharmacol. **61:** 247–262.

33. CAMPBELL, N. S. P., J. G. KELLY, A. A. J. ADGET & R. G. SHANKS. 1978. The clinical pharmacology of mexiletine. Br. J. Clin. Pharmacol. **6:** 103–108.

34. HARRISON, D. C. & E. L. ALDERMAN. 1972. The pharmacology and clinical use of lidocaine as an antiarrhythmic drug. Mod. Treat. **9:** 139–175.
35. KOCH-WESER, J. & S. W. KLEIN. 1971. Procainamide dosage schedules, plasma concentrations and clinical effects. JAMA **215:** 1454–1460.
36. WINKLE, R. A., P. J. MEFFIN & D. C. HARRISON. 1978. Long-term tocainide therapy for ventricular arrhythmias. Circulation **57:** 1008–1016.
37. BIGGER, J. T., D. H. SCHMIDT & H. KUTT. 1968. Relationship between the plasma level of diphenylhydantoin sodium and its cardiac antiarrhythmic effects. Circulation **38:** 363–374.
38. GREENSPAN, A. M., L. N. HOROWITZ, S. R. SPIELMAN & M. E. JOSEPHSON. 1980. Large-dose procainamide therapy for ventricular tachyarrhythmia. Am. J. Cardiol. **46:** 453–492.
39. MYERBURG, R. J., K. M. KESSLER, I. KIEM, K. C. PEFKAROS, C. A. CONDE, D. COOPER & A. CASTELLANOS. 1981. Relationship between plasma levels of procainamide, suppression of premature ventricular complexes and prevention of recurrent ventricular tachycardia. Circulation **64:** 280–290.
40. NARAHASHI, T., D. T. FRAZIER & M. YAMADA. 1970. The site of action and active form of local anesthetics. I. Theory and pH experiments with tertiary compounds. J. Pharmacol. Exp. Ther. **171:** 32–44.
41. ALMERS, W. 1978. Gating currents and charge movements in excitable membranes. Rev. Physiol. Biochem. Pharmacol. **82:** 96–100.
42. HENRY, P. D. 1980. Comparative pharmacology of calcium antagonists, nifedipine, verapamil and diltiazem. Am. J. Cardiol. **46:** 1047–1058.
43. GALEAZZI, R. L., L. Z. BENET & L. B. SHEINER. 1976. Relationship between the pharmokinetics and pharmacodynamics of procainamide. Clin. Pharmacol. Ther. **20:** 278–289.
44. KUPERSMITH, J., E. M. ANTMAN & B. F. HOFFMAN. 1975. In vivo electrophysiologic effects of lidocaine in canine acute myocardial infarction. Circ. Res. **36:** 84–91.
45. SARTO, S., C. CHEN, J. BUCHANAN, JR., L. S. GETTES & M. N. LYNCH. 1978. Steady-state and time-dependent slowing of conduction in canine hearts: Effects of potassium and lidocaine. Circ. Res. **42:** 246–256.
46. GRANT, A. O., L. J. STRAUSS, A. G. WALLACE & H. C. STRAUSS. 1980. The influence of pH on the electrophysiological effects of lidocaine in guinea pig ventricular myocardium. Circ. Res. **47:** 542–550.
47. PATTERSON, R. E., W. S. WEINTRAUB, D. A. HALGASH, J. MIAO, J. R. ROGERS & J. KUPERSMITH. 1982. Spatial distribution of [14C]-lidocaine and blood flow in transmural and lateral border zones of ischemic canine myocardium. Am. J. Cardiol. **50:** 63–73.
48. KUPERSMITH, J. 1979. Electrophysiologic and antiarrhythmic effects of lidocaine in canine acute myocardial ischemia. Am. Heart J. **97:** 320–327.
49. WENGER, T. L., C. E. MASTERTON, M. B. ABOU-DONIA, K. L. LEE, R. J. BACHE & H. C. STRAUSS. 1978. Relationship between regional myocardial procainamide concentration and regional myocardial blood flow during ischemia in the dog. Circ. Res. **42:** 846–851.
50. LEAHEY, E. B., JR., J. A. REIFFEL, R. E. DRUSIN, R. M. HUSSENBUTEL, W. P. LOVEJOY & J. T. BIGGER, JR. 1978. Interaction between quinidine and digoxin. JAMA **240:** 533–534.
51. DOHERTY, J. E., K. D. STRAUB, M. L. MURPHEY, N. DE SOYZO, J. K. BISSETT & J. J. KANE. 1980. Digoxin-quinidine interaction. Am. J. Cardiol. **45:** 1196–1200.
52. BALL, W. J., JR., D. TSE-ENG, E. T. WALLICK, J. P. BILEZIKIAN, A. SCHWARTZ & V. P. BUTLER, JR. 1981. Effect of quinidine on the digoxin receptor in vitro. J. Clin. Invest. **68:** 1065–1074.
53. SCHENCK-GUSTAFSSON, D. & R. DOHLQUIST. 1981. Pharmacokinetics of digoxin in patients subjected to the quinidine-digoxin interaction. Br. J. Clin. Pharmacol. **11:** 181–186.
54. MOGENSEN, L. 1970. Ventricular tachyarrhythmias: Lidocaine prophylaxis in acute myocardial infarction. Acta Med. Scand. (Suppl. 513): 1–80.
55. ROZANSKI, J. J., I. DIMICH, L. STEINFELD & J. KUPERSMITH. 1979. Maximal exercise

testing in the evaluation of arrhythmias in children: Results and reproducibility. Am. J. Cardiol. **43:** 951–957.

56. MYERBURG, R. J., C. CONDE, D. S. SHEPS, R. A. APPEL, I. KIEM, R. J. SUNG & A. CASTELLANOS. 1979. Antiarrhythmic drug therapy in survivors of prehospital cardiac arrest: Comparison of effects on chronic ventricular arrhythmias and recurrent cardiac arrest. Circulation **59:** 855–863.

57. KATES, R. E. 1980. Therapeutic monitoring of antiarrhythmic drugs. Therapeutic Drug Monitoring **2:** 119–126.

58. SQUIRE, A., M. GOLDMAN, J. KUPERSMITH, J. MORGAN, V. FUSTER & P. SCHWEITZER. Chronic antiarrhythmic therapy: A problem of low serum drug levels and patient non-compliance. Am. J. Med. In press.

# Invasive Electrophysiologic Testing: A Critical Appraisal

MELVIN M. SCHEINMAN,[a] FRED MORADY, AND
EDWARD N. SHEN

*Department of Medicine and
Cardiovascular Research Institute
University of California, San Francisco
San Francisco, California 94143*

Over the past decade, the use of intracardiac recording and pacing techniques has allowed for a much deeper understanding of both the mechanisms of cardiac arrhythmias and the action of antiarrhythmic drugs. These techniques are currently being widely applied in the clinical evaluation of patients with cardiac arrhythmias, conduction disturbances, syncope, and sudden death. The purpose of this essay is to place electrophysiologic testing in reasonable perspective. Obviously, in this young, developing arena much remains to be learned and much will undoubtedly change with the test of time.

## DISORDERS OF SINOATRIAL FUNCTION

Sinoatrial function is evaluated in the laboratory by means of both atrial overdrive pacing as well as decremental atrial stimulation during spontaneous sinus rhythm. These pacing modalities allow for measurement of the sinus node recovery time[1] (post-pacing pause) or sinoatrial conduction time.[2,3] While abnormalities in the sinus node recovery time or sinoatrial conduction time are specific indicators of the sick sinus syndrome, these tests are insensitive and therefore generally not helpful in clinical decision-making (such as in determining the need for permanent pacemaker insertion).[4] A new technique to evaluate sinus node function is catheter electrode detection of the sinus node electrogram for direct measurement of the sinoatrial conduction time.[5] While this technique allows for greater understanding of sinoatrial disorders (post-pacing pauses)[6] and the site of drug effects, it has not yet been demonstrated to have any clinical utility. In practical terms, the decision to implant a permanent pacemaker in patients with symptomatic sinus node disorders is based on clinical grounds, often after the use of multiple continuous electrocardiographic recordings. When continuous monitoring cannot demonstrate whether a patient's symptoms are due to sinus node dysfunction, atrial overdrive pacing may tilt the clinician towards permanent pacemaker insertion if a markedly prolonged post-pacing pause is found, especially if the patient experiences typical symptoms during the pause.

[a] Address for correspondence: Melvin M. Scheinman, M.D., Room 573, Moffitt Hospital, University of California, San Francisco, San Francisco, California 94143.

155

## ATRIOVENTRICULAR CONDUCTION DISTURBANCES

Perhaps the most useful application of intracardiac recordings is the precise localization of atrioventricular (AV) conduction disturbances.[7] Currently available techniques allow for the localization of these conduction disturbances within the atria, at the level of the AV node, within the His bundle, or between the His bundle and the bundle branches. From the clinical standpoint, the most important differentiation is whether a supraventricular impulse is blocked at the node or below the node. While the former situation is usually benign, the latter often requires permanent cardiac pacing to avert Stokes-Adams attacks.

Block in the AV node is diagnosed when the atrial impulse fails to elicit a His bundle response. Conversely, infranodal block is diagnosed when block occurs distal to the recorded His bundle potential. Two possible pitfalls must be kept in mind. Firstly, one must be certain that the recorded potential originates in the His bundle and not in the atrium or from the right bundle branch. Late atrial depolarizations can usually be diagnosed on the basis of response to atrial overdrive pacing, which should result in minimal or no delay of the atrial potentials, particularly if several areas of the atria are paced. In contrast, there is no universally agreed upon method for differentiating the His bundle from the right bundle branch potentials. The available criteria with respect to morphology, amplitude of the low atrial electrogram, and direct His bundle pacing are all subject to criticism.[8]

A second pitfall relates to catheter position when recording the His bundle potential. If the catheter is positioned such that the distal His bundle potential is registered, an atrial impulse that blocks in the proximal His bundle will not result in a His bundle depolarization and may be misinterpreted as blocking in the AV node. Similarly, an atrial impulse conducted with sufficient delay in the proximal His bundle may not result in a deflection, even if the catheter is properly positioned. These limitations must be kept in mind when using His bundle recordings to localize the site of AV block.[9]

## SUPRAVENTRICULAR TACHYCARDIA

Invasive electrophysiologic techniques have been applied fruitfully to patients with supraventricular tachycardia (SVT) with respect to assessment of drug therapy,[10] antitachycardia pacing,[11] and cardiac electrosurgery.[12] For patients with recurrent SVT who are resistant to or intolerant of empiric drug therapy or those in whom SVT is associated with serious symptoms, invasive electrophysiologic testing has been suggested in order to rapidly obtain an effective drug regimen. The basic technique involves use of programmed stimulation for tachycardia induction and serial testing with drugs until a regimen is established that prevents tachycardia induction. In this technique, an artificial premature stimulus is applied; therefore, a drug that may actually be effective by eliminating premature beats may incorrectly be judged ineffective by this technique. Furthermore, the importance of changes in autonomic tone cannot be minimized, in terms of both tachycardia induction in the laboratory as well as effects on chronic oral efficacy. The clinical electrophysiologist frequently finds that sustained tachycardia cannot be induced (even in patients with frequent episodes of spontaneous tachycardia) unless atropine or isoproterenol is administered. Moreover, while intravenous verapamil has been shown to be effective in terminating SVT in well over 90% of patients,[13] results with chronic oral verapamil therapy are less spectacular.[14,15] This is probably due to changes in spontaneous sympathetic tone which are not present in the laboratory and which serve to override the direct effects of this drug. Assessment of drug efficacy on the basis of acute intravenous dosing at one point in time is fraught with the possibility of erroneous conclusions. More promising is the technique of repeated testing after oral drug titration in which the arrhythmia is noninducible at trough blood drug levels.[16,17]

Similar problems relate to use of these techniques with regard to finding an optimal "antitachycardia pacing prescription." In the majority of patients with paroxysmal supraventricular tachycardia (PSVT) a reentrant mechanism is operative. The basic objective of antitachycardia pacing is the insertion of a critically timed impulse which blocks antidromic conduction in the reentrant circuit while also producing orthodromic block owing to refractoriness of a portion of this circuit. The same principle applies whether one uses burst overdrive, underdrive, or so-called scanning pacemakers. The tachycardia termination zone may be quite different under laboratory conditions as compared with the usual stresses of daily life. This factor demands use of protocols in which the proposed antitachycardia system is tested during various manipulations of autonomic tone (that is, changes in body posture, exercise, and so forth).

Careful invasive studies are required prior to cardiac electrosurgical procedures (such as, His bundle or accessory pathway ablation). These studies must be carefully designed to prove not only the existence of accessory pathways, but also their involvement in the tachycardia circuit. For example, patients with AV nodal reentrant tachycardia may have an accessory pathway which is not a necessary link in the tachycardia circuit (bystander pathway).[18] Surgical ablation of this pathway would be inappropriate. A more serious challenge is the patient with dual accessory pathways in whom one pathway may be masked by exclusive utilization of the other pathway during tachycardia.[19] This situation should always be kept in mind during operative interventions in these patients.

## VENTRICULAR TACHYCARDIA

Serial electropharmacologic testing is used for the management of patients with ventricular tachycardia.[20] This approach involves tachycardia induction by means of programmed ventricular stimulation and serial testing of antiarrhythmic drugs until a regimen is found that prevents tachycardia induction. This technique has proven to be especially useful in patients with malignant ventricular arrhythmias. Nevertheless, many problems still exist in the application of this technique to clinical practice.

One problem is the lack of standard stimulation protocol. This problem is of more than academic interest since the sensitivity and specificity of ventricular tachycardia induction varies greatly with the aggressiveness of the stimulation protocol used.[21,22] For example, use of double ventricular extrastimuli results in a sensitivity of approximately 85% with a high degree of specificity. The use of triple ventricular extrastimuli results in a significantly higher sensitivity (that is, 95% for patients with coronary artery disease), but a much lower specificity. In addition to variations in the number of stimuli, the role of other variables, such as current strength of the stimuli, the number of ventricular sites, and the number of basic drive rates, has not been completely assessed. At this time, every laboratory must rigorously establish the sensitivity and specificity of its own stimulation protocol, and the clinician referring patients for these studies must be aware of the specific protocol used in order to draw meaningful clinical conclusions from the derived data.

Another problem relates to different endpoints used by laboratories in the course of such testing. There is general agreement, for example, that the suppression of inducible sustained ventricular tachycardia is a beneficial response. Somewhat less clear are responses in which sustained ventricular tachycardia becomes nonsustained or when inducible ventricular tachycardia becomes more difficult to provoke after drug treatment. Our own experience has shown that patients left with nonsustained ventricular tachycardia are still at risk for recurrent ventricular tachycardia.[23] Moreover, in studies in which ventricular tachycardia is repeatedly provoked (that is, when antitachycardia pacing is being evaluated), one often notes substantial variation in the number of extrastimuli needed for ventricular tachycardia induction; this casts doubt on the contention that making the arrhythmia more difficult to provoke is a valid criterion for a beneficial response to a drug trial. In addition, in the course of induction studies, one may at times induce ventricular arrhythmias that were never apparent spontaneously. In patients with documented ventricular tachycardia, these nonclinical arrhythmias can be clearly identified as such. However in patients whose clinical arrhythmia is undocumented (as, for example, in patients with unexplained syncope), it may be unclear whether induced ventricular tachycardia is clinically significant or a laboratory artifact. For example, in our experience with a group of 57 patients with recurrent syncope of unknown cause, we found that using a stimulation protocol consisting of up to triple extrastimuli from both right and left ventricles produced a varied response.[24] Those in whom sustained unimorphic ventricular tachycardia could be induced (nine patients) were treated on the basis of serial testing and none had a recurrence of syncope. On the other hand, the incidence of relief of syncope for those with nonsustained ventricular tachycardia (usually polymorphic ventricular tachycardia) was similar to that of patients with negative electrophysiologic studies who were left untreated. Thus with this protocol the induction of nonsustained polymorphic ventricular tachycardia appears to be a relatively nonspecific response, and great caution must be used before embarking on specific antiarrhythmic therapy for these patients. There is no question that symptoms of syncope or dizziness may be due to nonsustained rapid ventricular tachycardia; the ability of ventricular tachycardia induction studies to discern these patients is still unknown.

Serial invasive electrophysiologic testing for patients with ventricular tachycardia involves significant patient discomfort as well as risk of morbidity due to the catheterization. Lown and associates[32] have suggested the use of serial noninvasive testing in order to define a treatment regimen that prevents recurrence of ventricular arrhythmias. This regimen involves continuous electrocardiographic recordings before and after exercise stress testing in order to assess the effects of drugs on premature ventricular complex frequency and complexity. The patient is discharged with at least two drugs that prove effective in suppressing ventricular ectopic activity. This regimen has been shown by this group to be very effective for arrhythmia control. The drawbacks in using this technique involve: (1) the length of time required to devise an effective regimen (2 to 3 weeks); (2) the inability to use this approach in patients with recurrent ventricular tachycardia or ventricular fibrillation who show few or no ectopic beats (20%), and (3) the finding in some patients of a dissociation between premature ventricular complex suppression and tachycardia suppression. Since no direct comparison has been made between invasive versus noninvasive testing, no recommendations with regard to preference for either approach are possible.

Another problem in the assessment of a beneficial drug response relates to the number of ventricular sites tested. As originally described, ventricular tachycardia induced from a right ventricular site that was no longer inducible after drug testing was judged to be a beneficial response.[20] We and others have shown that ventricular tachycardia that is noninducible from the right ventricle after drug therapy may still be inducible when testing is applied to the left ventricle.[23,25] Moreover, those patients in whom tachycardia cannot be induced by both right and left ventricular stimulation after drug therapy appear to have a better chronic therapeutic response compared with those in whom the tachycardia cannot be induced after right ventricular stimulation alone. Conceivably, drugs may affect either conduction or refractoriness of intervening myocardial tissue so that stimuli induced in the right ventricle are no longer able to penetrate and initiate a reentrant circuit in the left ventricle.

The limitations discussed earlier in relationship to SVT induction studies are equally valid for ventricular tachycardia induction studies; namely, a drug deemed ineffective may prove effective by abolishing the extrasystoles that trigger the arrhythmia. Differences in autonomic tone between the laboratory and "real life" may confound the interpretation of results. In addition, it is unreasonable to expect that the electrophysiologic milieu operative at one point in time will remain immutable forever. For example, in patients with coronary artery disease, progression of the disease is very common. These factors may explain in part the differences obtained between the earlier electropharmacologic studies which showed rather dramatic positive responses[26,27] over relatively short follow-up times compared with the somewhat more sobering results obtained in later studies in which patients were followed for longer periods.[28,29]

The available data suggest that while serial electropharmacologic testing with conventional drugs appears to be predictive of the clinical response, at least over a short-term follow-up period, this does not apply to serial testing with amiodarone.[30,31] With this drug, ventricular tachycardia induction is the rule, even in patients who have a beneficial clinical response. In view of this finding, the predictive value of electropharmacologic testing must be determined for each new drug.

In addition, it is now clear that ventricular tachycardia inducibility will vary greatly depending on the underlying pathologic process. For example, ventricular tachycardia is almost always inducible in those with ventricular tachycardia associated with coronary artery disease, but seldom inducible in those with the congenital long Q-T syndrome. The incidence of provocable ventricular tachycardia in patients with spontaneous ventricular tachycardia associated with mitral valve prolapse, cardiomyopathy, or coronary arterial spasm or in those without structural heart disease appears to be lower than in patients with coronary artery disease.

In conclusion, the use of electrophysiologic studies has added enormous insights into the mechanisms of cardiac arrhythmias and antiarrhythmic drug action. However, these studies, especially as they apply to patients with ventricular arrhythmias, are still in their infancy. The criticisms detailed in this essay are not meant to be destructive, but rather are meant to highlight the need for continued clinical research in order that electrophysiologists may supply techniques for effective methods of arrhythmias management.

## REFERENCES

1. MANDEL, W., H. HAYAKAWA, R. DANZIG & H. S. MARCUS. 1971. Evaluation of sinoatrial node function in man by overdrive suppression. Circulation **44**: 59–66.
2. STRAUSS, H. C., A. L. SAROFF, J. T. BIGGER, JR. & E. G. V. GIARDINA. 1973. Premature atrial stimulation as a key to the understanding of sinoatrial conduction in man. Circulation **47**: 86–93.
3. NARULA, O. S., N. SHANTO, M. VASQUEZ, W. D. TOWNE & J. W. LINHART. 1978. A new method for measurement of sinoatrial conduction time. Circulation **58**: 706–714.
4. SCHEINMAN, M. M., H. C. STRAUSS & J. A. ABBOTT. 1979. Electrophysiologic testing for patients with sinus node dysfunction. J. Electrocardiol. **12**(2): 211–216.
5. REIFFEL, J. A., E. GANG, J. GLIKLICH, M. B. WEISS, J. C. DAVIS, J. N. PATTON & J. T. BIGGER. 1980. The human sinus node electrogram: A transvenous catheter technique and a comparison of directly measured and indirectly estimated sinoatrial conduction time in adults. Circulation **62**: 1324–1334.
6. ASSEMAN, P., B. BERZIN, D. DESRY, D. VILAREM, P. DURAND, C. DELMOTTE, E. H. SARKIS, J. LEKIEFFRE & C. THERY. 1983. Persistent sinus nodal electrograms during abnormally prolonged post pacing atrial pauses in sick sinus syndrome in humans. Circulation **68**: 33–41.
7. NARULA, O. S. 1975. Current concepts of atrioventricular block. *In* His Bundle Electrocardiography. O. S. Narula, Ed.: 143–155. F. A. Davis. Philadelphia, PA.
8. JOSEPHSON, M. E. & S. SEIDES. 1979. Electrophysiologic investigation: General concepts. *In* Cardiac Electrophysiology: Techniques and Interpretations.: 23–57. Lea & Febiger. Philadelphia, PA.
9. PEUCH, P. 1975. Atrioventricular block: The value of intracardiac recordings. *In* Cardiac Arrhythmias. D. Krikler & J. F. Goodwin, Eds.: 88–95. W. B. Saunders. London.
10. WU, D., F. AMAT-Y-LEON, R. J. SIMPSON, P. LATIF, C. R. C. WYNDHAM, P. DENES, & K. M. ROSEN. 1977. Electrophysiologic studies with multiple drugs in patients with atrioventricular reentrant tachycardia utilizing an extranodal pathway. Circulation **56**: 727–736.
11. CAMM, J. & P. WARD. 1983. Suppression and prevention of tachycardia by pacemakers. *In* Pacing for Tachycardia Control.: 43–57. Butler & Tanner. Fromme and London.
12. GALLAGHER, J. J. 1978. Surgical treatment for arrhythmias: Current status and future directions. Am. J. Cardiol. **41**: 1035–1044.
13. SUNG, R. J., B. ELSER, & R. G. MCALLISTER, JR. Intravenous verapamil for termination of reentrant supraventricular tachycardias. Ann. Int. Med. **93**: 682–689.
14. RINKENBERGER, R. L., E. N. PRYSTOWSKY, J. J. HEGER, P. J. TROUP, W. M. JACKMAN & D. P. ZIPES. 1980. Effects of intravenous and chronic verapamil administration in patients with supraventricular tachyarrhythmias. Circulation **62**: 996–1010.
15. GONZALEZ, R. & M. M. SCHEINMAN. 1981. Treatment of supraventricular arrhythmias with intravenous and oral verapamil. Chest **80**: 465–470.
16. WU, D., H. C. KOU, S. J. WYEH, F. C. LIN & J. S. HUNG. 1983. Effects of oral verapamil in patients with atrioventricular reentrant tachycardia incorporating an accessory pathway. Circulation **67**: 426–433.
17. YEH, S. J., H. C. KOU, F. C. LIN, J. S. HUNG & D. WU. 1983. Effects of oral diltiazem in paroxysmal supraventricular tachycardia. Am. J. Cardiol. **52**: 271–278.
18. SMITH, W., A. BROUGHTON, M. J. REITER, W. BENSON, JR., A. O. GRANT & J. J. GALLAGHER. 1983. Bystander accessory pathway during AV node reentrant tachycardia. PACE **6**: 537–547.
19. GALLAGHER, J. J., M. GILBERT & R. H. SVENSON. 1975. Wolff-Parkinson-White syndrome. The problem, evaluation and surgical correction. Circulation **51**: 767–785.
20. JOSEPHSON, M. E. & L. N. HOROWITZ. 1979. An electrophysiologic approach to the therapy of recurrent sustained ventricular tachycardia. Am. J. Cardiol. **43**: 631–642.
21. MASON, J. W. & R. A. WINKLE. 1978. Electrode-catheter arrhythmia induction in the selection and assessment of antiarrhythmic drug therapy for recurrent ventricular tachycardia. Circulation **58**: 971–985.

22. SWERDLOW, C. D., J. BLUM, R. A. WINKLE, J. C. GRIFFIN, D. L. ROSS & J. W. MASON. 1983. Decreased incidence of antiarrhythmic drug efficacy at electrophysiologic study associated with the use of a third extrastimulus. Am. Heart J. **104:** 1004–1011.
23. MORADY, F., D. HESS & M. M. SCHEINMAN. 1982. Electrophysiologic drug testing in patients with malignant ventricular arrhythmias: Importance of stimulation at more than one ventricular site. Am. J. Cardiol. **50:** 1055–1060.
24. MORADY, F., E. SHEN, A. SCHWARTZ, D. HESS, A. BHANDARI, R. J. SUNG & M. M. SCHEINMAN. 1984. Long-term follow-up of patients with recurrent unexplained syncope evaluated by electrophysiologic testing. Am. J. Cardiol.: in press.
25. HENTHORN, R. W., V. J. PLUMB, J. G. ARCINIEGAS, S. H. ZIMMERN & A. L. WALDO. 1983. Significance of the mode and site of ventricular tachycardia inducibility to assure adequate electrophysiologic study. J. Am. Coll. Cardiol. **1**(2): 594.
26. FISHER, J. D., H. L. COHEN & R. MEHRA. 1977. Serial electrophysiologic-pharmacologic testing for control of recurrent tachyarrhythmias. Am. Heart J. **93:** 658–668.
27. HOROWITZ, L. N., M. E. JOSEPHSON, A. FARSHIDI, S. R. SPIELMAN, E. L. MICHELSON & A. M. GREENSPAN. 1978. Recurrent sustained ventricular tachycardia. 3. Role of electrophysiologic study in selection of antiarrhythmic regimens. Circulation **58:** 186–997.
28. MORADY, F., M. M. SCHEINMAN, D. HESS, R. J. SUNG, E. SHEN & W. SHAPIRO. 1982. Electrophysiologic testing in the management of survivors of out-of-hospital cardiac arrest. Am. J. Cardiol. **51:** 85–89.
29. MASON, J. W. & R. A. WINKLE. 1980. Accuracy of the ventricular tachycardia induction study for predicting long-term efficacy and inefficacy of antiarrhythmic drugs. N. Engl. J. Med. **303:** 1075–1077.
30. MORADY, F., M. J. SAUVE, P. MALONE, E. N. SHEN, A. B. SCHWARTZ, A. BHANDARI, E. KEUNG, R. J. SUNG & M. M. SCHEINMAN. 1984. Long-term efficacy and toxicity of high-dose amiodarone therapy in patients with ventricular tachycardia or ventricular fibrillation. Am. J. Cardiol.: in press.
31. HEGER, J. J., E. N. PRYSTOWSKY, W. M. JACKMAN, G. V. NACCARELLI, K. A. WARFEL, R. L. RICKENBERGER & D. P. ZIPES. 1981. Amiodarone: Clinical efficacy and electrophysiology during long-term therapy for recurrent ventricular tachycardia and ventricular fibrillation. N. Engl. J. Med. **305:** 539–545.
32. GRABOYS, T. B., B. LOWN, P. J. PODRID & R. DESILVA. 1982. Long-term survival of patients with malignant ventricular arrhythmia treated with antiarrhythmic drugs. Am. J. Cardiol. **50:** 437–443.

# Quinidine

JAY W. MASON

Cardiology Division
University of Utah School of Medicine
Salt Lake City, Utah 84112

LUC M. HONDEGHEM

Department of Pharmacology
University of California, San Francisco
San Francisco, California 94143

Quinidine is by far the oldest and most frequently used antiarrhythmic drug, and was the first agent developed solely for its antiarrhythmic effect. Quinidine is an alkaloid derived from cinchona bark (FIG. 1). The compound was prepared by Pasteur in the 1850s and was first applied as a therapeutic agent by Wenckebach in the second decade of this century. Remarkably, despite its many untoward effects, and despite prolific efforts of pharmaceutical houses around the world to produce improved antiarrhythmic agents, quinidine continues to be the first choice of most physicians in the United States for treatment of the widest spectrum of cardiac arrhythmias. The purpose of this article is to briefly summarize the electrophysiology and pharmacology of quinidine in the context of recent developments in treatment of cardiac arrhythmias.

## BASIC ELECTROPHYSIOLOGY OF QUINIDINE

Therapeutic concentrations of quinidine, that is, those that reduce ventricular conduction in normal tissue less than 30 percent,[1] have small direct effects upon the sinoatrial (SA) and atrioventricular (AV) nodes.[2,3] Healthy (well-polarized negative resting potential) atrial, His-Purkinje, and ventricular myocardial tissues are, at normal heart rates, only minimally affected by such a dose: their upstroke and conduction velocity are somewhat decreased, excitability is slightly reduced, and effective refractory period may be lengthened.[4] In contrast, these changes are much more marked in tissues stressed by hypoxia,[5] ischemia,[6] depolarization by potassium[7] or electrical current,[8,9] and tachycardias.[10] Thus, quinidine selectively depresses conduction and excitability of depolarized tissue, especially at fast heart rates. For example, at $-85$ mV and 60 beats/min, the effect of quinidine is much less marked than at 200 beats/min or at $-70$ mV (FIG. 2).

Also, therapeutic concentrations of quinidine do not reduce resting membrane potential, but markedly reduce spontaneous phase-4 depolarization, especially in ectopic pacemakers.[11] The aforementioned actions of quinidine are thought to occur as a result of blockade of transmembrane ionic channels, primarily the fast inward sodium channel.

Hondeghem and Katzung[12] proposed a modulated receptor hypothesis (FIG. 3) that can nicely account for the just-listed drug actions. Basically, sodium channels exist in three states[13]: rested (R), activated (A), and inactivated (I). Each state has

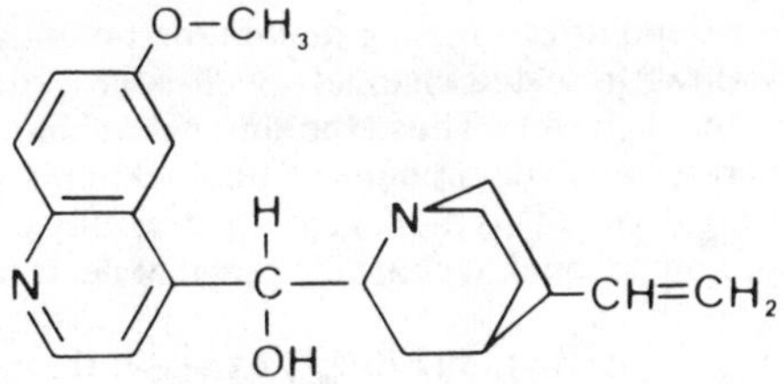

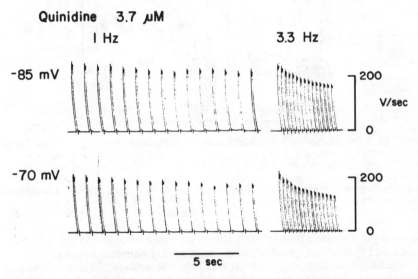

**FIGURE 1.** The structure of 6'-methoxy cinchonine (quinidine). (From Hondeghem and Mason.[1] Reproduced by permission.)

a characteristic affinity for quinidine and rate of interaction with the drug. Channels blocked by quinidine behave similarly to drug-free channels, except that they do not conduct and they behave as if they are more depolarized by about 40 mV. As a result, at $-90$ mV, drug-free channels are rested (R), while blocked channels behave as if they were at $-50$ mV, that is, they remain inactivated (I.D.). The rested and inactivated states have a low affinity for quinidine, while the activated, or open channel, has a high affinity.[14,15] Thus, with each action potential upstroke, a fraction of the sodium channels become blocked. For the duration of the inacti-

**FIGURE 2.** Rate- and voltage-dependence of sodium channel blockade by quinidine. The tracings show dV/dt of the action potential upstroke recorded by standard glass microelectrode techniques in guinea pig papillary muscle exposed to quinidine. In the *upper tracings* the preparation is voltage-clamped at $-85$mV, except during the action potential. At a stimulation rate of 1 Hz, there is minimal depression of dV/dt. At the faster stimulation of 3.3 Hz, dV/dt is progressively reduced during the stimulus train. In the *lower tracings,* the membrane is voltage-clamped at a less-polarized level of $-70$mv. At the 1-Hz stimulation rate, greater reduction in dV/dt is seen compared to that of the normally polarized state, and at 3.3-Hz stimulation, the extent of depression of dV/dt is even more striking.

vated state (plateau or depolarized resting membrane potentials), the rate of unblocking is relatively slow. In rested channels (well-polarized resting potentials), unblocking proceeds much faster. Thus, the amount of block that develops is proportional to heart rate, and the amount of unblocking is proportional to the diastolic time and its negativity. This model can successfully predict the actions of quinidine upon the sodium channel over a wide range of heart rates and membrane potentials.[9]

Quinidine, like most antiarrhythmic drugs, exists in the neutral and cationic forms. Cationic quinidine blocks open channels, while neutral quinidine diffuses away from closed-channel receptors through the lipid phase of the membrane.[12,16] Thus, acidosis, which promotes the cationic drug form, is expected to slow recovery from block,[17,18] thereby promoting accumulation of block. Conversely, alkalosis promotes the neutral drug form, but also reduces external potassium (resulting

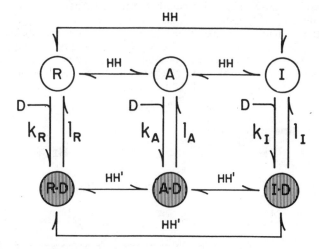

**FIGURE 3.** Modulated-receptor hypothesis of Hondeghem and Katzung. R, A and I refer to the rested, activated, and inactivated states. HH indicates standard Hodgkin-Huxley kinetics determining the state of the sodium channels. The *shaded circles* indicate the three channel states associated with or blocked by drug (D), in this case, quinidine. K and l are the rate constants of drug association and dissociation for the three channel states. The model is explained further in the text.

in hyperpolarization). Both of these effects are expected to hasten recovery from block and hence to be beneficial in the treatment of quinidine toxicity.

Quinidine can also lengthen the action potential duration,[19] which can be seen as an increase of the Q-T interval in the ECG. The longer action potential duration can also contribute to a longer effective refractory period, which in turn reduces the maximum reentry frequency. The longer action potential duration probably results from the drug's effect upon potassium currents. It should be noted that the longer action potential duration will result in shorter diastolic time and will therefore enhance the sodium-blocking activity of quinidine or any other sodium channel blocker. In addition, if the drug also blocks inactivated sodium channels, then development of block may be potentiated. Such potentiation was predicted by the modulated receptor hypothesis[9] and has been observed clinically.[20,21]

## CLINICAL ELECTROPHYSIOLOGY OF QUINIDINE

The most obvious electrophysiologic effects of quinidine in humans are those detected by surface electrocardiography. The most prominent change in the electrocardiogram seen at therapeutic concentrations is lengthening of the Q-T interval. Increases in the corrected Q-T interval of 25% are commonly seen in patients with therapeutic concentrations of the drug and without toxicity. A small proportion of patients are especially sensitive to this effect of quinidine, and they show dramatic Q-T prolongation by as much as 100% or more. Some of these patients develop quinidine syncope (see below).

The second most discernible electrocardiographic change is an increase in the sinus rate. Generally, quinidine does not increase the sinus rate beyond the physiologic range, and it may cause a decrease in sinus rate in some individuals, for reasons that will become clear below.

The third common electrocardiographic effect of quinidine is an increase in QRS duration. While this change may be detected in most patients receiving quinidine, the change is usually less than 0.04 sec, and it is unusual to see an increase in QRS duration of more than 25% in patients without manifestations of electrophysiologic toxicity of quinidine.

In a minority of patients a small increase in the P-R interval may be noted. In even fewer patients without conduction abnormalities prior to quinidine administration, a complete right bundle branch block or left bundle branch block pattern may develop with quinidine. This effect of quinidine does not appear to occur in patients without conduction system disease.

Quinidine's electrophysiologic effects are a result of the combined influence of direct and autonomically mediated actions. These distinct effects were recently separately identified in humans.[22] Cardiac transplant recipients were studied by means of intracardiac electrophysiologic techniques before and after intravenous administration of quinidine. Transplant recipients were studied because the cardiac heterograft remains denervated chronically. Thus, transplant recipients lack cardiac autonomic innervation. Their hearts would be expected to respond only to the direct electrophysiologic effects of quinidine while failing to manifest its autonomically mediated actions.

Evaluation of the sinoatrial nodal effects of quinidine was additionally benefited in this study by virtue of the simultaneous presence in cardiac transplant recipients of the donor, denervated atria, and the viable, innervated, remnant atria. This dual presence is a result of the surgical technique developed by Shumway, which entails attachment of the posterior portions of the right and left atria of the donor heart to residual right and left atrial tissue left in place during excision of the diseased recipient organ. Furthermore, both donor and recipient atria retain their sinus nodes. As a result, the investigators were able to assess the effects of quinidine upon an innervated sinus node and a denervated sinus node within the same patient. The results are shown in the left and middle pannels of FIGURE 4. As expected from the known actions of quinidine in intact man, the recipient sinus node cycle length decreased after an intravenous infusion of quinidine consisting of 10 mg/kg delivered over 20 minutes. The donor heart sinus nodes, however, acted differently. These denervated sinus nodes slowed down by an average of 5%. This portion of the experiment demonstrated that the direct action of quinidine slows sinus node automaticity, but that its autonomically mediated acceleratory effect, via vagolysis, overrides the direct effect and produces a net increase in heart rate in normally innervated hearts.

The AV nodal effects of quinidine paralleled its sinoatrial nodal effects in this

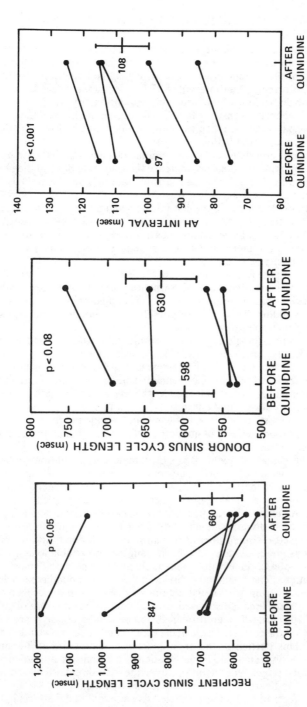

**FIGURE 4.** Electrophysiologic effects of quinidine in the transplanted human heart.[22] All three panels show electrophysiologic values before and after administration of quinidine, 10 mg/kg over 20 minutes, to healthy cardiac transplant recipients. The panel on the *left* shows a decrease in the recipient sinus node cycle length. The *middle panel* shows an increase in the donor sinus cycle length in the same patients. The panel on the *right* shows an increase in atrioventricular conduction time after quinidine administration. See the text for further explanation. (From Mason *et al.*[22] Reproduced by permission.)

study. It is known from earlier studies in intact man[23] that parenterally administered quinidine causes enhancement of AV nodal conduction. In the denervated
donor hearts, however, the A-H interval was increased by quinidine (FIG. 4, *right*
panel). Again, the autonomic influence of quinidine overrides its direct effect
upon the atrioventricular node. Since quinidine is a potent vagolytic agent, it is
not surprising that the sinoatrial and atrioventricular nodes, which receive rich
autonomic innervation, manifest this antivagal action.

In this study the other electrophysiologic actions of quinidine were similar to
those seen in intact man. Specifically, the His-Purkinje conduction time was
significantly increased, the atrial effective refractory period was increased, and
the blood pressure fell significantly.

A new aspect of the clinical electrophysiology of any antiarrhythmic drug is
the applicability of inducing arrhythmias in order to assess drug efficacy. Arrhythmia induction has become a widely used technique for predicting chronic antiarrhythmic drug efficacy.[24] It is quite clear that quinidine, perhaps in a prototypical
fashion, is accurately evaluable by the arrhythmia-induction method. It may well
turn out that quinidine is atypical in this regard since it has become apparent in
recent years that certain new antiarrhythmic drugs may be effective during
chronic therapy, despite continued inducibility of the clinical arrhythmia.

## ANTIARRHYTHMIC EFFICACY OF QUINIDINE

Quinidine can be considered a broad-spectrum antiarrhythmic agent because it
has been used to treat both ventricular and supraventricular arrhythmias of various types. Its earliest, and perhaps its currently most prevalent use, was in the
conversion of atrial fibrillation to sinus rhythm or in the maintenance of sinus
rhythm in patients with paroxysmal atrial fibrillation. Quinidine has also been
used for treatment of atrial flutter and atrial ectopic depolarizations. Surprisingly,
a controlled study of the efficacy of quinidine in treatment of most atrial arrhythmias has never been carried out. However, there is little doubt in most experienced clinicians' minds that quinidine is effective. Quinidine has been studied in
comparison with other antiarrhythmic drugs in treatment of the circus movement
tachycardia associated with the Wolff-Parkinson-White syndrome.[25] This study
documented quinidine's efficacy, although a placebo control was lacking.

Sound, placebo-controlled, comparative studies of quinidine versus other
compounds in treatment of ventricular arrhythmias have appeared recently in the
literature. Interestingly, it was not until comparison trials were required by the
Food and Drug Administration for introduction of new antiarrhythmic drugs that
these studies of quinidine were carried out.

In a multicenter trial, quinidine was compared to flecainide for treatment of
chronic, but generally not immediately life-threatening, ventricular arrhythmias.[26]
Although flecainide was uniformly superior to quinidine in its ability to suppress
various types of ventricular arrhythmias, quinidine was highly efficacious, and
might conceivably have been as efficacious as flecainide in a trial permitting
greater range in dosing. In this trial, which included 139 patients treated with
quinidine, either 300 or 400 mg were administered every 6 hours. Seventy-five
percent of the patients sustained greater than a 50% reduction in PVC frequency.
Fifty-seven percent had greater than 80% suppression, and one-third of the patients had 95% suppression of PVCs by quinidine. Episodes of unsustained ventricular tachycardia and of pairs of ventricular beats were more thoroughly sup-

pressed by quinidine. Thus, in this placebo-controlled trial, quinidine was found to be highly effective in suppressing ventricular arrhythmias.

In another trial quinidine was compared to encainide in a longitudinal cross-over trial in which both treadmill exercise tests and 24-hour ambulatory electro-cardiograms were used to measure ventricular arrhythmia frequency.[27] Once again, in this study, dosing was rigidly limited. A single dose of quinidine, 300 mg every 6 hours, was used. Twenty patients were studied. Encainide was found to be superior to quinidine. However, quinidine was highly effective. It reduced the mean frequency of PVCs from approximately 50 per hour to less than 10 per hour on the ambulatory electrocardiogram. It also significantly reduced the frequency of ventricular ectopic beats on treadmill tests.

Thus, quinidine is unquestionably effective in suppressing atrial and ventricular arrhythmias. It may be less effective than new antiarrhythmic drugs, but dose equivalency in comparative trials is nearly impossible to achieve with confidence. As with all antiarrhythmic drugs, it is not yet clear whether quinidine can substantially improve survival in patients with immediately or potentially life-threatening arrhythmias.

## PHARMACOKINETICS

Quinidine is given orally as the sulfate or gluconate. An aqueous solution of the gluconate is used for parenteral therapy. Usual therapeutic oral doses of quinidine sulfate range from 300 to 600 mg every 6 hours. The daily dose of the gluconate preparation is 30% greater. Both the sulfate and gluconate are about 70% bioavailable after oral dosing. While the sulfate preparation reaches a peak plasma concentration about 90 minutes after oral ingestion, peak concentration occurs 3 to 4 hours after ingestion of the gluconate form. Thus, the gluconate form can be administered three rather than four times a day.

Quinidine is frequently given intramuscularly, but the injections are painful and occasionally produce sterile abscesses.

There has been a longstanding bias against the use of quinidine by the intravenous route because of reports of adverse hemodynamic effects. Recently, however, it has been shown that quinidine can be given safely by vein if appropriate precautions are taken.[28] Specifically, blood pressure must be carefully monitored, either by frequent cuff determinations or by direct intraarterial recording. Any fall in blood pressure should be promptly treated with saline infusion and, if necessary, a decrease in the quinidine infusion rate. With these precautions, quinidine can be infused at a rate of 0.5 mg/kg/min to a total dose of 10 mg/kg in most patients, even in individuals with congestive heart failure.

Quinidine has an elimination half-life of 5 to 8 hours during oral therapy. Quinidine is eliminated largely by hepatic metabolism and less importantly by the kidneys. The major metabolites of quinidine are mono- and dihydroxy-quinidine. These and other quinidine metabolites are not believed to have significant antiarrhythmic activity. However, the hydroxy metabolites are measured along with the parent compound by the single, and less extensively by the double, extraction assay techniques.[29,30] The presence of these metabolites may confuse interpretation of the plasma concentration level since metabolites may constitute a larger portion of the assayed material in certain situations, such as renal failure.

## TOXICITY OF QUINIDINE

Quinidine syncope, a term coined by Selzer and Wray,[31] is the best known, although not the most common side effect of quinidine. The presenting symptom is paroxysmal syncope and presyncope, usually in patients who recently began therapy with quinidine or in whom the dose was recently adjusted. Syncope is caused by paroxysmal, usually self-limited, episodes of a rapid ventricular tachyarrhythmia. The rhythm itself has been termed "torsade de pointes" because of the characteristic electrocardiographic pattern seen in one or more leads (FIG. 5). The QRS complexes first "point" in one direction, and then twist around the baseline to point in the opposite direction. The rhythm is frequently interrupted by sinus beats. The Q-T interval of sinus beats is prolonged, often markedly.

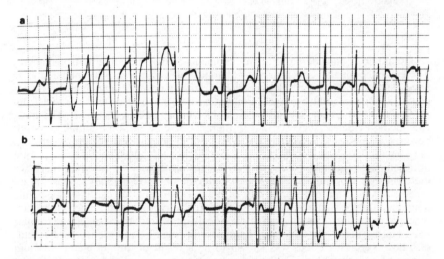

**FIGURE 5.** Torsade de pointes. This pleomorphic rhythm was a result of quinidine toxicity. In both panels the main QRS axis rotates through 180 degrees during rapid ventricular tachycardia, and the tachyarrhythmia is frequently interrupted by sinus beats. From Anderson and Mason.[33] Reproduced by permission.)

Reynolds and Van der Ark[32] have estimated that as many as 4% of patients given large doses of quinidine develop this complication.

There are two distinct varieties of this complication. The first variety is a manifestation of drug overdose, and is associated with high plasma concentrations, usually in excess of 10 $\mu$g/ml. The other variety of the syndrome is apparently an idiosyncratic reaction since it occurs in patients with low plasma concentrations, often after the first few doses of the drug. In both varieties, the syndrome usually lasts for 12 to 24 hours after discontinuation of quinidine. Many antiarrhythmic drugs have been tried in treatment of this disorder, but none has been unequivocably effective. However, overdrive cardiac pacing often dramatically controls the paroxysmal tachyarrhythmia.[33] Pacing rates between 100 and 150 beats/min are usually required.

**TABLE 1.** Results of Studies of the Effects of Quinidine on Myocardial Contractility

| Finding | In vivo | In vitro |
|---|---|---|
| *Studies in animals:* | | |
| +Inotropy or no change | Angelakos and Hastings[34] Pruett and Woods,[35] Markiewicz et al.[36] | Kruta et al.,[39] Kennedy and West,[40] Chiba,[41] Himori and Taira[42] |
| −Inotropy | Angelakos and Hastings,[34] Pruett and Woods,[35] Stern[43] | Kruta et al.,[39] Tomoda et al.,[44] Chiba,[41] Himori and Taira[42] |
| *Studies in man:* | | |
| +Inotropy or no change | Ferrer et al.[45] Mason et al.[46] | |
| −Inotropy | Sokolow,[47] Samet and Surawicz[48] | |

Quinidine is considered by many clinicians to be a negative inotropic agent. The evidence for this conclusion is not solid. *In vitro* and *in vivo* animal studies have yielded conflicting results because of varying doses of quinidine and differences in experimental protocol. Conflicting data have also been derived from studies in man. These several studies are summarized in TABLE 1. The most convincing evidence suggests that in therapeutic concentration quinidine is not negatively inotropic, although it does exert potent hemodynamic effects. Markiewicz and associates[36] rigidly controlled preload, afterload, and cardiac rate in an animal experiment (FIG. 6) and found that there was no direct, negative inotropic effect of quinidine, although quinidine did alter hemodynamics. In another study at Stanford University in human recipients of cardiac transplants quinidine did not significantly alter indices of contractility determined from fluoroscopic recording of the motion of previously implanted, midwall left ventricular tantalum markers.[46] In this study quinidine did significantly reduce cardiac output, however. This effect was shown to be a result of the peripheral vascular effects of quinidine (FIG. 7). Quinidine reduced stroke volume by markedly decreasing the end-diastolic left ventricular volume, presumably a result of peripheral venodilatation. The systemic arterial pressure also fell, but quinidine did not cause a significant decrease in systemic vascular resistance. Thus, quinidine reduces blood pressure and cardiac output by venous vascular dilatation, not through a negative inotropic action. Walsh and Horowitz[37] also found that quinidine exerted no negative inotropic effect in conscious "instrumented" dogs, and O'Rourke and Horowitz[38] were unable to demonstrate any depression in left ventricular performance by quinidine in this model even during an acute pressure load induced by phenylephrine infusion. Thus, the clinician should recognize that quinidine is not a negative inotrope in therapeutic dosage. The clinician should also be aware, however, that quinidine may reduce systemic pressure and cardiac output, largely by reducing preload. Thus, the deleterious hemodynamic effects of quinidine can be properly managed with volume expansion, although frequently no therapeutic intervention is required.

Three excellent studies are available in the literature detailing the additional adverse effects of quinidine. The Boston Collaborative Drug Surveillance program provides data from 652 hospitalized patients taking quinidine.[49] There was an adverse reaction in 91 or 14% of the patients. Half of the adverse reactions were gastrointestinal, predominately diarrhea. What appeared to be an exacerbation of arrhythmia developed in 2.5% of the patients: either new onset of bradyarrhythmia, increased ventricular response rate to atrial fibrillation, increase in ventricular ectopy, or the new appearance of ventricular tachycardia or fibrillation. In 1.7% of the patients a febrile reaction was reported.

In the flecanide-quinidine trial[26] 65% of the 139 patients who received quinidine developed a side effect. In 21 of these patients quinidine had to be discontinued: The most frequent side effect was diarrhea, which was reported in 40% of the patients. Twenty-one percent of the patients developed nausea. Fourteen percent of the patients complained of headache and 11 percent reported dizziness. In the encainide-quinidine[27] comparison, 12 of 18 patients had gastrointestinal complaints that were severe enough to require dose reduction in 3. Three of the patients developed a fever and one a rash. A significant proarrhythmic effect was not reported in the two drug comparison trials. The incidence of side effects in these two studies was similar for the comparison, experimental agent. Thus, the most common side effects of quinidine are gastrointestinal, neurologic, and febrile responses. The most serious, although relatively uncommon, side effect of quinidine is arrhythmia exacerbation, especially that characterized by torsade de pointes.

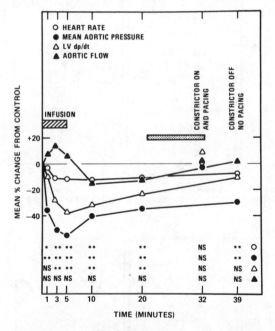

**FIGURE 6.** Hemodynamic effects of quinidine in the dog. The results of one experiment of Markiewicz et al.[36] are shown. The change in heart rate, aortic pressure, left ventricular dP/dt, and aortic flow after quinidine administration are graphed. Although all four variables decreased in response to quinidine, initiation of aortic constriction to return afterload to the baseline level, as well as cardiac pacing to return the heart rate to baseline, resulted in normalization of both ventricular dP/dt and aortic flow. Thus quinidine did not exert a negative inotropic effect. (From Markiewicz et al.[36] Reproduced by permission.)

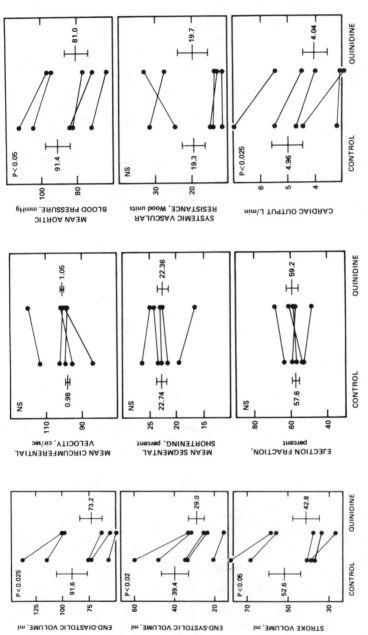

**FIGURE 7.** Hemodynamic effects of quinidine in the transplanted human heart.[46] Hemodynamic response of quinidine was assessed using previously implanted midwall left ventricular markers. Heart rate was controlled by atrial pacing. Quinidine reduced the stroke volume by causing a greater fall in end-diastolic volume than in end-systolic volume, as shown in the graphs on the *left*. The graphs in the *center* show no significant change in three measures of left ventricular contractility. The end result of these effects, shown on the *right*, was a decrease in cardiac output and mean aortic blood pressure and no significant change in systemic vascular resistance. (From Mason *et al.*[46] Reproduced by permission.)

## THE QUINIDINE-DIGOXIN INTERACTION

In both animals and man quinidine causes an increase in digoxin concentration when it is administered in addition to a stable dose of digoxin.[50-54] Details regarding the mechanism of this interaction are still controversial. However, a number of points can be made. First, the digoxin concentration rises proportionately with the quinidine dose. Second, quinidine does not cause an increase in gastrointestinal absorption of digoxin. Third, quinidine probably decreases the volume of distribution of digoxin. Fourth, it significantly decreases the renal clearance of digoxin. Fifth, quinidine may also decrease nonrenal clearance of digoxin. Sixth, in the brain and myocardium, the sites in which a change in digoxin concentration might have the most serious consequences, it remains controversial whether concentrations of digoxin increase, decrease, or remain the same during quinidine administration. Nonetheless it does appear that the inotropic effect of digoxin is preserved during quinidine administration, suggesting the possibility that myocardial levels do not fall. Finally, although the issue remains controversial, it seems likely that digoxin toxicity can be precipitated by the increase in digoxin concentration caused by quinidine.

## RECOMMENDATIONS FOR USE OF QUINIDINE

Quinidine continues to be one of the most useful antiarrhythmic drugs available because of its wide spectrum of activity and because of the current paucity of more effective agents. Appropriate indications for quinidine are as follows.

1. Prophylaxis against paroxysmal atrial fibrillation or flutter. It is inappropriate to continue administration of quinidine in patients who have developed permanent atrial fibrillation or flutter.

2. Control of premature atrial contractions.

3. Control of the circus movement tachycardia in the Wolff-Parkinson-White syndrome.

4. Suppression of premature ventricular contractions.

5. Prophylaxis against complex ventricular arrhythmias.

In patients who have significant congestive heart failure and in patients with complex ventricular arrhythmias, it is no longer appropriate to institute treatment with quinidine on an outpatient basis because of the risk of arrhythmia exacerbation in patients of that description. It is preferable to administer quinidine to such patients in the hospital under continuous cardiac monitoring.

It is even more important to hospitalize and monitor any patient who is given very large doses of quinidine for rapid conversion of atrial fibrillation or flutter, regardless of his or her cardiovascular status.

In the intensive care situation, where blood pressure can be carefully monitored, quinidine can be used intravenously as a second-line agent for control of serious ventricular arrhythmias.

Whenever quinidine is used, the plasma concentration should be monitored so that the concentration is brought into the therapeutic range, and toxic levels, especially those above 10 $\mu$g/ml, are avoided. When quinidine is instituted in patients taking digoxin, it appears wise to halve the dose of digoxin initially, or at least to monitor frequently its concentration and signs of toxicity.

## REFERENCES

1. HONDEGHEM, L. M. & J. W. MASON. 1982. Agents used in cardiac arrhythmias. *In* Basic and Clinical Pharmacology. B. G. Katzung, Ed.: 138–54. Lange Medical Publications. Los Altos, CA.
2. WATANBE, Y. & L. S. DREIFUS. 1967. Interactions of quinidine and potassium on artioventricular transmission. Circ. Res. **20:** 434–446.
3. HOFFMAN, B. F. 1958. The action of quinidine and procainamide on single fibers of dog ventricle and specialized conduction system. An. Acad. Bras. Cienc. **29:** 365–368.
4. VAUGHAN WILLIAMS, E. M. 1958. The mode of action of quinidine on isolated rabbit atria interpreted from intracellular records. Br. J. Pharmacol. **13:** 276–287.
5. HONDEGHEM, L. M. 1976. Effects of lidocaine, phenytoin, and quinidine on the ischemic canine myocardium. J. Electrocardiol. **9:** 203–209.
6. HONDEGHEM, L. M., A. D. GRANT & R. A. JENSEN. 1974. Antiarrhythmic drug action: Selective depression of hypoxic cardiac cells. Am. Heart J. **87:** 602–605.
7. WATANBE, Y., L. S. DREIFUS & W. LIKOFF. 1963. Electrophysiologic antagonism and synergism of potassium and antiarrhythmic agents. Am. J. Cardiol. **12:** 702.
8. WEIDMANN, S. 1955. The effect of the cardiac membrane potential on the rapid availability of the sodium-carrying system. J. Physiol. **127:** 213–224.
9. HONDEGHEM, L. M. & B. G. KATZUNG. 1980. Test of a model of antiarrhythmic drug action. Effect of quinidine and lidocaine on myocardial conduction. Circulation **61:** 1217–1224.
10. JOHNSON, E. A. & M. G. MCKINNON. 1957. The differential effect of quinidine and pyrilamine on the myocardial action potential at various rates of stimulation. J. Pharmacol. Exp. Ther. **120:** 460–468.
11. WEIDMANN, S. 1955. Effects of calcium ions and local anesthetics on electrical properties of Purkinje fibers. J. Physiol. **129:** 568–582.
12. HONDEGHEM, L. M. & B. G. KATZUNG. 1977. A unifying model for the interaction of antiarrhythmic drugs with cardiac sodium channels: Application to quinidine and lidocaine. Proc. West Pharmacol. Soc. **20:** 253–256.
13. HODGKIN, A. L. & A. F. HUXLEY. 1952. A quantitative description of membrane current and its application to conduction and excitation in nerve. J. Physiol. **117:** 500–544.
14. COLATSKY, T. J. 1982. Quinidine block of cardiac sodium channels is rate- and voltage-dependent. Biophys. J. **37:** 343a.
15. WELD, F. M., J. COROMILAS, J. N. ROTTMAN & J. T. BIGGER, JR. 1982. Mechanism of quinidine-induced depression of maximum upstroke velocity in ovine cardiac Purkinje fibers. Circ. Res. **50:** 369–376.
16. HILLE, B. 1977. The pH-dependent rate of action of local anesthetics on the node of Ranvier. J. Gen. Physiol. **69:** 475–496.
17. GRANT, A. O., J. L. TRANTHAM, K. K. BROWN & H. C. STRAUSS. 1982. pH-dependent effects of quinidine on the kinetics of dV/dt-max in guinea pig ventricular myocardium. Circ. Res. **50:** 210–217.
18. NATTELL, S., V. ELHARRAR, D. P. ZIPES & J. C. BAILEY. 1981. pH-dependent electrophysiological effects of quinidine and lidocaine on canine cardiac Purkinje fibers. Circ. Res. **48:** 55–61.
19. COLATSKY, T. J. 1982. Mechanisms of action of lidocaine and quinidine on action potential duration in rabbit cardiac Purkinje fibers. Circ. Res. **50:** 17–27.
20. BREITHARDT, G., L. SEIPEL & R. R. ABENDROTH. 1981. Comparison of antiarrhythmic efficacy of disopyramide and mexiletine against stimulus-induced ventricular tachycardia. J. Cardiovasc. Pharmacol. **3:** 1026–1037.
21. DUFF, H. J., D. RODEN, R. K. PRIMM, J. A. OATES & R. L. WOOSLEY. 1983. Mexiletine in the treatment of resistant ventricular arrhythmias: Enhancement of efficacy and reduction of dose-related side effects by combination with quinidine. Circulation **67:** 1124–1128.
22. MASON, J. W., R. A. WINKLE, A. K. RIDER, E. B. STINSON & D. C. HARRISON. 1977.

The electrophysiologic effects of quinidine in the transplanted human heart. J. Clin. Invest. **59:** 481–489.

23. JOSEPHSON, M. E., S. F. SEIDES, W. P. BATSFORD, G. M. WEISFOGEL, M. AKHTAR, A. R. CARACTS, S. H. LAU & A. N. DAMATO. 1974. The electrophysiologic effects of intramuscular quinidine on the atrioventricular conducting system in man. Am. Heart J. **87:** 55–64.

24. SWERDLOW, C. D., R. A. WINKLE & J. W. MASON. 1983. Determinants of survival in patients with ventricular tachyarrhythmias. N. Engl. J. Med. **308:** 1436–1442.

25. SELLERS, T. D., R. W. F. CAMPBELL, T. M. BASHORE & J. J. GALLAGHER. 1977. Effects of procainamide and quinidine sulfate in the Wolff-Parkinson-White syndrome. Circulation **55:** 15–22.

26. FLECAINIDE-QUINIDINE RESEARCH GROUP. 1983. Flecainide versus quinidine for treatment of chronic ventricular arrhythmias: A multicenter clinical trial. Circulation **67:** 1117–1123.

27. SAMI, M., D. C. HARRISON, H. KRAEMER, N. HOUSTON, C. SHIMASKI & R. F. DE-BUSK. 1981. Antiarrhythmic efficacy of encainide and quinidine: Validation of a model for drug assessment. Am. J. Cardiol. **48:** 147–156.

28. SWERDLOW, C. D., J. O. YU, E. JACOBSON, S. MANN, R. A. WINKLE, J. C. GRIFFIN, D. L. ROSS & J. W. MASON. 1983. Safety and efficacy of intravenous quinidine. Am. J. Med. **75:** 36–41.

29. BRODIE, B. B., J. E. BAER & L. C. CRAIG. 1951. Metabolic products in cinchona alkaloids in human urine. J. Biol. Chem. **188:** 567.

30. SOKOLOW, M. & A. L. EDGAR. 1950. Blood quinidine concentrations as guide in the treatment of cardiac arrhythmias. Circulation **1:** 576.

31. SELZER, A. & H. W. WRAY. 1964. Quinidine syncope: Paroxysmal ventricular fibrillation occurring during treatment of chronic atrial arrhythmias. Circulation **30:** 17–26.

32. REYNOLDS, E. W. & C. R. VAN DER ARK. 1976. Quinidine syncope and the delayed repolarization syndromes. Mod. Concepts Cardiovasc. Dis. **45:** 117–122.

33. ANDERSON, J. L. & J. W. MASON. 1978. Successful treatment by overdrive pacing of recurrent quinidine syncope due to ventricular tachycardia. Am. J. Med. **64:** 715–718.

34. ANGELAKOS, E. T. & E. P. HASTINGS. 1960. The influence of quinidine and procaine amide on myocardial contractility in vivo. Am. J. Cardiol. **6:** 791–798.

35. PRUETT, J. K. & E. F. WOODS. 1967. The relationship of intracellular depolarization rates and contractility in the dog ventricle in situ: Effects of positive and negative inotropic agents. J. Pharmacol. Exp. Ther. **157:** 1–7.

36. MARKIEWICZ, W., R. WINKLE, G. BINETTI, R. KERNOFF & D. C. HARRISON. 1976. Normal myocardial contractile state in the presence of quinidine. Circulation **53:** 101–106.

37. WALSH, R. A. & L. D. HOROWITZ. 1979. Adverse hemodynamic effects of intravenous disopyramide compared with quinidine in conscious dogs. Circulation **60:** 1053–1058.

38. O'ROURKE, R. A. & L. D. HOROWITZ. 1981. Effects of chronic oral quinidine on left ventricular performance. Am. Heart J. **101:** 769–773.

39. KRUTA, V., P. BRAVENY, J. HLAVKOVA-STEJSKALOVA, et al. 1963. Réstitution de la contractilité du myocarde et effets inotropes ouabaine, quinidine, tyramine, theophylline et acetylcholine chez la labaye et le rat. Cripta Medica Facultatum Medicinae Universitatum Brunensis et Olomucensis **36:** 1–26.

40. KENNEDY, B. J. & T. C. WEST. 1969. Factors influencing quinidine-induced changes in excitability and contractility. J. Pharmacol. Exp. Ther. **163:** 47–59.

41. CHIBA, S. 1976. Effects of quinidine, procainamide, lidocaine and phenytoin on inotropic responses to acetylcholine and norepinephrine. Jpn. J. Pharmacol. **26:** 276–278.

42. HIMORI, N. & N. TAIRA. 1976. Effects of quinidine on blood flow rate and developed tension in blood-perfused canine papillary muscle. Clin. Exp. Pharm. Physiol. **3:** 1–7.

43. STERN, S. 1971. Hemodynamic changes following separate and combined administration of beta-blocking drugs and quinidine. Eur. J. Clin. Invest. **1:** 432–436.

44. TOMODA, H., L. CHUCK & W. W. PARMLEY. 1972. Comparative myocardial depressant effects of lidocaine, ajmaline, propranolol and quinidine. Jpn. Circ. J. **36:** 433–437.
45. FERRER, M. I., M. HARVEY, L. WERKO, D. T. DRESDALE, A. COURNAND & D. W. RICHARDS. 1948. Some effects of quinidine sulfate on the heart and circulation in man. Am. Heart J. **36:** 816–837.
46. MASON, J. W., R. A. WINKLE, N. B. INGELS, G. T. DAUGHTERS, D. C. HARRISON & E. B. STINSON. 1977. Hemodynamic effects of intravenously administered quinidine on the transplanted human heart. Am. J. Cardiol. **40:** 99–104.
47. SOKOLOW, M. 1951. The present status of therapy of the cardiac arrhythmias with quinidine. Am. Heart J. **42:** 771–797.
48. SAMET, J. M. & B. SURAWICZ. 1974. Cardiac function in patients treated with phenothiazines. Comparison with quinidine. J. Clin. Pharmacol. **14:** 588–596.
49. COHEN, I. S., J. HERSHEL & S. I. COHEN. 1977. Adverse reactions to quinidine in hospitalized patients: Findings based on data from the Boston Collaborative Drug Surveillance Program. Prog. Cardiovasc. Dis. **20:** 151–163.
50. LEAHEY, E. B., J. A. REIFFEL, R. H. HEISSENBUTTEL, R. E. DRUSIN, W. P. LOVEJOY & J. T. BIGGER. 1979. Enhanced cardiac effect of digoxin during quinidine treatment. Arch. Intern. Med. **139:** 519–521.
51. BIGGER, J. T. 1982. The quinidine-digoxin interaction. Am. Heart J. **51:** 73–78.
52. BELZ, G. G., P. E. AUST, W. DOERING, M. HEINZ & B. SCHNEIDER. 1982. Pharmacodynamics of a single dose of quinidine during chronic digoxin treatment. Eur. J. Clin. Pharmacol. **22:** 117–122.
53. BELZ, G. G., W. DOERING, P. E. AUST, M. HEINZ, J. MATHEWS & B. SCHNEIDER. 1982. Quinidine-digoxin interaction: Cardiac efficacy of elevated serum digoxin concentration. Clin. Pharmacol. Ther. **31:** 548–554.
54. WARNER, N. J., E. B. LEAHEY, T. J. HOUGEN, J. T. BIGGER & T. W. SMITH. 1983. Tissue digoxin concentrations during the quinidine-digoxin interaction. Am. J. Cardiol. **51:** 1717–1721.

# Procainamide: Clinical Pharmacology and Efficacy against Ventricular Arrhythmias[a]

ELSA-GRACE V. GIARDINA

*Department of Medicine*
*College of Physicians & Surgeons*
*Columbia University*
*New York, New York 10032*

## INTRODUCTION

Procainamide has been in clinical use for more than 30 years and millions of patients have been exposed to it. That it is effective against ventricular arrhythmias and relatively well tolerated has been documented. The purpose of this report is to review and update information on the electrophysiology, mechanism of action, efficacy, clinical pharmacology, and adverse effects of procainamide (PA).

## ELECTROPHYSIOLOGY AND PHARMACOLOGY

Procainamide, like other drugs with a local anesthetic action, depresses the responsiveness of cardiac cells (TABLE 1).[1-4] It will decrease maximum rate of depolarization, amplitude, and overshoot of the action potential upstroke recorded from atrial and ventricular muscle fiber and Purkinje fibers.[1-4] These effects become more intense as PA concentration increases and are not accompanied by a significant change in resting membrane potential. Conduction velocity and excitability are also decreased progressively as drug concentration rises. Procainamide also delays repolarization and increases the duration of refractoriness in atrial and ventricular muscle fibers and Purkinje fibers. The effective refractory period (ERP) of all cell types increases more than would be expected from changes in duration of the action potential. Moreover, PA decreases the slope of phase-4 depolarization, which is associated with normal automaticity. The effect of PA on sinus node function is dependent on preexisting function of the sinus node. In patients with normal sinus function, PA probably has no adverse effects; on the other hand, with preexisting sinus node dysfunction, PA prolongs the corrected sinus node recovery time and enhances conduction[5] in the sinoatrial junction.

[a] This work was supported in part by Grant HL 27206 from the National Heart, Lung, and Blood Institute of the National Institutes of Health.

**TABLE 1.** Electrophysiologic and Electrocardiographic Effects of PA and NAPA

| Effects | PA | NAPA |
|---|---|---|
| Electrophysiologic (Purkinje fibers) | | |
| Normal automaticity | ↓ | NC[a] |
| Membrane responsiveness | ↓ | NC |
| Action potential duration | ↑ | ↑ |
| Effective refractory period | ↑ | NC/↑ |
| Conduction velocity | ↓ | NC |
| Afterdepolarizations | NC | ↑ |
| Electrocardiographic | | |
| P-R | ↑ | NC |
| QRS | ↑ | NC |
| Q-Tc | ↑ | ↑ |

[a] NC = no change.

## Effect on the Heart and Circulation

As might be expected from its effects on electrical activity of single cardiac cells, PA causes dose-dependent changes which may be observed from a standard 12-lead electrocardiogram. Within the therapeutic plasma concentration range, prolongation of the P-R, QRS, and Q-Tc intervals can be expected; on the other hand, PA has no significant effect on the R-R interval (TABLE 1).[6] In contrast to some new antiarrhythmic agents, such as encainide[7] and flecainide,[8] procainamide does not exert a very marked effect on P-R and QRS duration. Clinical electrophysiologic studies reveal that PA prolongs the ERP of the atrium, may shorten the A-H interval, and usually prolongs the H-V interval (His-Purkinje conduction).[4] High plasma PA concentrations have been associated with atrioventricular block, asystole, intraventricular conduction defects, and ventricular arrhythmias including VPDs, ventricular tachycardia and ventricular fibrillation. Progressive prolongation of the QRS as plasma PA concentration increases is frequently used to assess myocardial effect; and widening of the QRS interval >25 percent has been recommended as an endpoint to PA dosing.

## MECHANISM OF ACTION

The mechanism of action of PA against ventricular arrhythmias has been inferred from its electrophysiologic properties. PA increases the effective refractory period of atrial and ventricular fibers (by decreasing the ability of incompletely repolarized fibers to generate an active response and by delaying completion of repolarization), which may in part account for its antifibrillatory effects.[1-4] Since the atrial rate in fibrillation and flutter decrease, PA probably slows the maximum repetition rate for a cell until it is not possible for a circulating wave front of excitation to find a mass of excitable cells.[4]

The mechanism of action of PA against ventricular premature depolarizations (VPDs) is dependent on the genesis of the arrhythmia (TABLE 2). Arrhythmias due to altered automaticity may be interrupted by suppression of phase-4 depolarization in conjunction with a shift in the level of threshold potential toward zero.[2,4] Arrhythmias which have their genesis in depressed conduction and unidirectional block, that is, reentrant arrhythmias, may be suppressed by other mechanisms. If premature depolarizations result from reentry, it is possible that PA depresses conduction in a reentrant circuit such that unidirectional block is converted to bidirectional block.[9] In support of this view, we showed that as the plasma PA concentration rises, the coupling interval of reentrant VPDs progressively lengthen until VPDs are completely abolished. This clinical observation is a compelling piece of evidence that reentrant arrhythmias are suppressed by converting unidirectional to bidirectional block. Termination might also result from prolongation of the effective refractory period in tissues proximal to the site of reentry.

## EFFICACY OF PROCAINAMIDE

Procainamide is a broad-spectrum agent that has been in clinical use for more than 30 years[10-12] for treating ventricular arrhythmias. Patients with chronic stable VPDs[13-15] and patients with post myocardial infarction[6,16,17] as well as patients with sustained ventricular arrhythmias have all been exposed to PA.[18,19] It has been shown to reduce or abolish ventricular arrhythmias in the acute setting in up to 90% of patients with VPDs and 80% of patients with ventricular tachycardia[6,10,11] (TABLE 3). In a double-blind study by Koch-Weser et al.,[17] the prophylactic effect of PA was evaluated in 70 patients with uncomplicated myocardial infarction. PA gave significant protection against all types of ventricular arrhythmias without major adverse effects. On the other hand, there are also studies that do not support these beneficial findings. Kosowsky et al.[20] found no statistically significant difference in VPD frequency between control and treated groups (39 patients), although advanced grades of arrhythmia were diminished.[20] Koch-Weser and Klein[16] found an antiarrhythmic effect in 65% of 218 patients with chronic ventricular arrhythmias treated with PA. Other studies have shown similar results in patients with chronic ventricular arrhythmias.[21,22] In a study to evaluate the efficacy of a sustained-release PA formulation we found that 76% of the patients had at least a 75% reduction in VPD frequency (FIG. 1) and complex features. More than 50% of the patients responded at doses between 3.0 and 4.5 g/day (FIG. 2).

One dilemma about procainamide's efficacy relates to the fact that it was marketed before strict criteria for judging antiarrhythmic efficacy were established. Recently, investigators have commented on the length of drug-free moni-

TABLE 2. Mechanism of Action of PA

| Mechanism Responsible for Ventricular Arrhythmia | Mechanism of Action of Procainamide |
| --- | --- |
| *Abnormality of automaticity* | |
| Altered normal automaticity | Suppression of phase-4 depolarization; shifts threshold potential towards zero |
| Early afterdepolarizations | |
| Delayed afterdepolarizations | |
| Triggered arrhythmias | Prevents inciting of premature depolarizations |
| *Reentry* | |
| Altered fast responses | Decreases responsiveness; decreases conduction velocity |
| Slow responses and very slow conduction | Prolongs ERP; decreases responsiveness; decreases conduction velocity |

**TABLE 3.** Procainamide's Efficacy against VPDs

| Author | Number of Patients | Number Success-fully Treated | Percentage | Daily Dose | Plasma Concentration ($\mu$g/ml) |
|---|---|---|---|---|---|
| Kayden et al.[11] (1957) | 185 | 162 | 88 | 1–6 g/day | 10–20[a] |
| Koch-Weser et al.[17] (1969) | 37 | 23 | 62 | 2–4 g/day | 4–6[a] |
| Giardina et al.[6] (1973) | 20 | 17 | 85 | 300–1000 mg | 4–10[a] |
| Jelinek et al.[22] (1974) | 23 | 8 | 35 | 3–6 g/day | 3–12[a] |
| Winkle et al.[45] (1978) | 10 | 6 | 60 | 3 g/day | — |
| Giardina et al.[15] (1980) | 33 | 25 | 76 | 3–7.5 g/day | 2–17[a] 2–25[b] |

[a] Procainamide
[b] NAPA.

toring and percentage of VPD suppression required to judge antiarrhythmic efficacy.[23-25] Since many data regarding the antiarrhythmic effect of procainamide antedated these recent reports, PA has not been subjected to as rigorous testing as have many antiarrhythmic drugs in clinical trials.[7,8,26,27] Although millions of patients have been treated successfully with PA, studies using PA versus newer antiarrhythmic agents will have to address this issue in the future.

The value of PA in managing patients with sustained ventricular arrhythmias has been reported.[18,19] In one study PA was found to prevent initiation of VT in 45% of patients, and where arrhythmia was not prevented, resultant VT was slower.[18] In other laboratories, however, this has not been the case, and a number

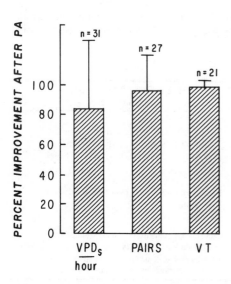

FIGURE 1. Percent improvement in frequency of VPDs per hour and complex features after PA. The numbers above each of the bars refer to the number of patients with each event.

of variables including patient population, method of drug administration, number of repetitive stimuli required to evaluate inducible arrhythmia, and use of other drugs (beta blockers, nitrates, calcium channel antagonists) may all account for this.

The therapeutic antiarrhythmic plasma concentration range of PA against acute VPDs has been determined and spans from 4 to 10 mg per liter.[6,16] This range may vary among patients and in different clinical situations, and to achieve and maintain an effective concentration requires individualization of dosage. The typical or average dose may lead to ineffective arrhythmia control in some patients and untoward adverse effects in others or result in a wide range of plasma drug concentration (FIG. 3). The average plasma concentration of drug required for suppression of chronic stable VPDs is higher than that for acute arrhythmias and those seen after myocardial infarction, that is, the range is 2 to 17 mg per liter (TABLE 3, FIG. 3).[15] The average plasma concentration that prevents initiation of sustained ventricular tachyarrhythmias is high, and in some cases higher than

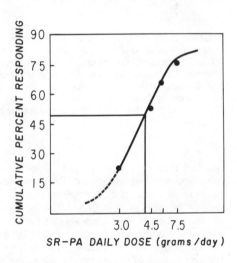

FIGURE 2. Cumulative percent of patients who responded to sustained-release procainamide (SR-PA) with arrhythmia suppression (75 percent or more reduction in VPD frequency) in relation to the effective dose of the drug. Arrhythmia was suppressed in more than half of the patients with a dosage of < 4.5 grams per day.

SR−PA DAILY DOSE (grams /day )

previously considered acceptable.[18] The average PA concentration required to prevent initiation of ventricular tachycardia is about 14.0 mg per liter, with a range of 5 to 32 mg per liter.[18] However, Myerburg et al.[28] suggested that even when drug levels are not very high and mean VPD suppression is less than 70% (mean = 36%), there is a beneficial effect from PA which may be important in preventing sudden death. We noted that even relatively low plasma concentrations of PA are associated with reduction in frequency of complex ventricular arrhythmias, including ventricular tachycardia, before VPD frequency is significantly reduced.[15] It may be that suppression of complex features with PA is sufficient to protect against malignant outcome in some patients.

## PHARMACOKINETICS

TABLE 4 summarizes the pharmacokinetics of PA. The bioavailability of orally administered PA ranges from 75 to 95 percent.[13,14] Peak plasma concentration is

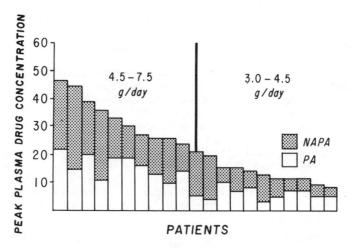

**FIGURE 3.** *Peak* plasma NAPA concentration in patients with greater than 75 percent VPD suppression after SR-PA; the *vertical line* represents the median. All patients received from 3.0 to 7.5 grams SR-PA per day. Wide variation in peak plasma PA and peak plasma NAPA is noted. Dose size, different rates of gastrointestinal absorption of sustained-release PA, variable rates and extent of metabolism, diminished renal function, or an altered volume of distribution could all account for the variability observed. Bars 1–6 (from left) show very high plasma peak PA and NAPA concentration and these patients received between 6 and 7.5 grams SR-PA daily.

reached relatively rapidly, that is, within 1.5 to 2 hours. An advantage of sustained-release formulations of PA is that the "peak" concentration is attenuated because of prolonged absorption from the gastrointestinal tract.[13,14,29] A small amount of PA is protein-bound (that is, 10 to 20 percent) and the apparent volume of distribution is very large (about 1.5 to 2.5 liters per kg body weight).[13] However, the volume of distribution can be significantly reduced under conditions such as congestive heart failure or cardiogenic shock, resulting in higher concentrations from a dose. At steady state, the myocardium-to-plasma PA concentration ratio is 3 : 1. The $t_{1/2}$ elimination of the parent compound is reported to range from 3 to 5 hours; however, this time can be significantly prolonged in patients with diminished renal function or low output states. The active metabolite, $N$-acetylprocainamide (NAPA), which is renally excreted, accumulates to an even greater extent in renal failure.[30,31] In contrast to quinidine, PA does not interact with digoxin.[32]

**TABLE 4.** Clinical Pharmacology of Procainamide

|  |  |
|---|---|
| Bioavailability | 75–95% |
| Half-time for absorption | 0.5 hr |
| Volume of distribution | 1.5–2.5 liter/kg |
| Plasma protein-binding | 15–25% |
| Effective plasma concentration | 4–10 µg/ml |
| Half-time for elimination | 3–5 hr |
| Total body clearance | 300–700 ml/min |
| Excretion of unchanged drug | 30–60% |

## Intravenous Administration

Of all currently available antiarrhythmic agents, PA is the most versatile since it may be given intravenously, orally, or intramuscularly. In acute situations where a drug must be administered rapidly, *intermittent intravenous* PA can be given 100 mg over 5 minutes, through an indwelling intravenous catheter.[6] With this method, blood pressure is measured every 5 minutes after a dose, and continuous electrocardiographic monitoring of ECG intervals accompanies the intravenous injection. This method results in a graded decrease in frequency of VPDs and predictable increase of plasma PA concentration.[6] The formula: $y = 0.84 + 0.73x$ describes the relationship between plasma PA concentration ($y$) and dose of PA administered in milligrams per kilogram ($x$) and allows one to predict the plasma PA concentration after this method of drug administration if weight and total dose of PA are known. This method has been useful in treating patients with chronic stable VPDs as well as those with life-threatening ventricular arrhythmias. With intermittent intravenous injection of PA, significant hypotension is unusual in contrast to hypotension observed after intravenous injection of quinidine. Very high plasma concentrations of PA, however, can diminish myocardial performance and induce hypotension, particularly in patients with preexisting reduced left ventricular performance and low ejection fraction. An alternate method of PA administration for rapid control of arrhythmias would be to administer drug via a *rapid* constant rate infusion; thus, the same dose would be given, but at a constant-rate infusion, that is, 10–20 mg per minute.

After the acute arrhythmia has been controlled, we begin a constant-rate intravenous infusion to maintain effective plasma concentrations. Infusion rate can be estimated as the product of the desired plasma concentration (4 to 10 mg per liter) and estimated total clearance of PA (400 to 700 ml per min). For example, if PA clearance is estimated to be 500 ml per minute and the desired plasma concentration is 8 mg per ml, 4.0 mg per minute would be infused.

## Oral Administration

Oral administration is the most widely used method of giving PA for treatment of chronic stable VPDs. In general, 500 to 1000 mg every 4 to 6 hours has been shown to be a satisfactory schedule for many patients taking conventional PA.[16,17] This dosing interval was established on the basis of the half-life of elimination of PA, that is, 3 to 5 hours. However, many cardiac patients have significantly longer half-lives of elimination than do normal subjects because of decreased renal function and/or low cardiac output states. Moreover, since NAPA has antiarrhythmic effects,[33-36] it may contribute to a sustained antiarrhythmic effect, allowing longer dosing intervals than those predicted from the half-life of PA. To improve patient compliance, sustained-release formulations[14,15,29] that take account of delayed GI absorption have been developed to avoid peak and nadir plasma concentrations.

## Intramuscular Procainamide

Although not widely used, intramuscular administration of PA is possible.[4] Approximately 90 to 100% of an intramuscular dose will be absorbed, although intramuscular absorption offers little advantage over oral therapy since absorption time, time to peak, and plasma concentrations are approximately the same.

## ADVERSE EXTRACARDIAC EFFECTS

A number of extracardiac effects have been reported, including gastrointestinal symptoms (anorexia, nausea, vomiting), central nervous system symptoms (headache, dizziness, psychosis, hallucinations, and depression), fever, agranulocytosis, rash, myalgias, digital vasculitis, and Raynaud's phenomenon.[16,20,29,37]

The most worrisome adverse effect associated with PA is the systemic lupus-like syndrome.[38,39] This syndrome was reported to occur relatively late after administration of PA and to be associated with large doses. Kosowsky and associates[20] report that this complication develops in more than 50 percent of patients taking procainamide. We note that in approximately 60% of patients taking PA results of the antinuclear antibody test will convert from negative to positive, but that the SLE-like syndrome develops in fewer than 15 percent.

Efforts have been made by a number of investigators to determine whether the potential for developing the SLE-like syndrome is predictable.[40-43] Investigators have focused on rate of acetylation to assess whether slow or fast acetylators are more likely to develop adverse effects. In large part, this approach was based on the observation that the drug hydralazine (acetylated by the enzyme with a bimodal distribution) is more likely to cause SLE in slow than in fast acetylators. The relationship between the fraction of NAPA in urine and plasma samples versus acetylation phenotype determined with isoniazid (INH) or dapsone has been reported. However, acetylation phenotype determined from the fraction of NAPA recovered in timed urine or plasma samples has limitations. For example, a subject who is a phenotypic slow acetylator but who has a prolonged rate of renal excretion due to congestive heart failure or renal disease can excrete a very large fraction as NAPA. We compared the metabolism of PA to sulfamethazine (SMZ), which is controlled by the hepatic N-acetyltransferase enzyme with a bimodal distribution. We could not be certain that the enzyme accounting for acetylation of PA is the same as for SMZ or dapsone.[40]

Woosley and associates[42] investigated the relation between acetylator phenotype and development of PA-induced adverse effects. They observed that 18 of 20 subjects had a positive antinuclear antibody test after 1 year on PA and, moreover, that slow acetylators developed positive antinuclear antibody more rapidly and at a lower PA dose than did fast acetylators. They concluded that acetylator phenotype influences rate at which PA induces antinuclear antibodies and the SLE-like syndrome. We prospectively tested acetylation phenotype in patients taking PA. Acetylation phenotype did not reliably predict incidence of adverse effects, that is, fast acetylators developed adverse effects with the same frequency as did slow acetylators.[15] One patient who developed the SLE-like syndrome was a slow acetylator. While it is probably true that slow acetylators are more likely to be at risk for developing the SLE-like syndrome, fast acetylation phenotype does not offer protection from other adverse effects.

## N-ACETYLPROCAINAMIDE

In 1976, the metabolism of PA in man was studied[13] and NAPA was reported to be procainamide's major metabolite. Radioactive studies[13] indicate that NAPA is found in large quantities in plasma and urine of many patients and a small portion of PA is also metabolized to two unknown metabolites, Rf = 0.0 and Rf = 0.3.[13] There is wide interindividual variability in the amount of PA and NAPA recovered after a dose and this variability is dependent on genetic predisposition, factors that affect drug metabolism and excretion, and differences in volume of distribution, clearance, and so forth.

The discovery of NAPA was underscored by the finding that it had electrophysiological properties in animal models[44] and antiarrhythmic effects[33-35] in humans. NAPA's electrophysiological effects, however, are not identical to those of procainamide.[44] In isolated Purkinje fibers, NAPA does not alter phase-0 upstroke or phase-4 depolarization, but does prolong action potential duration (TABLE 1). In both dogs and humans, NAPA has no consistent effect on intraventricular or His-Purkinje conduction times, but does prolong ventricular refractoriness and Q-T intervals. The lack of effect on His-Purkinje conduction times at therapeutic concentrations makes the electrophysiological effects different from procainamide's. Findings in animals parallel changes on the electrocardiogram which show that NAPA prolongs the Q-Tc interval, but does not alter P-R or QRS duration.

Initial reports were optimistic about NAPA's antiarrhythmic effects, and NAPA's pharmacokinetics, with a mean half-life of elimination of 7.5 hours, suggested that NAPA might be useful in enhancing patient compliance. Long-term use, however, has been disappointing, not only because of recurrent arrhythmias, but also because of a relatively high incidence of minor adverse effects.

One area of particular interest has been the use of NAPA for patients who developed the SLE-like syndrome. A number of independent investigators[33-35] observed that NAPA could be used to treat patients unable to take PA because of the SLE-like syndrome. Roden and associates[33] suggested that NAPA might be useful in a subset of patients with ventricular arrhythmias in whom either the potential for developing the SLE-like syndrome was high or who had previously had the syndrome. Remission of PA-induced lupus when treatment is changed to NAPA and failure of NAPA to induce the SLE-like syndrome suggest that the aromatic amino group on the PA molecule may cause drug-induced lupus.

In summary, PA has been clinically useful for more than 30 years. Recent studies indicate that it continues to be an important agent for managing acute and chronic ventricular arrhythmias; doses and plasma concentrations must be individualized, depending on the clinical setting and patients' physiology as well as the genesis of the arrhythmia under consideration.

# SUMMARY

Procainamide (PA) has been a mainstay of treatment against acute and chronic supraventricular and ventricular arrhythmias for more than 30 years. PA's clinical pharmacology has been studied extensively and its bioavailability (75–95%); volume of distribution (1.5–2.5 liters per kg), plasma protein-binding (15–25%), half-time for elimination (3–7 hours), and metabolism are known. PA's efficacy against acute ventricular arrhythmias and chronic stable VPDs is associated with plasma drug concentrations of 4 to 10 $\mu$g per ml; but much higher plasma concentrations may be required against sustained ventricular arrhythmias. From 30 to 60% of a PA dose is excreted as the metabolite, $N$-acetylprocainamide (NAPA), and PA's metabolism is determined genetically (fast or slow acetylation phenotype). Studies in patients with VPDs indicate that NAPA is also antiarrhythmic, although the contribution of NAPA to the antiarrhythmic effect after PA is not known. Studies in patients with the systemic lupus-like syndrome from PA show that NAPA is not associated with this. Investigations comparing efficacy and adverse effects of PA with those of new antiarrhythmic agents available for clinical trials are indicated in the future.

## ACKNOWLEDGMENT

Grateful acknowledgment is made to Ms. May Louie for her assistance in preparation of this manuscript.

## REFERENCES

1. HOFFMAN, B. F. 1958. The action of quinidine and procaine amide on single fiber of dog ventricule and specialized conducting system. An. Acad. Bras. Cienc. **29:** 365.
2. HOFFMAN, B. F., M. R. ROSEN & A. L. WIT. 1975. Electrophysiology and pharmacology of cardiac arrhythmias. VII. Cardiac effects of quinidine and procaine amide. Am. Heart J. **90:** 117–122.
3. WOSKE, H., J. BELFORD, F. N. FASTIER & C. M. C. BROOKS. 1953. The effect of procaine amide on excitability, refractoriness and conduction in the mammalian heart. J. Pharmacol. Exp. Ther. **107:** 134–140.
4. HOFFMAN, B. F. & J. T. BIGGER, JR. 1971. Antiarrhythmic drugs. *In* Drill's Pharmacology in Medicine, Chapt. 40. J. Di Palma, Ed. McGraw-Hill. New York, NY.
5. GOLDBERG, D., J. A. REIFFEL, J. C. DAVIS, E. GANG, F. LIVELLI & J. T. BIGGER, JR. 1982. Electrophysiologic effects of procainamide on sinus node function in patients with and without sinus node disease. Am. Heart J. **103:** 75–79.
6. GIARDINA, E. G. V., R. H. HEISSENBUTTEL & J. T. BIGGER, JR. 1973. Intermittent intravenous procainamide to treat ventricular arrhythmias: Correlation of plasma concentration with effect on arrhythmia, electrocardiogram, and blood pressure. Ann. Intern. Med. **78:** 183–193.
7. RODEN, D. M., S. B. REELE, S. B. HIGGINS, R. F. MAYOL, R. E. GAMMANS, J. A. OATES & R. L. WOOSLEY. 1980. Total suppression of ventricular arrhythmias by encainide. N. Engl. J. Med. **302:** 877–882.
8. ANDERSON, J. L., J. R. STEWART, B. A. PERRY, D. D. V. HAMERSVELD, T. A. JOHNSON, G. J. CONARD, S. F. CHANG, D. C. KVAM & B. PITT. 1981. Oral flecainide for the treatment of ventricular arrhythmias. N. Engl. J. Med. **305:** 473–477.
9. GIARDINA, E. G. V. & J. T. BIGGER, JR. 1973. Procaine amide against reentrant ventricular arrhythmias. Circulation **48:** 959–968.
10. KAYDEN, H. J., J. M. STEELE, L. C. CLARK & B. B. BRODIE. 1951. The use of procainamide in cardiac arrhythmias. Circulation **4:** 13–22.
11. KAYDEN, H. J., B. B. BRODIE & J. M. SKELE. 1957. Procainamide: A review. Circulation **15:** 118–126.
12. MCCORD, M. C. & J. T. TAGUCHI. 1951. A study of the effect of procaine amide hydrochloride in supraventricular arrhythmias. Circulation **4:** 387–393.
13. GIARDINA, E. G. V., J. DREYFUSS, J. T. BIGGER, JR., J. M. SHAW & E. C. SCHREIBER. 1976. Metabolism of procainamide in normal and cardiac subjects. Clin. Pharmacol. Ther. **19:** 339–351.
14. GRAFFNER, C., G. JOHNSSON & J. SJOGREN. 1975. Pharmacokinetics of procainamide intravenously and orally as conventional and slow-release tablets. Clin. Pharmacol. Ther. **17:** 414–423.
15. GIARDINA, E. G. V., P. E. FENSTER, J. T. BIGGER, JR., M. MAYERSOHN, D. PERRIER & F. I. MARCUS. 1980. Efficacy, plasma concentrations and adverse effects of a new sustained release procainamide preparation. Am. J. Cardiol. **46:** 855–861.
16. KOCH-WESER, J. & S. M. KLEIN. 1971. Procainamide dosage schedules, plasma concentrations and clinical effects. JAMA **215:** 1454–1460.

17. KOCH-WESER, J., S. W. KLEIN, L. L. FOO-CANTO, J. A. KASTOR & R. W. DESANCTIS. 1969. Antiarrhythmic prophylaxis with procainamide in acute myocardial infarction. N. Engl. J. Med. **281:** 1253–1260.

18. HOROWITZ, L. N., M. E. JOSEPHSON & J. A. KASTOR. 1980. Intracardiac electrophysiologic studies as a method for the optimization of drug therapy in chronic ventricular arrhythmia. Prog. Cardiovasc. Dis. **23:** 81–98.

19. GREENSPAN, A. M., L. N. HOROWITZ, S. R. SPIELMAN & M. E. JOSEPHSON. 1980. Large-dose procainamide therapy for ventricular tachycardia. Am. J. Cardiol. **46:** 453–462.

20. KOSOWSKY, B. D., J. TAYLOR, B. LOWN & R. F. RITCHIE. 1973. Long-term use of procaine amide following acute myocardial infarction. Circulation **42:** 1204–1210.

21. KARLSSON, E. 1975. Procainamide and phenytoin. Comparative study of their antiarrhythmic effects at apparent therapeutic plasma levels. Br. Heart J. **3:** 731–740.

22. JELINEK, M. V., L. LOHRBAUER & B. LOWN. 1974. Antiarrhythmic drug therapy for sporadic ventricular arrhythmias. Circulation **49:** 659–666.

23. WINKLE, R. A. 1978. Antiarrhythmic drug effect mimicked by spontaneous variability of ventricular ectopy. Circulation **57:** 1116–1121.

24. MORGANROTH, J., E. L. MICHELSON, L. N. HOROWITZ, M. E. JOSEPHSON, A. S. PEARLMAN & W. B. DUNKMAN. 1978. Limitations of routine long-term electrocardiographic monitoring to assess ventricular ectopic frequency. Circulation **58:** 408–414.

25. SAMI, M., D. C. HARRISON, H. KRAMER, N. HOUSTON, C. SHIMASAKI & R. F. DEBUSK. 1981. Antiarrhythmic efficacy of encainide and quinidine: Validation of a model for drug assessment. Am. J. Cardiol. **48:** 147–156.

26. ZIPES, D. P. & P. J. TROUP. 1978. New antiarrhythmic agents. Am. J. Cardiol. **41:** 1005–1024.

27. PODRID, P. J., A. LYAKISHEV, B. LOWN & N. MAZUR. 1980. Ethmozin, a new antiarrhythmic drug for suppressing ventricular premature complexes. Circulation **61:** 450–457.

28. MYERBURG, R. J., K. M. KESSLER, I. KIEM, K. C. PEFKARAS, C. A. CONDE, D. COOPER & A. CASTELLANOS. 1981. Relationship between plasma levels of procainamide, suppression of premature ventricular complexes and prevention of recurrent ventricular tachycardia. Circulation **64:** 280–289.

29. KARLSSON, E. 1973. Plasma levels of procaine amide after administration of conventional and sustained-release tablets. Eur. J. Clin. Pharmacol. **6:** 245–250.

30. DRAYER, D. E., D. T. LOWENTHAL, R. L. WOOSLEY, A. S. NIES, A. SCHWARTZ & M. M. REIDENBERG. 1977. Cumulation of N-acetylprocainamide, an active metabolite of procainamide in patients with impaired renal function. Clin. Pharmacol. Ther. **22:** 63–69.

31. STRONG, J. M., J. S. DUTCHER, W.-K. LEE & A. J. ATKINSON, JR. 1975. Pharmacokinetics in man of the N-acetylated metabolite of procainamide. J. Pharmacokinet. Biopharm. **3:** 223–235.

32. LEAHEY, E. B., J. A. REIFFEL, E. G. V. GIARDINA & J. T. BIGGER, JR. 1980. The effect of quinidine and other oral antiarrhythmic drugs on serum digoxin: a prospective study. Ann. Int. Med. **92:** 605–608.

33. RODEN, D. M., S. B. REELE, S. B. HIGGINS, G. R. WILKINSON, R. F. SMITH, J. A. OATES & R. L. WOOSLEY. 1980. Antiarrhythmic efficacy, pharmacokinetics and safety of N-acetylprocainamide in human subjects: Comparison with procainamide. Am. J. Cardiol. **46:** 463–468.

34. ATKINSON, A. J., JR., W. K. LEE, M. L. QUINN, W. KUSHER, M. J. NEVIN & J. M. STRONG. 1977. Dose-ranging trial of N-acetylprocainamide in patients with premature ventricular contractions. Clin. Pharmacol. Ther. **21:** 575–587.

35. WINKLE, R. A., P. JAILLON, R. E. KATES & F. PETERS. 1981. Clinical pharmacology and antiarrhythmic efficacy of N-acetylprocainamide. Am. J. Cardiol. **47:** 123–130.

36. KLUGER, J., S. LEECH, M. M. REIDENBERG, V. LLOYD & D. E. DRAYER. 1981. Long-term antiarrhythmic therapy with acetylprocainamide Am. J. Cardiol. **48:** 1124–1132.

37.  BELLET, S., G. HAMDAN, A. SOMLYO & R. LARA. 1959. A reversal of the cardiotoxic effects of procaine amide by molar sodium lactate. Am. J. Med. Sci. **237:** 177–189.
38.  LADD, A. T. 1962. Procainamide-induced lupus erythematosus. N. Engl. J. Med. **267:** 1357–1358.
39.  LONDON, B. L. & I. PINCUS. 1966. Reversible lupus-like illness induced by procainamide. Am. Heart J. **71:** 806–808.
40.  GIARDINA, E. G. V., R. M. STEIN & J. T. BIGGER, JR. 1977. The relationship between the metabolism of procainamide and sulfamethazine. Circulation **55:** 388–394.
41.  REIDENBERG, M. M., D. E. DRAYER, M. M. LEVY & H. WARNER. 1975. Polymorphic acetylation of procainamide in man. Clin. Pharmacol. Ther. **17:** 722–730.
42.  WOOSLEY, R. L., D. E. DRAYER, M. M. REIDENBERG, A. S. NIES, K. CARR & J. A. OATES. 1978. Effect of acetylator phenotype on the rate at which procainamide induces antinuclear antibodies and the lupus syndrome. N. Engl. J. Med. **298:** 1157–1159.
43.  ALARCON-SEGOVIA, D. 1969. Drug-induced lupus syndromes. Mayo Clin. Proc. **44:** 664–681.
44.  DANGMAN, K. H. & B. F. HOFFMAN. 1981. In vivo and in vitro antiarrhythmic and arrhythmogenic effects of N-acetylprocainamide. J. Pharmacol. Exp. Ther. **217:** 851–862.
45.  WINKLE, R. A., A. H. GRADMAN, & J. W. FITZGERALD. 1978. Antiarrhythmic drug effect assessed from ventricular arrhythmia reduction in the ambulatory electrocardiogram and treadmill test: Comparison of propranolol, procainamide and quinidine. Am. J. Cardiol. **42:** 473–480.

# Disopyramide

E. M. VAUGHAN WILLIAMS

*Department of Pharmacology*
*Oxford University*
*Oxford, England*

Disopyramide was selected from more than 500 compounds synthesized for a research program designed to develop a new antiarrhythmic drug as an alternative to quinidine or procainamide, which were the main agents available in 1962. In FIGURE 1 the chemical structure of quinidine is compared with that of disopyramide, which bears some resemblance to the synthetic muscarinic antagonist lachesine.

## EFFECTS OBSERVED IN ANIMALS

### Normal Hearts

Mokler and Van Arman[1] found that atrial arrhythmias induced by aconitine in anesthetized dogs were suppressed by disopyramide at a mean dose of $2.7 \pm 0.5$ mg/kg (n = 9), and those electrically induced, at $5.8 \pm 0.9$ mg/kg ($n = 10$). The drug was orally active at a mean dose of 15 mg/kg. The effects of vagal stimulation in the anesthetized dog heart were abolished by 5 mg/kg of disopyramide intravenously. Cardiac output was depressed by more than 25% at 30 min, but blood pressure was not greatly affected. A substantial negative inotropic effect was demonstrated in isolated rabbit hearts also.[1,2] In the anesthetized animals disopyramide, 5 mg/kg, reduced heart rate by 17% at 30 min, but in conscious dogs the heart rate was more than doubled, illustrating at this early stage that the effects of disopyramide on the cardiovascular system depend critically upon the state of the autonomic background at the time the drug is administered.

The main electrophysiological effects of disopyramide were also established 20 years ago.[2] Like quinidine, procainamide, and several other agents then available,[3] disopyramide had no significant effect on resting potential, but the overshoot potential and maximum rate of depolarization were reduced, as illustrated in TABLE 1. In atrial muscle, action potential duration to 50% ($APD_{50}$) was not significantly altered, but the tail of the action potential was substantially prolonged. In Purkinje fibers (FIG. 2) $APD_{50}$ was actually shortened, an effect probably due to block of residually conducting sodium channels which fail to be inactivated at plateau potentials[4-6]; $APD_{90}$ was lengthened, as in the atrium.

In isolated rabbit atria, as in the anesthetized dog, disopyramide reduced the pacemaking frequency of the sinoatrial node in a dose-related manner. In spontaneously beating rabbit AV nodal pacemakers disopyramide also slowed the rate[7] by an effect largely due to prolongation of the APD, but there was also a reduction in the slope of the slow diastolic depolarization (FIG. 2). Both of these effects would be consistent with restriction of chloride current,[8-10] but no direct evidence concerning the effects of disopyramide in this context is available. Watanabe did observe, however, that disopyramide altered the clamp current required to hold the potential at $-40$ mV in these AV nodal pacemaking cells.[7]

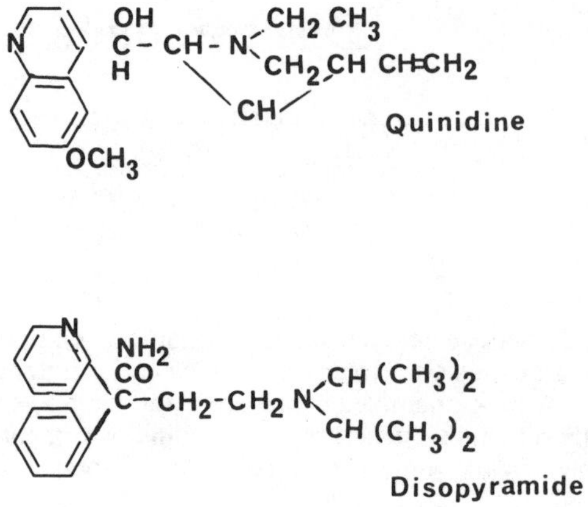

**FIGURE 1.** Chemical structures of quinidine and disopyramide.

Disopyramide had a definite and dose-related negative inotropic effect on rabbit isolated cardiac muscle.[2] The electrical threshold of normal muscle was raised, and conduction velocity slowed ($-20\%$ at a concentration of 4 $\mu g \cdot ml^{-1}$).

### Delayed Repolarization (Class 3 Action)

In the ventricular conduction system of dogs and rabbits the action potential duration in the bundle of His and ventricular muscle is much shorter than in the pre-terminal Purkinje cells. Lidocaine shortens APD throughout, but preferentially in the preterminal cells.[11] In contrast, amiodarone and its nonhalogenated congener, L9146, lengthened APD preferentially in those regions in which APD is normally shortest, the His bundle and ventricular muscle.[12] Indeed, if "false tendons" only had been used, as are customarily employed for electrophysiological studies, discovery of the APD-lengthening by amiodarone would have been missed. Kus and Sasyniuk[13] showed that $APD_{90}$ was prolonged by disopyramide

**TABLE 1.** Electrophysiological Effects of Disopyramide

| Concentration of Disopyramide ($\mu g \cdot ml^{-1}$) [$\mu mol \cdot l^{-1}$] | Resting Potential (mV) | Action Potential (mV) | Repolarization Times | | Maximum Rate of Depolarization (V·sec$^{-1}$) |
|---|---|---|---|---|---|
| | | | To 50% (msec) | To 95% (msec) | |
| 0.0 | 67.4 | 90.1 | 46.9 | 89.3 | 121 |
| 5.0 [14.8] | 64.1 | 84.0$^a$ | 47.8 | 111.0$^b$ | 51$^b$ |
| 8.0 [23.6] | 65.4 | 80.5$^b$ | 50.0 | 116.2$^b$ | 41$^b$ |

Statistical significance of differences:
$^a$ p < 0.05.
$^b$ p < 0.001.

in the ventricular pathway, with some preferential lengthening of $APD_{90}$ in proximal Purkinje cells and less lengthening in preterminal cells. In a subsequent paper by the same authors, however,[17] the lengthening $APD_{90}$ in the preterminal "gate" fibers was as great as in the His bundle; indeed, the increase (in the presence of 5 $\mu g \cdot ml^{-1}$ disopyramide in their Figure 1) was 41 msec in the regions in which the controls had both their shortest (at 4 mm from proximal end) and longest $APD_{90}$ (at 25 mm).

The effect of disopyramide on fast inward current was reduced when tissues were exposed to hyperpolarizing low K solutions[14] as has been observed with many other class 1 drugs.[15,16]

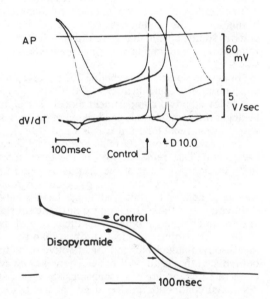

**FIGURE 2.** Effect of disopyramide 10 $\mu g \cdot ml^{-1}$, on intracellularly recorded potentials from a canine Purkinje fiber (*bottom*) and a spontaneously beating rabbit AV nodal pacemaker (*top*). The slowing of pacemaker rate was due partly to a reduction in the slope of the slow diastolic potential, partly to delayed repolarization, both of which effects would be consistent with restriction of chloride current. (Adapted from Watanabe.[7] Reproduced by permission.)

## Ischemic Muscle

In another group of experiments, in Purkinje fibers taken from experimentally infarcted regions in which $APD_{90}$ was already prolonged, disopyramide increased $APD_{90}$ from a mean of 365 to 373 msec, an increase of only 8 msec as compared with a mean increase of 18 msec (304 to 322) reported for normal fibers. It was thus suggested that disopyramide would reduce the disparities of APD between infarcted and normal regions, and that this could contribute to its antiarrhythmic action, but it seems doubtful whether this difference of only 10 msec could be of great importance.

In anesthetized dogs in which the left descending coronary artery was occluded for 10 minutes and then released,[18] treatment with disopyramide 3.3 $mg \cdot kg^{-1}$, just before occlusion, and with a further 2.2 $mg \cdot kg^{-1}$ in mid-occlusion, provided a significant protection against arrhythmias induced during and after the occlusion. It was of interest that in the control group none of the dogs in which arrhythmias did not occur during the occlusion (48%) suffered ventricular fibrillation on reperfusion. In the treated group 86% had no arrhythmias during occlusion, and again none of these had ventricular fibrillation on reperfusion.

Thus the evidence is clear from animal experiments that disopyramide is a potent antiarrhythmic agent in both fully oxygenated and ischemic cardiac muscle.

## EFFECTS OF DISOPYRAMIDE IN MAN

The first clinical studies of the antiarrhythmic action of disopyramide were reported 20 years ago,[19] but the drug was not widely used for more than a decade. It was not available in the United States until 1977. Recognition that the incidence of arrhythmias associated with myocardial infarction is high[20] and that ventricular fibrillation is the commonest cause of sudden death[21] led to a search for new antiarrhythmic agents that were orally active and suitable for out-of-hospital use. Interest in disopyramide was thus reawakened, and human studies were intensified.

In human volunteers receiving 200 mg disopyramide by mouth the mean peak concentration, occurring after $1.75 \pm 0.5$ hr, was $3.34 \pm 0.46$ $\mu g \cdot ml^{-1}$.[22] Elimination followed a two-compartment model. The alpha distribution phase was rapid, lasting a few minutes only, and the beta phase $4.35 \pm 1.3$ hr (but in two patients with chronic renal failure it was 8.3 and 8.9 hr).

In normal subjects 81% of an oral dose appeared in the plasma, and since first-pass metabolism removes 16% in the liver, total absorption may be assumed. Sixty to eighty percent of the drug is excreted unchanged in the urine, uninfluenced by pH. One of the isopropyl groups is removed from the amino nitrogen, leaving a metabolite which, although having only one-fifth the concentration of disopyramide in the plasma, may contribute substantially to side effects because it has an anticholinergic potency 24 times that of the drug itself.[23]

In an electrophysiological study in man by Josephson et al.[24] it was shown that disopyramide prolonged the effective refractory period (ERP) of the atrium, but reduced that of the AV node. There was no consistent effect on spontaneous heart rate. According to Josephson, "Several patients showed enhancement of AV nodal conduction during atrial pacing. Disopyramide does not depress AV nodal or His-Purkinje conduction, and might, therefore, be indicated in the treatment of arrhythmias which are associated with some degree of atrio-ventricular block"[24] Since in isolated preparations and anesthetised dogs disopyramide depresses nodal function by a direct action, the net effect in patients depends on the background vagal tone. When this was abolished by atropine, it was found that disopyramide always depressed sinus node automaticity and increased atrioventricular refractoriness.[25] Disopyramide was given to twelve patients with sinus node disease, resulting in deleterious effects in nine.[26]

Disopyramide prolonged ventricular refractoriness[27,28] and in the Wolff-Parkinson-White syndrome conduction through the accessory pathway was depressed or blocked. On the other hand, AV conduction was unaffected or improved, and it was suggested that the delay within the reentry circuit of conduction through the accessory pathway gave more time for the AV nodal part of the pathway to recover. The anticholinergic effect of disopyramide could also have contributed.

Disopyramide not only has proved effective in ventricular arrhythmias involving multiple ectopic beats, close-coupled extrasystoles, and ventricular tachycardias, but has also controlled some supraventricular arrhythmias.[28] The therapeutic plasma concentration required is in the range 2.5 to 4 $\mu g/ml$, which can usually be achieved with an initial dose of 200–300 mg, followed by 100–150 mg every 6 hours.

Two papers describing the effects of disopyramide in patients with recent myocardial infarction have aroused much comment. In the first[31] 49 patients were treated with placebo, and 46 with disopyramide, 100 mg 6-hourly, in the coronary care unit. In the treated patients there was a 50% reduction of ventricular arrhythmias, but little effect on atrial arrhythmias. In the second study[32] the patients were in open wards, and 30 were treated with placebo, 30 with disopyramide. There was a significant reduction in arrhythmias and mortality in the treated group. It was noteworthy, however, that in the *placebo* groups there were nine reinfarctions and five deaths in the first study, and eleven extensions of myocardial infarction and eleven deaths in the second (37%). In a comparative study of treatment of myocardial infarction in coronary care units and in open wards, Hill *et al.* found in the open ward a mortality of only 12% in patients under 65 and 25% in patients over 65.[33]

Proof of the beneficial effects of a drug in ischemic heart disease is notoriously difficult to obtain. The outcome is influenced by many factors, which include anxiety, exertion, tobacco, diet and life-style. Even in the acute phase in hospital after myocardial infarction, possibly relevant variables are hard to control, and the smaller the series, the greater the risk of mismatch between control and treated groups. In spite of much effort and the study of large numbers of patients, the prophylactic efficacy of sulfinpyrazone was hard to establish,[34] and the benefits of long-term beta blockade were proven only after several trials and the study of thousands of patients.[35-37] Nevertheless Zainal *et al.*[32] recommended that "oral disopyramide should be given for the first seven days to all patients not managed in an intensive care unit." The advice has not, however, been widely followed.

Disopyramide is not without side effects, some of which may be attributed to its anticholinergic action. Apart from dry mouth, which is transient, retention of urine may present a problem, and the drug should be administered with caution to patients who already have difficulty in passing urine. Skin rashes were observed in 1–3%, but agranulocytosis, and cholestatic jaundice have also been reported.[38] Many antiarrhythmic drugs can also initiate or exacerbate arrhythmias, and disopyramide is no exception. Ventricular tachycardia[39] and fibrillation[40] have been induced by the drug. The negative inotropic effect of disopyramide can represent a serious hazard in patients with impairment of myocardial function. In 11 such patients Jensen *et al.* found that disopyramide elevated pulmonary wedge pressure (mean + 2.7 mm) and left ventricular end-diastolic pressure, and caused a mean decrease in cardiac index of 28%.[41] In patients with atrial fibrillation disopyramide induced ventricular tachycardia. Podrid *et al.* also found disopyramide hazardous in patients with impaired cardiac function.[42] There was a 55% risk of inducing cardiac failure by disopyramide in subjects who had previously experienced an episode of such failure, and a 5% risk in those who had not.

The negative inotropic effect of disopyramide also has serious consequences in cases of poisoning. Death occurred in 12 of 16 patients admitted to the poisons unit at Guy's Hospital after overdoses of disopyramide.[43] In dogs the mean plasma concentration required to induce cardiac failure and death was 25 $\mu g \cdot ml^{-1}$ (range 19.3 to 41).

## RELEVANCE OF *IN VITRO* STUDIES TO CLINICAL CARDIOLOGY

Soon after the advent of techniques for intracellular recording with microelectrodes it was found that quinidine and several other antiarrhythmic drugs then available, of which disopyramide was one of the first to be studied,[2] had in common the property of reducing the maximum rate of depolarization without change of resting potential, and it was concluded that they interfered with the process by which the channels carrying fast inward sodium current were "reactivated in response to repolarization."[3] The concept that these drugs combined with the sodium channels in their inactivated form (that is, after depolarization) was supported by the very early finding that the compounds were more potent the faster the driving frequency.[44,45] That this, historically the first, class of action was responsible for the antiarrhythmic effects was not universally accepted, and indeed as late as 1970, Bigger and Mandel concluded from their studies that "the results caused us to reject the hypothesis that lidocaine exerts electrophysiological affects essentially like those of procainamide and quinidine."[46]

It is now widely accepted, from evidence discussed in detail elsewhere,[47] that the "membrane-stabilizing" or "local anesthetic" type of antiarrhythmic drugs do have in common the property of restricting fast inward current, but in addition have other actions that differ and so necessitate their division into subgroups. Lidocaine, mexiletine and tocainide (group 1B) shorten action potential duration *in vitro,* and shorten monophasic action potentials (MAPs) and Q-T intervals *in vivo,* do not lengthen H-V conduction time or QRS at sinus rhythm, but prolong effective refractory period (ERP) as measured by programmed stimulation. The most recently introduced class 1 drugs, flecainide, encainide and lorcainide (group 1C), have little effect on APD or Q-T interval, or on ERP measured by programmed stimulation, but increase H-V conduction time and widen QRS even in sinus rhythm. The oldest drugs, quinidine, procainamide and disopyramide (group 1A) are intermediate, moderately prolonging ERP, and lengthening Q-T and widening QRS at high concentrations (TABLE 2). The anticholinergic and APD-lengthening effects of quinidine and disopyramide are additional properties unrelated to their class 1 action. The shortening of APD by class 1B drugs, however, is thought to be due to elimination of some residual sodium channels which still remain open during the action potential plateau,[4,6] and not to an increased potassium conductance, as suggested by Arnsdorf and Bigger.[48]

An electrophysiological explanation for this subclassification into groups 1A, B and C has been proposed in a series of recent papers.[49-54] It was shown more than a quarter of a century ago that the sodium channels of Purkinje cells were similar to those of the squid axon, existing in at least three states: (1) closed, at potentials near the resting potential, but available to be opened by depolarization; (2) open, selectively permitting passage of sodium ions; and (3) closed, but not available to be opened, that is, inactivated.[55] Many models of sodium channels have been suggested, with more states than the minimal three, but there is much evidence, discussed in detail in the papers already cited, that antiarrhythmic drugs combine with sodium channels in their inactivated state and interfere with the process by which they recover from inactivation after repolarization of the membrane, as originally deduced.[3] The maximum rate of depolarization (MRD), upon stimulation at increasing intervals after repolarization has begun, can be taken as an approximate measure of the number of channels that have recovered (although simultaneous outward current complicates the picture to a small extent), as depicted diagrammatically in FIGURE 3. The heights of the columns in the left panel represent the magnitude of MRD in response to stimuli at various times after repolarization of an atrial action potential. The solid columns depict normal responses, the dashed columns the responses to be expected if 40% of the channels had been permanently eliminated by a drug. The remaining 60%, without drug attached, are normal, and so recover at the same time as the controls; that is, the electrical threshold would be raised, but there would be no increase in effective refractory period measured by programmed stimulation. On the right the dotted line depicts the "envelope" of normal responses. The columns represent responses to be expected if no channels had been permanently eliminated, but if all channels were temporarily out of action at the beginning of diastole, but recovered rapidly, (solid columns) or more slowly (dashed columns), as the drug became detached and allowed the channel to recover from inactivation. In both cases ERP would be prolonged, because no channels would be available at the start of diastole. At the end of diastole, however, all of the channels would have been freed from the rapidly dissociating drug, so that MRD (and conduction velocity) would be unaffected at sinus rhythm. The more slowly dissociating drug would depress MRD in sinus rhythm to some extent.

The action of disopyramide is frequency-dependent[52] ("use-dependent" and "rate-dependent" are synonymous terms). On initiating a train of stimuli, MRD decreases progressively until a steady state is reached, the degree of depression being a function of the frequency in the train. The time to reach a steady state can be measured as "τ-onset" because the frequency-dependent reduction of MRD follows a single exponential for each drug.

**TABLE 2.** Clinical Subdivision of Class 1 Antiarrhythmic Drugs

| Effect on: | Group B: Lidocaine Mexiletine Tocainide | Group A: Quinidine Procainamide Disopyramide (ORG 6001) | Group C: Lorcainide Encainide Flecainide (CCI 22277) |
|---|---|---|---|
| QRS | None in sinus rhythm | Widened at high concentration | Widened at low concentration |
| Conduction | None in sinus rhythm | Slowed at high concentration | Slowed at low concentration |
| ERP | Lengthened in relation to APD | Lengthened absolutely and relative to APD | Very little change |
| Action potential | Shortened | Lengthened at high concentration | Very little change |

Recovery from the frequency-dependent depression of MRD by the class 1 drugs also follows an exponential, the time constant of which (τ-re) can be measured by administering to cardiac muscle trains of stimuli long enough to produce a steady-state depression of MRD at a given frequency, and by then stopping stimulation, and measuring the recovery of MRD by single stimuli administered at intervals after the train.[49-54] The concentrations of drugs used were selected to achieve approximately a 50% depression of MRD at a frequency of 3.3 Hz within the train. TABLE 3 shows that flecainide, lorcainide, and encainide had time constants of recovery many times longer than a normal diastolic interval, so that the channels may be considered to have been "permanently" inactivated, as depicted on the left of FIGURE 3. Conversely, mexiletine was a rapidly dissociating drug (FIG. 3, right) and disopyramide a rather slowly dissociating drug (τ-re, 12.2 sec).

The onset kinetics gave the same grouping. Lidocaine, mexiletine, and tocainide had time constants for attachment of 0.5 sec or less, so that a steady-state depression of MRD was achieved within a couple of beats after the start of a train of stimuli. In contrast, with flecainide, lorcainide and encainide, a steady-state

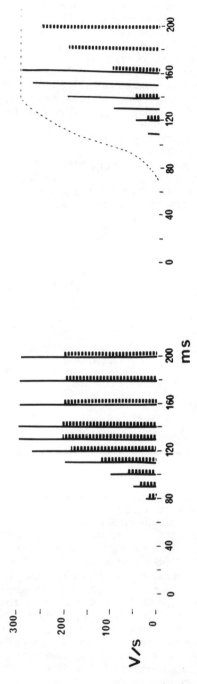

**FIGURE 3.** Recovery of the maximum rate of depolarization (MRD) in response to stimuli at increasing intervals after repolarization. Heights of columns are proportional to MRD in response to stimuli after the intervals indicated. (*Left*) **solid columns**, controls; **dashed columns**, responses expected if 40% of sodium channels had been permanently eliminated. (*Right*) **dotted line** depicts envelope of the normal responses. Columns represent MRD in response to stimuli (assuming that no channels were permanently eliminated, but that at the start of diastole all channels were attached to a drug, which kept them inactivated). MRD recovers as the drug rapidly (**solid columns**) or more slowly (**dashed columns**) becomes dissociated from the channels. (From Vaughan Williams.[47] Reproduced by permission.)

depression of MRD was not reached until 20 beats or more in a train. Quinidine, disopyramide, and procainamide were intermediate.

From the clinical viewpoint the main interest of this subdivision of class 1 antiarrhythmic drugs into those with fast, slow and intermediate onset-offset kinetics, made on the basis of purely objective electrophysiological measurements *in vitro,* is that the groups correspond exactly to 1B, C, and A respectively, as determined on clinical grounds. Furthermore the experiments support the view that the antiarrhythmic action of all class 1 drugs is fundamentally similar, involving attachment to sodium channels in their inactivated state. Quantitative disparities in the rapidity of attachment to and detachment from the channels can account for the observed differences in the clinical profiles of the various compounds.

In conclusion, it is apparent that disopyramide, from the recovery kinetics and molecular weight, is on the border between groups 1A and 1C. This is in agreement with the clinical finding that QRS may be widened, even in sinus rhythm.[26,28,38] All its other clinical effects are readily explicable by its dual action

**TABLE 3.** Some Class 1 Antiarrhythmic Drugs Arranged in Order of Magnitude of the Time Constant of Recovery of MRD[a]

| Compound | Molecular Weight (daltons) | Concentration ($\mu$mol·l$^{-1}$) | Depression of MRD (% of That of First Response in Train) | Time Constant of Recovery (sec) |
|---|---|---|---|---|
| Mexiletine | 179 | 20 | 49.2 | 0.47 |
| ORG 6001 | 305 | 30 | 57.7 | 4.6 |
| Disopyramide | 339 | 100 | 50.9 | 12.2 |
| Lorcainide | 358 | 5 | 45.0 | 13.2 |
| Flecainide | 408 | 2 | 50.7 | 15.5 |
| Encainide | 371 | 3 | 50.0 | 20.3 |

[a] After it had been depressed to a steady level during a train of stimuli at 3.3 Hz.

as a class 1 antiarrhythmic drug and an anticholinergic agent. The negative inotropic action may involve antagonism of the second slower inward (calcium) current, but the only evidence for this so far has been obtained in AV nodal cells.[7] It is possible that the lengthening of APD by disopyramide may also contribute to its antiarrhythmic effect (class 3), especially in ischemia. In any given patient the effects of disopyramide on heart rate and AV conduction depend on that patient's autonomic status. After removal of vagal tone by atropine, disopyramide causes bradycardia and delays AV conduction in all patients. It is of interest that it has recently been shown that although in untreated dogs, as in patients, disopyramide has no consistent effect on heart rate, in dogs chemically "sympathectomized" with 6-hydroxydopamine, disopyramide also causes bradycardia.[56]

## REFERENCES

1. MOKLER, C. M. & C. G. VAN ARMAN. 1962. Pharmacology of a new antiarrhythmic agent, $\gamma$-diisopropyl-amino-$\alpha$-phenyl-$\alpha$(2-pyridyl)-butyramide (SC-7031). J. Pharmacol. Exp. Ther. **136:** 114–124.

2. SEKIYA, A. & E. M. VAUGHAN WILLIAMS. 1963. A comparison of the antifibrillatory actions and effects on intracellular cardiac potentials of pronethalol, disopyramide and quinidine. Br. J. Pharmacol. **21:** 473–481.

3. SZEKERES, L. & E. M. VAUGHAN WILLIAMS. 1962. Antifibrillatory action. J. Physiol. London **160:** 470–482.

4. CARMELIET, E. & T. SAIKAWA. 1982. Shortening of the action potential and reduction of pacemaker activity by lidocaine, quinidine and procainamide in sheep cardiac Purkinje fibers. Circulation Res. **50:** 257–272.

5. ATTWELL, D., I. COHEN, D. A. EISNER, M. OHBA & C. OJEDA. 1979. The steady state TTX-sensitive ("window") sodium current in cardiac Purkinje fibres. Pfluegers Arch. **379:** 137–142.

6. CORABOEUF, E. & E. DEROUBAIX. 1978. Shortening effect of tetrodotoxin on action potentials of the conducting system in the dog heart. J. Physiol. **280:** 24P.

7. WATANABE, Y., M. NISHIMURA & S. YAMADA. 1984. Significance of a combination of different experimental approaches. In Lake Kawaguchi Conference of Cardiology, Japan. Heart **16:** 513–523.

8. DE MELLO, W. C. 1963. Role of chloride ions in cardiac action and pacemaker potentials. Am. J. Physiol. **205:** 567–575.

9. SEYAMA, I. 1979. Characteristics of the anion channel in the sino-atrial node cell of the rabbit. J. Physiol. **294:** 447–460.

10. MILLAR, J. S. & E. M. VAUGHAN WILLIAMS. 1981. Pacemaker selectivity. Influence on rabbit atria of ionic environment and of alinidine, a possible anion antagonist. Cardiovasc. Res. **15:** 335–350.

11. WITTIG, J. H., L. A. HARRISON, A. G. WALLACE. 1973. Electrophysiological effects of lidocaine on distal Purkinje fibers of canine heart. Am. Heart J. **86:** 69–78.

12. VAUGHAN WILLIAMS, E. M., L. SALAKO & J. H. WITTIG. 1977. The effect on atrial and ventricular intracellular potentials, and other pharmacological actions of L9146, a non-halogenated benzo(b) thiophene related to amiodarone. Cardiovasc. Res. **11:** 187–197.

13. KUS, T. & B. I. SASYNIUK. 1975. Electrophysiological actions of disopyramide phosphate on canine ventricular muscle and Purkinje fibers. Circ. Res. **37:** 844–853.

14. KUS, T. & B. I. SASYNIUK. 1978. The electrophysiological effects of disopyramide on the canine ventricular muscle and Purkinje fibers in normal and low potassium. Can. J. Physiol. Pharmacol. **56:** 139–149.

15. SINGH, B. N. & E. M. VAUGHAN WILLIAMS. 1971. The effect of altering potassium concentration on the action of lidocaine and diphenylhydantoin on rabbit atrial and ventricular muscle. Circ. Res. **29:** 286–296.

16. SALAKO, L. A., E. M. VAUGHAN WILLIAMS & J. A. WITTIG. 1975. Investigations to characterize a new anti-arrhythmic drug ORG 6001, including a simple test for calcium antagonism. Br. J. Pharmacol. **57:** 251–262.

17. SASYNIUK, B. I. & T. KUS. 1976. Cellular electrophysiologic changes induced by disopyramide phosphate in normal and infarcted hearts. J. Int. Med. Res. **4** (Suppl. 1): 20–25.

18. CHAGNAC, A., B. PELLEG, J. BELHASSEN, B. LUBLINER, B. WIDNE & S. LANIADO. 1983. Effects of disopyramide on reperfusion arrhythmias in dogs. J. Cardiovasc. Pharmacol. **5:** 994–998.

19. KATZ, M. J. & C. E. MEYER. 1963. Clinical evaluation of a new antiarrhythmic agent, SC-7031. Curr. Ther. Res. **5:** 343.

20. JULIAN, D. G., P. A. VALENTINE & G. G. MILLER. 1964. Disturbances of rate, rhythm and conduction in acute myocardial infarction. Am. J. Med. **37:** 915–927.

21. JULIAN, D. G. 1976. Toward preventing coronary death from ventricular fibrillation. Circulation **54:** 360–364.

22. WHITING, B., N. H. G. HOLFORD & L. B. SHIENER. 1980. Quantitative analysis of the disopyramide concentration-effect relationship. Br. J. Clin. Pharmacol. **9:** 67–75.

23. BAINES, M. W., J. E. DAVIES, D. N. KEILETT & P. L. MUNT. 1976. Some pharmacological effects of disopyramide and a metabolite. J. Int. Med. Res. **4** (Suppl. 1): 5–7.

24. JOSEPHSON, M. E., A. R. CARACTA, S. H. LAW, J. J. GALLACHER & A. N. DAMATO.

1973. Electrophysiological evaluation of disopyramide in man. Am. Heart J. **86:** 771–780.

25. BIRKHEAD, J. S. & E. M. VAUGHAN WILLIAMS. 1977. Dual effect of disopyramide on atrial and atrio-ventricular conduction and refractory periods. Br. Heart J. **33:** 657–660.
26. REID, D. S. & D. O. WILLIAMS. 1977. Disopyramide and sinoatrial node function. *In* Disopyramide Seminar. S. I. Ankier, Ed.: 31–36. Roussel. Wembley, England.
27. SPURRELL, R. A. J., C. W. THORNBURN, J. CAMM, E. SOWTON & D. C. DEUCHAR. 1975. Effects of disopyramide on electrophysiological properties of specialised conduction system in man and on accessory atrioventricular pathway in Wolff-Parkinson-White syndrome. Br. Heart J. **37:** 861–867.
28. MIZGALA, H. F. & P. R. HUVELLE. 1976. Acute termination of cardiac arrhythmias with intravenous disopyramide. J. Int. Med. Sci. **4** (Suppl. 1): 82–85.
29. WARD, J. W. & G. R. KINGHORN. 1976. The pharmacokinetics of disopyramide following myocardial infarction with special reference to oral and intravenous dose regimes. J. Int. Med. Res. **4** (Suppl. 1): 49–53.
30. RANGNO, R. E., W. WARNICA, R. I. OGILVIE, J. KREEFT & E. BRIDGER. 1976. Correlation of disopyramide pharmacokinetics with efficacy in ventricular tachyarrhythmia. J. Int. Med. Res. **4** (Suppl. 1): 54–58.
31. JENNINGS, G., D. G. MODEL, M. B. J. JONES, P. P. TURNER, E. M. M. BESTERMAN & P. H. KIDNER. 1976. Oral disopyramide in prophylaxis of arrhythmias following myocardial infarction. Lancet **i:** 51–54.
32. ZAINAL, N., D. J. S. CARMICHAEL, J. W. GRIFFITHS, E. M. M. BESTERMAN, P. H. KIDNER, A. D. GILLHAM & G. D. SUMMERS. 1977. Oral disopyramide for the prevention of arrhythmias in patients with acute myocardial infarction. Lancet **ii:** 887–889.
33. HILL, J. D., G. HOLDSTOCK & J. R. HAMPTON. 1977. Comparison of mortality of patients with heart attacks admitted to a coronary care unit and an ordinary medical ward. Br. Med. J. **ii:** 81–83.
34. ANTURANE REINFARCTION TRIAL POLICY COMMITTEE. 1982. The Anturane Reinfarction Trial: re-evaluation of anturane. N. Engl. J. Med. **306:** 1005–1008.
35. MULTICENTRE INTERNATIONAL STUDY. 1977. Reduction in mortality after myocardial infarction with long-term beta-adrenoceptor blockade. Br. Med. J. **2:** 419–421.
36. NORWEGIAN MULTICENTER STUDY GROUP. 1981. Timolol-induced reduction in mortality and reinfarction in patients surviving acute myocardial infarction. N. Engl. J. Med. **304:** 801–807.
37. BETA-BLOCKER HEART ATTACK TRIAL RESEARCH GROUP. 1982. A randomized trial of propranolol in patients with acute myocardial infarction. JAMA **247:** 1707–1714.
38. FENSTER, P. E. 1982. Clinical use of antidysrhythmic agents: procainamide, quinidine, disopyramide. *In* Cardiovascular Drugs and the Management of Heart Disease. G. A. Ewy & R. Bressler, Eds.: 115–129. Raven Press. New York, NY.
39. MELTZER, R. S., E. W. ROBERT & M. McMORROW. 1978. Atypical ventricular tachycardia as a manifestation of disopyramide toxicity. Am. J. Cardiol. **42:** 1049.
40. NICHOLSON, W. J., C. E. MARTIN, J. G. GRACEY & H. R. KNOCH. 1979. Disopyramide-induced ventricular fibrillation. Am. J. Cardiol. **43:** 1053–1055.
41. JENSEN, G., B. SIGURD & A. UHRENHOLT. 1976. Circulatory effects of intravenous disopyramide in heart failure. J. Int. Med. Res. **4** (Suppl. 1): 42–45.
42. PODRID, P. J., A. SCHOENBERGER & B. LOWN. 1980. Congestive heart failure caused by oral disopyramide. N. Engl. J. Med. **302:** 614–617.
43. O'KEEFE, B., A. M. HAYLER, D. N. HOLT & R. K. MEDD. 1979. Cardiac consequences and treatment of disopyramide intoxication. Experimental evaluation in dogs. Cardiovasc. Res. **13:** 630–634.
44. JOHNSON, E. A. & M. G. McKINNON. 1957. The differential effect of quinidine and pyrilamine on the myocardial action potential at various rates of stimulation. J. Pharmacol. Exp. Ther. **120:** 460–468.
45. VAUGHAN WILLIAMS, E. M. 1958. The mode of action of quinidine on isolated rabbit atria interpreted from intracellular potential records. Br. J. Pharmacol. **13:** 276–287.

46. BIGGER, J. T. & W. J. MANDELL. 1970. Effect of lidocaine on the electrophysiological properties of ventricular muscle and Purkinje fibres. J. Clin. Invest. **49:** 63–77.
47. VAUGHAN WILLIAMS, E. M. 1980. Antiarrhythmic Action. Academic Press. London.
48. ARNSDORF, M. F. & J. T. BIGGER. 1972. Effect of lidocaine hydrochloride on membrane conductance in mammalian cardiac Purkinje fibers. J. Clin. Invest. **51:** 2252–2263.
49. CAMPBELL, T. J. & E. M. VAUGHAN WILLIAMS. 1982. Electrophysiological and other effects on rabbit hearts of CCI 22277, a new steroidal antiarrhythmic drug. Br. J. Pharmacol. **76:** 337–345.
50. CAMPBELL, T. J. & E. M. VAUGHAN WILLIAMS. 1983. Voltage- and time-dependent depression of maximum rate of depolarisation of guinea-pig ventricular action potentials by two new antiarrhythmic drugs, encainide and lorcainide. Cardiovasc. Res. **17:** 251–258.
51. CAMPBELL, T. J. 1982. Voltage- and time-dependent depression of maximum rate of depolarisation of guinea-pig ventricular action potentials by two new antiarrhythmic drugs, CCI 22277 and ORG 6001. Br. J. Pharmacol. **77:** 541–548.
52. CAMPBELL, T. J. 1983. Resting and rate-dependent depression of maximum rate of depolarisation (Vmax) in guinea-pig ventricular action potentials by mexiletine, disopyramide and encainide. J. Cardiovasc. Pharmacol. **5:** 291–296.
53. CAMPBELL, T. J. 1983. Kinetics of onset of rate-dependent effects of class 1 antiarrhythmic drugs are important in determining their effects on refractoriness in guinea-pig ventricle, and provide a theoretical basis for their subclassification. Cardiovasc. Res. **17:** 344–352.
54. CAMPBELL, T. J. 1983. Importance of physico-chemical properties in determining the kinetics of the effects of class 1 antiarrhythmic drugs on maximum rate of depolarisation in the guinea pig ventricle. Br. J. Pharmacol. **80:** 33–40.
55. WEIDMANN, S. 1955. The effect of the cardiac membrane potential on the rapid availability of the sodium-carrying system. J. Physiol. **127:** 213–224.
56. GUIMOND, C., C. VASSEUR, D. GODIN, B. PELLETIER, A. R. LEBLANC & R. NADEAU. 1982. Intracardiac electrophysiological study of disopyramide in intact and chemically sympathectomized dogs. Eur. Heart J. **3:** 553–563.

# Electrophysiology and Pharmacology of Aprindine, Encainide, and Propafenone[a]

DOUGLAS P. ZIPES, ERIC N. PRYSTOWSKY, AND
JAMES J. HEGER

*Krannert Institute of Cardiology*
*Department of Medicine*
*Indiana University School of Medicine; and the*
*Veterans Administration Medical Center*
*Indianapolis, Indiana 46202*

## APRINDINE

Aprindine, an antiarrhythmic agent with prominent local anesthetic effects, was developed and used initially in Belgium. It is available clinically in many parts of Europe and was evaluated as an investigational agent at a number of centers in the United States. It has not been approved by the FDA and further clinical research with the drug has been suspended in the United States.

Aprindine is well absorbed, has high systemic availability, and is 85% to 95% protein-bound. Approximately 95% of the hydroxylated metabolites undergo glucuronidation in the liver. Sixty-five percent of aprindine and its metabolites are found in the urine, with the remaining 35% in the feces.[1] Elimination half-life has ranged from 13 to 50 hours (mean = 27.9 hours) in one study[1] and 20 to 30 hours in another.[2] The $N$-desethyl metabolite is present in small amounts in the plasma of patients treated chronically with aprindine and exerts some antiarrhythmic actions.[2] Clinically, the antiarrhythmic effect of aprindine may not occur for several days, even when the drug is initially administered in a loading dose.

Hemodynamic studies have revealed that therapeutic doses of aprindine mildly depressed myocardial function.[3] In humans, aprindine (200 mg orally) slightly decreased systolic and mean aortic blood pressure during exercise in one study[4] and slightly depressed myocardial contractility when given intravenously (100 mg) in another.[5] At a total dose of 140 or 150 mg intravenously, aprindine produced a moderate and dose-related decrease in peak left ventricular dP/dt and $V_{max}$.[6]

In isolated cardiac preparations, aprindine shortened the duration of the action potential and effective refractory period of Purkinje fibers; the former was short-

[a] This work was supported in part by the Herman C. Krannert Fund, Indianapolis, Indiana; by Grants HL-06308 and HL-07182 from the National Heart, Lung and Blood Institute of the National Institutes of Health, Bethesda, Maryland; by the Attorney General of Indiana Public Health Trust and the Roudebush Veterans Administration Medical Center, Indianapolis, Indiana; and by a Grant-in-Aid from the American Heart Association, Indiana Affiliate, Inc., Indianapolis, Indiana.

ened more than the latter.[7,8] In cardiac muscle fibers, however, action potential duration was only slightly reduced and the duration of the effective refractory period was lengthened.[7] The rate of rise of phase 0 was depressed, more so at rapid rates, at higher potassium levels, and to a greater degree than that seen with comparable amounts of lidocaine.[7,8] Diastolic depolarization and spontaneous firing were depressed or abolished by aprindine. Aprindine also reduced digitalis-induced increases in potassium permeability[7] and suppressed transient depolarizations caused by acetylstrophanthidin in canine Purkinje fibers.[9] Aprindine does not appear to affect slow-channel activity[7,9] of canine Purkinje fibers at aprindine concentrations of $3 \times 10^{-6}$ to $1 \times 10^{-5}$ M.

The effects of aprindine on transmembrane currents in frog (*Rana ridibunda*) atrial trabeculae have been studied using a voltage clamp technique.[10] Aprindine $(1 \times 10^{-6}$ g/ml) reduced maximum inward sodium current by $38.6 \pm 7.2\%$ (mean = $\pm$S.E.M., n = 6), but had no effect on the slow inward current or outward current. A higher dose of aprindine $(2.8 \times 10^{-5}$ g/ml) suppressed both the fast inward current and the slow inward current. Aprindine $(2.8 \times 10^{-5}$ g/ml) also depressed slow-channel-dependent membrane oscillations induced in atrial trabeculae by injection of current pulses. These data indicated that aprindine possesses fast- and slow-channel-blocking properties in the frog, the latter being more apparent with high concentrations of the drug.

Aprindine is an effective antiarrhythmic agent against a variety of supraventricular[11] and ventricular arrhythmias[12] occurring in patients with different types of heart disease.

Our total current experience includes 203 patients treated with aprindine for a variety of tachyarrhythmias, including 179 patients with ventricular tachycardia, 16 patients with supraventricular tachycardia, 4 patients with premature ventricular complexes, 3 patients with atrial fibrillation, and 1 patient with atrial tachycardia. Fifty-four patients continued to receive aprindine (range, 1 to 64 months) for ventricular arrhythmias (50 patients) and supraventricular arrhythmia (4 patients). Reasons for discontinuing the drug included inadequate control of ventricular arrhythmias (84 patients) or of supraventricular arrhythmias (13 patients) or exacerbation of ventricular arrhythmias (5 patients). In two patients, the arrhythmia resolved, and the drug was stopped in two patients for noncompliance. Twenty-one patients discontinued aprindine because of side effects, and 22 patients died while receiving the drug, although in none was the drug implicated as a cause of death.

The toxic-therapeutic ratio for aprindine is rather narrow, and side effects, particularly during the initial loading period and adjustment of the maintenance dose, are common. These side effects, related to the dose and serum concentration of aprindine, include most commonly a tremor of the hands and fingers. As the serum concentration increases, dizziness, intention tremor, ataxia, hallucinations, diplopia, nervousness, memory impairment, or seizures may also occur. Neurologic side effects are minimal or absent at serum aprindine concentrations of less than 1 $\mu$g/ml.[12] Gastrointestinal side effects are more infrequent than neurologic side effects.

Cholestatic jaundice and agranulocytosis have been reported to occur in association with the use of aprindine and are thought to be idiosyncratic reactions as opposed to dose-related toxicity. The problems have generally occurred between the fourth and sixteenth weeks of aprindine therapy. Transient abnormalities in liver function tests have been noted in some patients, but no abnormality has persisted or has led to discontinuation of the drug in our group of patients.

Studies in intact dogs have revealed that aprindine, injected into the sinus nodal (SN) artery, decreased the spontaneous sinus rate and, injected into the atrioventricular (AV) nodal artery, prolonged the functional refractory period and conduction time of the AV node. Given intravenously (1.4, 2.8, and 4.2 mg/kg cumulative dose), aprindine prolonged the AV interval, H-V interval, transmural left ventricular conduction time, and the effective refractory period of the ventricle.[13] It appears that aprindine slows conduction in all cardiac tissue.

Aprindine has effectively suppressed digitalis-induced arrhythmias including a specific type exhibiting overdrive acceleration.[14] Aprindine has been very effective against certain ischemia-induced arrhythmias, such as those ventricular arrhythmias occurring 24 hours after coronary arterial ligation.[15] Aprindine has also been found to elevate the ventricular fibrillation threshold in the nonischemic canine heart, but not during ischemia.[16]

Results of aprindine given intravenously immediately before coronary arterial ligation are conflicting because of differences in dose and methodology.[3,15,17] To investigate further the effects of coronary artery occlusion on the distribution and actions of aprindine, we[18] administered aprindine to open-chest dogs immediately before, 5 minutes after, and 24 hours after one-stage left anterior descending coronary artery (LAD) occlusion. Aprindine concentrations were measured in the serum and in ventricular myocardial samples at various times after LAD occlusion.

Coronary artery occlusion performed after aprindine administration slowed the rate of disappearance of aprindine from ischemic zone, so that concentrations of aprindine in the ischemic zone decreased more slowly than they did in the normal zone and averaged more than twice those in the normal zone 1 hour after LAD occlusion. When LAD occlusion was performed before aprindine administration, aprindine concentrations in the ischemic zone were initially less than 15% of those in the normal zone and increased with time to approach half of the normal zone concentration 70 minutes after LAD occlusion. Aprindine concentrations in the border zone were intermediate between those in the normal and ischemic zones. Seventeen of 35 dogs (49%) receiving aprindine before LAD occlusion experienced sustained ventricular tachycardia or ventricular fibrillation, compared with 5 of 34 (14%) receiving aprindine immediately after LAD occlusion ($p < 0.01$), 1 of 10 (10%) undergoing LAD occlusion without receiving aprindine ($p < 0.05$), and none of 16 receiving aprindine without LAD occlusion ($p < 0.01$). Aprindine administered 24 hours after coronary occlusion reduced premature ventricular complexes from a mean of 35 to 12 per 100 beats ($p < 0.01$). The results of these studies indicated that the temporal relationship between aprindine administration and LAD occlusion significantly modifies the regional myocardial distribution of aprindine and its effects on ventricular arrhythmias after coronary artery occlusion.

Studies in humans have demonstrated that aprindine increased the A-H and H-V intervals and QRS duration, increased the effective refractory period of the atria and ventricles, and increased the functional and effective refractory period of the AV node.[11]

## ENCAINIDE

Encainide HCl, a new benzanilide derivative, is reported to be more potent than quinidine or procainamide in abolishing a variety of experimental atrial and ventricular arrhythmias.[19-21] In human beings, encainide administered either intravenously[22,23] or orally[23-25] effectively suppresses premature ventricular complexes, and preliminary data in selected patients who have ventricular tachycardia demonstrated that encainide can prevent recurrence of the arrhythmia.[26-29]

In both dogs[30] and human subjects,[31] a single intravenous dose (0.6 to 0.9 mg/kg) of encainide substantially lengthens H-V and QRS intervals without affecting atrioventricular (AV) nodal conduction or refractoriness of atrium, ventricle, or atrioventricular node. Recent data[21,23,24] suggest that encainide may have active metabolites, whose effects might not be observed in electrophysiologic studies performed after a single intravenous dose. On the basis of those observations, we compared the electrophysiological effects of encainide and two recently identified metabolites (MJ14030, MJ9444) on canine Purkinje and ventricular fibers *in vitro*.[32] Standard microelectrode techniques were used to measure the resting potential, action potential amplitude and duration at 90% of repolarization (APD$_{90}$), maximum upstroke velocity (V$_{max}$), and propagation velocity. Rheobasic current was determined by intracellular ejection of constant-current pulses of 100 msec in duration. Current injection through a single sucrose gap was used to determine the voltage threshold and the voltage dependency of cellular automaticity in shortened Purkinje fibers. In Purkinje fibers, the relative potency of these compounds was 9 : 1 : 1 for MJ9444, MJ14030, ranged between $10^{-8}$ and $10^{-7}$ M, and that for MJ9444 ranged between $10^{-9}$ and $10^{-8}$ M. At a concentration of $10^{-6}$ M, these compounds significantly (p < .05) decreased APD$_{90}$, V$_{max}$ and propagation velocity. Resting potential was not altered. Only MJ9444 significantly decreased action potential amplitude. The effects on V$_{max}$ and APD$_{90}$ were markedly rate-dependent. Rheobasic current was increased from 280 ± 20 nA to 360 ± 35, 375 ± 32, and 645 ± 40 nA (mean ± S.E.M., n = 5) by encainide, MJ14030, and MJ9444, respectively. None of the compounds altered voltage threshold for all-or-none depolarization and all failed to suppress slow-channel-dependent action potentials induced in Purkinje fibers by superfusion with KCl (22 mM) and isoproterenol ($10^{-5}$ M). Similar findings were obtained in ventricular fibers except that none of these compounds reduced APD$_{90}$. In sucrose gap experiments, cellular automaticity arising from the high level of transmembrane potential was markedly slowed by MJ9444 ($10^{-6}$ M) but not by encainide or MJ14030 ($10^{-6}$ M). Automaticity arising from the low level of transmembrane potential was not altered by any compound. We concluded that the metabolites have electrophysiological profiles similar to those of encainide and that MJ9444 is most potent. These metabolites may contribute to the antiarrhythmic action of encainide. However, they do not account for the effects of chronic oral administration of encainide, in particular for the prolongation of the AV nodal and ventricular refractory periods. Thus, additional metabolite(s) to be identified may also be involved in the electrophysiological effects of encainide.

Oral encainide therapy in humans substantially depresses conduction in the AV node and His-Purkinje system and lengthens refractoriness of atrium, ventricle, and accessory AV muscle connections. In association with these changes, encainide suppresses supraventricular tachycardia utilizing an accessory AV pathway and due to AV nodal reentry. The electrophysiologic effects of oral encainide therapy differ considerably from those found after single intravenous dose of encainide.[27,30,31] Although H-V and QRS intervals increased to nearly the same extent as that with oral therapy, a single intravenous dose (0.6 to 0.9 mg/kg) of encainide had no significant effect on atrial or ventricular refractoriness of AV nodal conduction. In studies[30,31] using intravenous encainide, maximal H-V and

QRS prolongation occurred immediately after the 15-min infusion, and the percent change in H-V and QRS intervals correlated well with peak plasma encainide concentration.[30] During oral therapy no significant relation was found between plasma encainide concentration obtained at the time of electrophysiologic study and the degree of change in atrial or ventricular effective refractory period, shortest atrial pacing cycle length sustaining 1 : 1 AV nodal conduction, H-V interval, or QRS interval.[27] Our data can be explained by one or more metabolites of encainide that exert electrophysiologic effects different from those of the parent compound. Furthermore, one of the active metabolites could have slow-channel-blocking effects, accounting for the substantial effects on AV nodal function caused by oral encainide therapy. Alternatively, the effects of oral encainide therapy might result from tissue accumulation of the parent compound. However, the rapid metabolism of encainide (half-life, approximately 3 hours[23,24]) makes the latter explanation unlikely.

Recent reported data support the hypothesis that one or more metabolites are responsible for many of the electrophysiologic effects of oral encainide therapy. In a study of 11 patients who had frequent premature ventricular complexes, the investigators[24] found an unusually wide range of minimal effective (antiarrhythmic) plasma encainide concentration in the 10 responding patients. One patient had no change in electrocardiographic intervals or frequency of premature ventricular complexes with encainide therapy. That patient eliminated encainide much more slowly than did the other patients (half-life, 13.6 hours) and was the only patient who had no detectable plasma *O*-demethyl encainide. Investigators in the same laboratory subsequently demonstrated that doses of *O*-demethyl encainide one-tenth as large as encainide lengthened the QRS interval and prevented aconitine-induced ventricular tachycardia in rats.[21] In another study[23] involving patients who had frequent premature ventricular complexes, the minimal effective plasma encainide concentration was lower and duration of antiarrhythmic activity longer when encainide was administered orally than when administered intravenously. The investigators also found a longer elimination half-life for several demethylated metabolites of encainide than for the parent compound.

Because of the apparent striking effect of encainide in patients with Wolff-Parkinson-White syndrome by lengthening refractoriness of both the AV node and accessory pathway, we performed electrophysiologic studies in 19 patients with accessory pathways before and during encainide therapy with a mean daily dose of 197 mg.[33] Fourteen patients had manifest and five patients had concealed accessory atrioventricular connections. The patients had recurrent atrioventricular reentrant tachycardia for a mean of 15.8 years and had received a mean of 3.6 drug trials without successful suppression of recurrent arrhythmias. Encainide caused complete antegrade conduction block in the accessory pathway in 8 of 14 patients with manifest accessory atrioventricular connections. The shortest atrial pacing cycle length maintaining 1 : 1 conduction over the accessory pathway in the control study was 328 ± 66 msec in patients in whom antegrade conduction block occurred and was 247 ± 21 msec (p < 0.01) in patients in whom conduction remained during encainide therapy. Retrograde conduction over accessory atrioventricular connections could be evaluated in 14 patients, and complete block occurred in 7 patients during encainide therapy. There was no correlation between control retrograde effective refractory period or conduction in the accessory pathway and subsequent development of conduction block with encainide therapy. Of note, five patients who developed drug-related retrograde block over the accessory pathway had initial accessory pathway retrograde effective refractory periods of less than 270 msec. Nineteen patients had atrioventricular reentrant tachycardia initiated at control electrophysiologic study. Encainide prevented induction of tachycardia in 10 patients, and in the other 9 patients tachycardia cycle length increased during drug treatment from $313.9 \pm 53.1$ to $418.3 \pm 80.9$ msec (p < 0.001), primarily because of an increase in ventriculo-atrial conduction time from $162.2 \pm 43.8$ to $238.3 \pm 87.9$ msec (p < 0.01). Fifteen patients continued encainide treatment for a mean of 18.0 months (range, 7 to 38), and all but one patient remains asymptomatic. Encainide is well tolerated and very effectively prevents recurrence of reentrant tachycardia in patients with the Wolff-Parkinson-White syndrome.

We have initiated encainide treatment in 130 patients with recurrent ventricular tachycardia or ventricular fibrillation unsuccessfully treated by conventional drugs. During initial in-hospital treatment, encainide was discontinued in 78 of 130 patients because of failure to prevent spontaneous ventricular tachycardia in 49 patients, failure to prevent ventricular tachycardia induced during electrophysiologic testing in 16 patients, exacerbation of ventricular tachycardia during encainide therapy in 9 patients, and other adverse side effects in 4 patients. Of 52 patients discharged from hospital care receiving encainide, 16 had a recurrence of nonfatal ventricular tachycardia. Of these 16 patients, encainide was discontinued in 6 patients, continued alone in 5 patients, and continued following the addition of another antiarrhythmic drug in 5 patients. During long-term follow-up, 6 patients had sudden cardiac death and 7 patients died because of heart failure from progression of underlying heart disease. At present, 33 patients continue to receive encainide for prevention of recurrent ventricular tachycardia or ventricular fibrillation.

Encainide has been associated with exacerbation of ventricular arrhythmias. We found that 9 patients developed incessant ventricular tachycardia requiring multiple electrical cardioversions and resuscitative measures over several hours while they received encainide. Encainide-induced arrhythmias were not associated with excessive prolongation of QRS or Q-T intervals and were not dose-related. The occurrence of encainide-induced arrhythmias within 36 hours of initiation of a dose regimen or within 2 hours of a single large dose has been noted by others.[34] It is recommended that the ECG be monitored continuously and dosages changed only after 48 hours of electrocardiographic monitoring at a given dosage level during encainide treatment in order to detect and treat immediately encainide-induced arrhythmias.

In 22 patients who had recurrent ventricular tachycardia, we compared the antiarrhythmic efficacy of encainide and aprindine by means of a crossover trial.[35] Continuous electrocardiographic recording showed the decrease in frequency of PVCs from control levels to be statistically significant while patients received encainide but not during treatment with aprindine. Effectiveness of the drug regimen was defined as greater than 80% decrease in PVC frequency compared to control values, prevention of spontaneous ventricular tachycardia, and prevention of ventricular tachycardia induction at electrophysiologic testing. Encainide was an effective antiarrhythmic drug in 9 of 22 patients, while aprindine was effective in 5 of 22 patients, not a statistically significant difference. Both drugs appeared to have an equivalent degree of efficacy, and successful therapy with either drug could not be predicted on the basis of type of heart disease or other clinical characteristics.

As mentioned, encainide has significant potential to exacerbate or induce arrhythmias. In our series, 9 (7%) of 130 patients with ventricular arrhythmias had encainide-induced arrhythmia and in other reports encainide-induced arrhythmias have occurred in 11% of patients treated for ventricular tachycardia and 2% of patients treated for chronic PVCs.[34] Encainide routinely produced prolongation of P-R, QRS, and Q-T intervals during oral treatment, usually at dosages that are effective and not associated with toxic manifestations. The increase in P-R and QRS intervals averaged 30%, and corrected Q-T intervals increased by 12% in patients we have studied. During chronic treatment encainide has generally been tolerated well, for the drug was discontinued because of symptomatic side effects in only 4 of 130 patients treated for recurrent ventricular tachycardia. These side effects included nausea, headaches, weakness, and dizziness. Encainide has not been associated with significant changes in left ventricular function, measured by rest and exercise radionuclide ventriculograms.[36] However, the potential for adverse hemodynamic effects does exist.

Encainide is administered orally in daily dosages of 75 to 240 mg/day in 3 or 4 divided doses. We usually begin treatment at 25 mg every 6 hours and maintain a constant dose regimen for at least 48 hours. Doses are increased incrementally to 35, 50, and 60 mg, given every 6 hours. If QRS duration is <0.10 sec at control, a maximal increase of 50% in QRS is accepted; if QRS is prolonged, the maximal accepted increase is 30%.

## PROPAFENONE

Propafenone is a new antiarrhythmic agent that has cellular electrophysiologic properties similar to those of quinidine and procainamide. Propafenone has been reported to be effective in significantly reducing PVC frequency even in patients not successfully treated with other antiarrhythmic drugs.[37]

We have tested the antiarrhythmic efficacy of propafenone in patients who had recurrent ventricular tachycardia or ventricular fibrillation not successfully prevented by conventional drugs.[38] Of 26 patients treated, 13 patients who continued to exhibit spontaneous ventricular tachycardia and 3 patients who had limiting side effects had the drug discontinued. In 11 patients, electrophysiologic studies were performed during the drug-free control period and were repeated while the patients received 900 mg of propafenone a day. Propafenone treatment resulted in significant increase in H-V interval and in atrial and ventricular refractory periods, but did not change the sinus nodal recovery time. Ventricular tachycardia was induced at control study in all 11 patients, and propafenone treatment prevented induction of ventricular tachycardia in 2 of 11 patients. In the 9 patients who still had inducible ventricular tachycardia, the cycle length of ventricular tachycardia lengthened from a mean of 245 msec at control to 340 msec during treatment. In a double-blind placebo crossover study to examine change in PVC frequency, 4 of 8 patients had a greater than 90% reduction in PVC frequency during propafenone treatment, as compared with the control and placebo groups.

Propafenone has been continued for long-term treatment in 10 patients. After a mean follow-up period of 6 months, 9 of 10 patients have remained free of symptomatic arrhythmia and 1 patient had had recurrence of ventricular tachycardia after 3 months of treatment. Therefore, propafenone appears to have some promise for preventing recurrent ventricular tachycardia and ventricular fibrillation.

Adverse side effects have generally been mild. By other reports, 3% of patients have required discontinuation because of side effects, whereas 12% (3 of 26 patients) in our series had limiting side effects.[37,38] The side effects most commonly observed have been paresthesia, nausea, vomiting, anorexia, and blurred vision. In our patients the QRS duration has increased usually in the range of 15 to

25% without other cardiac side effects. Other reports have noted hypotension, AV block, sinus arrest, and negative inotropic effects during propafenone administration. The recommended dosage is 300 to 900 mg, administered every 8 to 12 hours.

## REFERENCES

1. FASOLA, A. F. & R. CARMICHAEL. 1974. The pharmacology and clinical evaluation of aprindine—a new antiarrhythmic agent. Acta Cardiol. 18 (Suppl.): 317–333.
2. MURPHY, P. J. 1974. Metabolic pathways of aprindine. Acta Cardiol. 18 (Suppl.): 131–142.
3. VERDOUW, P. D., W. J. REMME & P. G. HUGENHOLTZ. 1977. Cardiovascular and antiarrhythmic effects of aprindine (AC-1802) during partial occlusion of a coronary artery in the pig. Cardiovasc. Res. 11: 317–321.
4. BREITHARDT, G. et al. 1974. Long-term oral antiarrhythmic therapy with aprindine (AC-1802). Acta Cardiol. 18 (Suppl.): 341–353.
5. BESSE, P. & A. CHOUSSAT. 1974. Effects de l'aprindine (AC-1802) sur la fonction myocardique chez l'homme. Acta Cardiol. 18 (Suppl.): 217–231.
6. PIESSENS, J. et al. 1974. Effects of aprindine on left ventricular contractility in man. Acta Cardiol. 18 (Suppl.): 203–216.
7. CARMELIET, E. & F. VERDONCK. 1974. Effects of aprindine and lidocaine on transmembrane potentials and radioactive K efflux in different cardiac tissues. Acta Cardiol. 18 (Suppl.): 73–90.
8. STEINBERG, M. I. & K. GREENSPAN. 1976. Intracellular electrophysiological alterations in canine cardiac conducting tissue induced by aprindine and lidocaine. Cardiovasc. Res. 10: 236–244.
9. ELHARRAR, V. et al. 1978. Effects of aprindine HCl on slow channel action potentials and transient depolarizations in canine Purkinje fibers. J. Pharmacol. Exp. Ther. 205, 410–417.
10. GILMOUR, R. F. et al. 1979. Effects of aprindine on transmembrane currents and contractile force in frog atria (abstract.) Circulation 59–60 (Suppl. 2): 209.
11. ZIPES, D. P., W. E. GAUM, P. R. FOSTER, K. M. ROSEN, D. WU, F. AMAT-Y-LEON & R. J. NOBLE. 1977. Aprindine for treatment of supraventricular tachycardias with particular application to Wolff-Parkinson-White syndrome. Am. J. Cardiol. 40: 586–596.
12. FASOLA, A. F., R. J. NOBLE & D. P. ZIPES. 1977. Treatment of recurrent ventricular tachycardia and fibrillation with aprindine. Am. J. Cardiol. 39: 903–909.
13. ELHARRAR, V. et al. 1975. Effects of aprindine HCl on cardiac tissues. J Pharmacol. Exp. Ther. 195: 201–205.
14. FOSTER, P. R. et al. 1976. Suppression of ouabain-induced ventricular rhythms with aprindine HCl. A comparison with other antiarrhythmic agents. Circulation 53: 315–321.
15. ZIPES, D. P. et al. 1977. Effects of various drugs on ventricular conduction delay and ventricular arrhythmias during myocardial ischemia in the dog. In Re-entrant Arrhythmias. H. E. Kulbertus, Ed.: 312. MTP Press. London.
16. GAUM, W. E. et al. 1977. Influence of excitability on the ventricular-fibrillation threshold in dogs. Am. J. Cardiol. 40: 929–935.
17. ELHARRAR, V., W. E. GAUM & D. P. ZIPES. 1977. Effect of drugs on conduction delay and incidence of ventricular arrhythmias induced by acute coronary occlusion in dogs. Am. J. Cardiol. 39: 544–549.
18. NATTEL, S., D. H. PEDERSEN & D. P. ZIPES. 1981. Alterations in regional myocardial distribution and arrhythmogenic effects of aprindine produced by coronary artery occlusion in the dog. Cardiovasc. Res. 15: 80–85.
19. BYRNE, J. E., A. W. GOMOLL & G. R. MCKINNEY. 1977. Antiarrhythmic properties of MJ 9067 in acute animal models. J. Pharmacol. Exp. Ther. 200: 147–154.

20. ENCAINIDE: INVESTIGATOR'S BROCHURE. 1979.: 3–9. Mead Johnson Pharmaceutical Division. Evansville, IN.
21. RODEN, D. M., H. J. DUFF, T. WANG & R. L. WOOSLEY. 1980. Contribution of a metabolite to the ECG and antiarrhythmic actions of encainide (abstract). Circulation **62** (Suppl. III): III–141.
22. KESTELOOT, H. & R. STROOBANDT. 1979. Clinical experience of encainide (MJ 9067), a new antiarrhythmic drug. Eur. J. Clin. Pharmacol. **16:** 323–326.
23. WINKLE, R. A., F. PETERS, R. E. KATES, C. TUCKER & D. C. HARRISON. 1981. Clinical pharmacology and antiarrhythmic efficacy of encainide in patients with chronic ventricular arrhythmias. Circulation **64:** 290–296.
24. RODEN, D. M., S. B. REELE, S. B. HIGGINS, R. F. MAYOL, R. E. GAMMANS, J. A. OATES & R. L. WOOSLEY, 1980. Total suppression of ventricular arrhythmias by encainide: Pharmacokinetic and electrocardiographic characteristics. N. Engl. J. Med. **302:** 877–882.
25. SAMI, M., R. DEBUSK, H. KRAEMER, N. HOUSTON & D. HARRISON. 1979. Evaluation of antiarrhythmic efficacy of encainide and quinidine (abstract.) Circulation **60** (Suppl. II): II–184.
26. HEGER, J. J., S. NATTEL, R. RINKENBERGER & D. P. ZIPES. 1979. Encainide therapy in patients with drug-resistant ventricular tachycardia (abstract). Circulation **60** (Suppl. II): II–185.
27. JACKMAN, W. M., D. P. ZIPES, G. V. NACCARELLI, R. L. RINKENBERGER, J. J. HEGER & E. N. PRYSTOWSKY. 1982. Electrophysiology of oral encainide. Am. J. Cardiol. **49:** 1270–1278.
28. RAHILLY, G. T. JR., E. N. PRYSTOWSKY, D. P. ZIPES, G. V. NACCARELLI, W. M. JACKMAN & J. J. HEGER. 1982. Clinical and electrophysiologic findings in patients with repetitive monomorphic ventricular tachycardia and otherwise normal electrocardiograms. Am. J. Cardiol. **50:** 459–468.
29. MASON, J. W. & F. A. PETERS. 1981. Antiarrhythmic efficacy of encainide in patients with refractory recurrent ventricular tachycardia. Circulation **63:** 670–675.
30. SAMI, M., J. W. MASON, G. OH & D. C. HARRISON. 1979. Canine electrophysiology of encainide, a new antiarrhythmic drug. Am. J. Cardiol. **43:** 1149–1154.
31. SAMI, M., J. W. MASON, F. PETERS & D. C. HARRISON. 1979. Clinical electrophysiologic effects of encainide, a newly developed antiarrhythmic agent. Am. J. Cardiol. **44:** 526–532.
32. ELHARRAR, V. & D. P. ZIPES. 1982. Effects of encainide metabolites (MJ14930) and (MJ19444) on canine Purkinje and ventricular fibers. J. Pharm. Exp. Ther. **220:** 440–447.
33. PRYSTOWSKY, E. N., R. L. RINKENBERGER, G. KLEIN *et al.* 1982. Encainide in Wolff-Parkinson-White syndrome: Electrophysiologic alterations of accessory pathways and clinical efficacy. Circulation **66** (Suppl. II): II–271.
34. WINKLE, R. A., J. W. MASON, J. C. GRIFFIN *et al.* 1981. Malignant ventricular tachyarrhythmias associated with the use of encainide. Am. Heart. J. **102:** 857–864.
35. HEGER, J. J., E. N. PRYSTOWSKY, G. V. NACCARELLI *et al.* 1981. Comparison of encainide and aprindine in patients with ventricular tachycardia. Clin. Res. **29:** 694.
36. DIBIANCO R., R. D. FLETCHER, A. I. COHEN *et al.* 1982. Treatment of frequent ventricular arrhythmia with encainide: Assessment using serial ambulatory electrocardiograms, intracardiac electrophysiologic studies, treadmill exercise tests, and radionuclide cineangiographic studies. Circulation **65:** 1134–1147.
37. PROPAFENONE. INVESTIGATOR'S BROCHURE. 1981. Medical Research Department, Knoll Pharmaceutical Co.
38. CHILSON, D. A., D. P. ZIPES, J. J. HEGER *et al.* 1982. Propafenone, clinical and electrophysiologic effects in patients with ventricular tachycardia. Clin. Res. **30:** 706A.

# The Electrophysiology and Pharmacology of Verapamil, Flecainide, and Amiodarone: Correlations with Clinical Effects and Antiarrhythmic Actions[a]

BRAMAH N. SINGH,[b] KOONLAWEE NADEMANEE,
MARTIN A. JOSEPHSON, NOBUO IKEDA,
NAGAMMAL VENKATESH, AND RAMASWAMY KANNAN

*Department of Cardiology*
*Wadsworth Veterans Administration Hospital; and*
*Department of Medicine*
*UCLA School of Medicine*
*Los Angeles, California 90024*

An understanding of the electrophysiologic and pharmacologic properties of antiarrhythmic compounds is central to the definition of their clinical utility in the control of dysrhythmias. Verapamil, flecainide, and amiodarone represent three pharmacodynamically distinct antiarrhythmic compounds. The spectrum of antiarrhythmic activity of verapamil is reasonably well defined; it is the prototype of compounds now designated as slow-channel inhibitors.[1] Flecainide typifies a new subclass of antiarrhythmic agents which, in common with encainide and its metabolites, has a potent depressant effect on cardiac conduction and on the suppression of ventricular ectopy.[2,3] Amiodarone, while not being a new compound, has attracted widespread experimental and clinical interest recently because of its many remarkable pharmacologic properties[4] in addition to its extreme potency in the suppression of most supraventricular and ventricular tachyarrhythmias. In this paper, the electropharmacology of verapamil, flecainide, and amiodarone are discussed relative to their established and expanding clinical indications as antiarrhythmic compounds.

## VERAPAMIL

In isolated cardiac muscle, verapamil produces a concentration-dependent inhibition of the "slow response"[5–7]; it inhibits excitation-contraction coupling[8] and produces negative inotropic effect[5] which is competitively antagonized by cal-

[a] This work was supported by grants from the Medical Research Service of the Veterans Administration and from the American Heart Association (the Greater Los Angeles affiliate).

[b] Address for correspondence: Bramah N. Singh, M.D., Section of Cardiology 691/111E, Wadsworth Veterans Administration Hospital, Wilshire and Sawtelle Boulevards, Los Angeles, California 90073.

cium. In isolated vascular smooth muscle, both from peripheral vessels as well as in those from the coronary circulation, the drug inhibits $K^+$-depolarized contractions[9] and depresses the slow-response action potentials from helical strips of canine small and large coronary arteries exposed to tetraethylammonium.[10] These experimental observations in cardiac and vascular smooth muscle provide the basis for interpreting the hemodynamic and electrophysiologic actions of verapamil in intact animals and in man.[11]

When given intravenously or orally, verapamil produces a complex interplay of simultaneous changes in preload, afterload, contractility, heart rate, and coronary blood flow.[11] Except in patients with severely depressed ventricular ejection fraction, the intrinsic negative inotropic effect of the drug is nullified by its impedance-reducing properties,[11,12] although the net effect is also influenced significantly by inhibitory effect on the sympathetic nervous system.[1] Of particular interest is the fact that verapamil, a weak coronary vasodilator under resting conditions producing little or no increase in coronary sinus flow measured by the thermodilution technique,[13] reverses the ergonovine-induced and sympathetically mediated coronary vasoconstriction in man.[14]

### *Electrophysiologic Actions of Verapamil*

From the standpoint of the antiarrhythmic actions of verapamil, its electrophysiologic actions are the most relevant. The drug has little effect on the upstroke velocity in atrial, ventricular, and Purkinje fibers. For example, in rabbit atrial and ventricular fibers, Singh and Vaughan Williams[5] found that 1–6 $\mu$g/ml of verapamil abolished isometric contractions and accelerated phases 1 and 2 of the action potential, but without effect on the upstroke velocity of phase 0 or on the resting membrane voltage. Similar effects on Purkinje fibers were reported by Cranefield *et al.*[6] as well as by Rosen and his associates.[7] Cranefield *et al.*[6] also demonstrated that Purkinje fibers that were spontaneously active in a media containing zero Na and 4.0 mM Ca were markedly depressed in rate and amplitude on exposure to low concentrations of verapamil; similarly, fibers exposed to low Na concentrations and developing repetitive activity after bursts of sustained depolarizing impulses could be inhibited by verapamil.[6] Rosen *et al.*[7] have also shown that spontaneous activity in diseased human atria, undoubtedly mediated by slow-channel activity, was suppressed by verapamil, and Spear *et al.*[15] have found that the slow-response potentials in human ventricular tissue removed during aneurysmectomy were sensitive to the depressant effects of verapamil. Perhaps also of significance are the observations that catecholamine-induced delayed afterdepolarization of simian mitral valve fibers and "triggered"[16] sustained rhythmic activity may both be abolished by low concentrations of verapamil, as are also the afterdepolarizations induced by digitalis in human atria.[7] The clinical significance of these observations at present is unknown. In contrast, the observed effect of verapamil on nodal tissues (SA and especially AV nodes) is best defined; the drug depresses phase-4 depolarization in these slow-channel-dependent tissues[17,19] and in the case of the AV node, produces a marked increase in its effective refractory period (ERP) and the functional refractory period (FRP)[17] as well as in intranodal (but not infranodal) conduction (FIG. 1).

The clinical electrophysiological studies with verapamil are in substantial agreement with the experimental data. The data are summarized in TABLE 1 and provide the basis for predicting the antiarrhythmic spectrum of the drug in man. It will be evident that the drug has no effect on the ERP of the atria, ventricle, His-

CONTROL                          VERAPAMIL    0,2 µg/ml

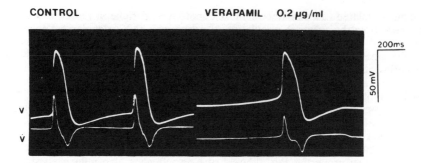

**FIGURE 1.** Effects of verapamil on slow-channel-dependent pacemaker potential from the AV node. Note that both the amplitude as well as phase 4 of the action potential is depressed by verapamil; the threshold potential is also elevated. (From Tritthart.[8] Reproduced by permission.)

**TABLE 1.** Electrophysiological Effects of Verapamil: Experimental and Clinical Correlations

|  | Effect of Verapamil |
| --- | --- |
| *Isolated Tissues (Animals):* | |
| Fast-response potentials (atria, ventricle, His-Purkinje fibers) | Accelerate phases 2 and 3 of the action potential; no effect on ERP or conduction velocity |
| Sinoatrial node | Depress phase 4; reduce amplitude and overshoot |
| Atrioventricular node | Depress phase 4; reduce amplitude and overshoot; reduce conduction velocity; increase ERP and FRP (antegrade and retrograde) |
| Abnormal slow response | Inhibited |
| *Man:* | |
| R-R cycle length | ± |
| P-R interval | Lengthened + + |
| QRS duration | No change |
| Q-Tc interval | No change |
| Atrial ERP | No change |
| A-H interval | Lengthened + + + |
| AVN ERP antegrade | Lengthened + + + |
| AVN ERP retrograde | Lengthened + + + |
| Ventricular ERP | No change |
| His-Purkinje ERP | No change |
| Accessory Pathway ERP (antegrade/retrograde) | ± |
| SNRT[a] | No change |

[a] Increases in patients with conduction system disease.

Purkinje tissue, or the accessory tracts in the heart. In patients in sinus rhythm, intravenous verapamil has no effect on the R-R, QRS and Q-Tc intervals of the ECG,[20] but predictably increases the PR interval. During His bundle studies, verapamil was found to impede AV conduction proximal to the His bundle without having an effect on intraatrial or intraventricular conduction. The conduction delay was in the AV node and was largely independent of autonomic influences (see Singh *et al.*[20]). The drug's effect on AV conduction is of clinical significance since it represents the fundamental mechanism through which the ventricular response in atrial fibrillation and flutter is controlled and AV nodal reentrant PSVT is abolished.[20] Two further features need emphasis. First, the drug's pharmacologic effects are accentuated by the presence of underlying disease. For example, while it has little or no effect on sinus node function in normal subjects, a markedly depressant effect may become apparent in patients with conduction system disease.[11] Second, the electrophysiologic changes in the normal ventricular myocardium that the drug produces differ from those found in the ischemic myocardium.[11] Here, it may ameliorate depressed conduction and lengthen refractoriness, presumably as a consequence of a salutary effect on ischemia itself. Such an indirect effect is clearly of relevance in patients with ventricular tachyarrhythmias triggered by transient myocardial ischemia, especially coronary artery spasm.[20,21]

### Clinical Role of Verapamil in Cardiac Arrhythmias

The most significant effect of verapamil appears to be due largely to its direct electrophysiologic actions.[11] However, in contrast to the experimental data, clinical experience with verapamil has indicated a somewhat narrow antiarrhythmic spectrum.[20] Indeed, intravenous verapamil (5–15 mg, average 10 mg) has been found to promptly terminate 90–100% of the paroxysms of PSVT, a success rate of reversion unmatched by any other drug regimen. The efficacy of verapamil in this context does not depend on whether reciprocation occurs within the AV node or whether it involves an anomalous tract, provided the ventricular activation occurs orthodromically, that is, the impulse traverses the AV node anterogradely.[21] Various electrophysiologic modes of termination of PSVT have been reported.[21] In this setting, when the drug is given intravenously, the onset of action is rapid; sinus rhythm is restored within 2–3 min. The success rate of conversion of PSVT to sinus rhythm by verapamil may be improved to nearly 100% by carotid sinus massage or the addition of 5–10 mg edrophonium chloride given in rapid succession after verapamil. The success of prompt conversion appears to be related to high transient plasma verapamil concentrations, usually exceeding 100 ng/ml.[22]

The bulk of the clinical experience in PSVT in verapamil has been in AV nodal and orthodromic PSVT.[20,21] It is unclear whether the drug is effective in other forms of reentrant PSVT (such as the sinoatrial and intraatrial); however, increasing experience suggests that ectopic PSVT does not respond to intravenous verapamil,[23] although PAT with block has been reported to be reversible by the drug.[24]

It should be emphasized that in contrast to intravenous verapamil, which is extremely potent in terminating PSVT, the orally administered drug may not have comparable efficacy in preventing recurrences of PSVT. For example, Rinkenberger *et al.*[23] found that when verapamil was given orally (180–480 mg/day) to patients who had responded to intravenous verapamil, 10 of 19 patients discontinued therapy within 1 month either because of side effects or lack of response.

Another approach that appears somewhat promising is suggested by the use of programmed electrical stimulation. It has been reported that patients in whom electrically inducible PSVT is inhibited by verapamil tend to have uniformly successful prophylactic response to long-term oral therapy[25,26]; this approach, however, needs further validation whether verapamil is used alone or in combination with digoxin and beta blockade.

The inhibitory effects of verapamil on AV conduction is of clinical value in the control of ventricular response in atrial fibrillation and flutter.[20] Moreover, recent data have clearly suggested that oral verapamil may effectively control the ventricular response in atrial flutter and fibrillation,[27] not only at rest but with exercise,[28] an effect that may be additive to those of beta-blockers in the control of the ventricular response in atrial flutter-fibrillation in patients with bronchospastic disease, diabetes mellitus, and peripheral vascular disease.

The role of verapamil in preexcitation syndromes is reasonably well defined. In the cases of orthodromic tachycardias, the drug is effective electively and prophylactically.[21] It is without effect in antidromic tachycardia, in which the decrease in blood pressure may produce serious hemodynamic sequelae. The drug is contraindicated in patients with atrial flutter and fibrillation complicating the Wolff-Parkinson-White syndrome, in which AV nodal blockade by the drug may preferentially increase the ventricular response, possibly with potentially lethal consequences.[23,29]

Currently, there are few data to indicate that calcium antagonists are effective in the treatment of ventricular arrhythmias,[20] except in those instances in which such dysrhythmias arise in the wake of coronary vasospasm with transmural myocardial ischemia. The role of the slow response in the genesis of ventricular arrhythmias still remains somewhat controversial,[30] but it is conceivable that slow-channel inhibitors may improve electrical conduction in ischemic myocardium, an action that may produce salutary effects on dysrhythmias after coronary occlusion. This action may provide the basis for evaluating the role of verapamil in the prevention of sudden death in the survivors of acute myocardial infarction.

## FLECAINIDE

Flecainide (R-818), a new investigational antiarrhythmic compound, has recently been shown to be effective in controlling various experimental tachyarrhythmias, especially those induced by aconitine, ouabain, and chloroform-epinephrine and by coronary arterial occlusion.[31,32] On a milligram per kilogram basis, the drug is 7–12 times more potent than quinidine, procainamide, and lidocaine in suppressing chloroform-epinephrine-induced ventricular arrhythmias in mice.[31] In the intact canine heart, it was[33] found that flecainide increased the ventricular fibrillation threshold of supraventricular beats and ventricular premature beats as a function of plasma drug concentration. The electrophysiologic, inotropic, and hemodynamic effects have been evaluated in our laboratories.[34,35] These are briefly discussed herein relative to the findings of other investigators and the potential clinical utility of this potent new compound.

### Inotropic and Hemodynamic Effects

Flecainide is known to have no vagomimetic or vagolytic properties, nor does the compound appear to produce presynaptic or postsynaptic adrenergic block-

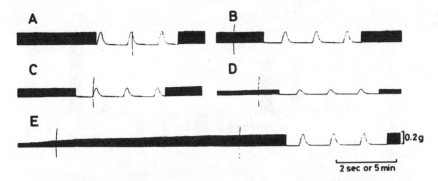

**FIGURE 2.** Representative records from an experiment with rabbit right ventricular papillary muscle driven at 1 Hz and subjected to varying concentrations of flecainide. **(A)** Control recording at slow and fast speeds; **(B)** after superfusion with 1 $\mu$g/ml flecainide; **(C)** after 5 $\mu$g/ml flecainide; **(D)** after 10 $\mu$g/ml flecainide; **(E)** after 10 $\mu$g/ml flecainide plus an increase of external calcium from 1.8 to 5.4 mM. Note the concentration-dependent decrease in developed tension and the reversal of the depressant effect by the elevation of the calcium concentration in the physiologic medium. (From Josephson *et al.*[35] Reproduced by permission.)

ade. However, in isolated cardiac muscle, it produces a concentration-dependent depression of contractile force in rabbit papillary muscle (FIG. 2), the threshold concentration being 1 $\mu$g/ml. A 30% reduction in contraction amplitude was found with 10 $\mu$g/ml of the drug and 50% with 20 $\mu$g/ml, the overall effect being nullified by the elevation of calcium ion concentration (FIG. 3). These *in vitro* data, which

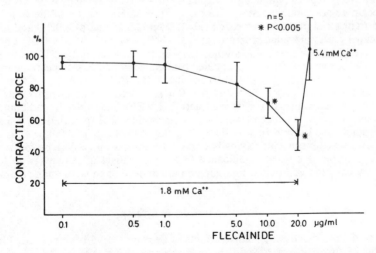

**FIGURE 3.** Summary of data from rabbit papillary muscles driven at 1 Hz and superfused with varying concentrations of flecainide at 2 concentrations of calcium in the physiologic medium (see FIGURE 1). The data shown are means ($\pm$S.D.) from five preparations. Again, note the concentration-dependent decrease in the amplitude of contraction induced by flecainide and its reversal by additional calcium in the physiologic medium.

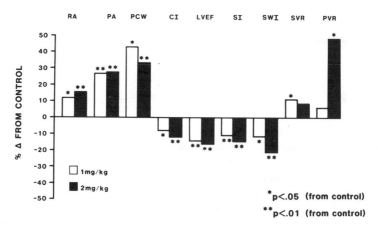

**FIGURE 4.** Summary of the hemodynamic changes and the effects on ventricular ejection fraction induced by two doses of intravenously administered flecainide in patients with coronary artery disease. Eleven patients were studied at each dose. The data shown represent changes compared to control values. The overall changes were similar after the two doses of flecainide and are consistent with a moderate but significant inotropic propensity of the compound. (From Josephson et al.[35] Reproduced by permission.)

have been confirmed by others also,[36–38] were found to be consistent with the changes effected by the drug when it was given intravenously to patients with coronary artery disease who had varying levels of left ventricular ejection fraction and who were undergoing diagnostic cardiac catheterization.[35] The salient findings in two groups of patients given 1 mg/kg (n = 11) and 2 mg/kg (n = 11) doses of flecainide are summarized in FIGURE 4. After administration of the drug, the mean right atrial pressure increased (12–15%, $p < 0.05$ and $p < 0.01$) and mean preliminary arterial wedge pressure rose (33–44%, $p < 0.05$ and $p < 0.01$) with an associated increase in the mean pulmonary arterial pressure (25–27%, both $p < 0.01$). These changes were accompanied by significant decreases in cardiac index (8–12%; $p < 0.05$ and $p < 0.01$), stroke index (11–15%; $p < 0.01$), and stroke-work index (12–21%; $p < 0.05$ and $p < 0.01$). Particularly noteworthy was the effect on the left ventricular ejection fraction (LVEF) determined by radionuclide ventriculography. The mean LVEF was depressed by 15% ($p < 0.01$) by 1 mg/kg of flecainide and by 16% ($p < 0.01$) by 2 mg/kg of the drug ($p < 0.01$). Thus, the drug exerts significant but modestly depressant effects on cardiac performance, which may be of clinical significance in a small subset of patients who have severely impaired ventricular function and are in need of antiarrhythmic therapy.

### Electrophysiologic Effects

The *in vitro* electrophysiologic effects of flecainide have been evaluated by a number of investigators[36–38] and the data are concordant. Over a wide range of concentrations (1–30 μg/ml), the drug produces a concentration-dependent reduction in the maximum rate of rise of phase 0 of the action potential ($V_{max}$) in fast-channel-dependent myocardial fibers (atria, ventricles, and His-Purkinje tissues) with a concomitant reduction in the action potential amplitude and overshoot potential, but without effect on resting membrane voltage. However, differences in the effects of flecainide on ventricular muscle and Purkinje fibers were noted particularly in our own studies (FIGS. 5 and 6). For example, in ventricular muscle, after 1 $\mu$g/ml, $\dot{V}_{max}$ fell by 52.5% (p < 0.01) and by 79.8% after 10 $\mu$g/ml (p < 0.01). The corresponding values for Purkinje fibers were 18.6% (p < 0.01) and 70.8% (p < 0.01), respectively, but in these fibers the ERP was shortened at the lower concentration and restored to control value at the higher concentration. The depression of $\dot{V}_{max}$ was frequency-dependent. The $APD_{50}$ and $APD_{90}$ in ventricular muscle were lengthened (17.6% and 12.7% at 1.0 $\mu$g/ml, p < 0.01, and 28.2% and 23.6% at 10 $\mu$g/ml, p < 0.01). In Purkinje fibers they were markedly shortened ($APD_{90}$ by 25.7% at 1 $\mu$g/ml and 47.5% at 10 $\mu$g/ml), and modestly reversed by high $(Ca^{2+})_o$. Slow-response potentials induced by high K and isoproterenol were attenuated by flecainide at high (10 $\mu$g/ml) concentrations only. Automatic firing induced by isoproterenol in Purkinje fibers was slowed by flecainide by an elevation of the threshold potential rather than by the depression of the slope of phase-4 depolarization. Thus, the dominant effects of flecainide in various isolated cardiac tissues studied here are consistent with a potent inhibitory action on the fast sodium current, as indicated by the decrease in $\dot{V}_{max}$[15] and the shift of the membrane responsiveness curve in the hyperpolarizing direction. In this respect, then, the actions of flecainide resemble those of the broad category of compounds that appear to exert their salutary effects on arrhythmias predominantly by prolonging sodium-mediated time-dependent refractoriness in cardiac muscle.[39–41] In contrast to the complex actions of flecainide on canine

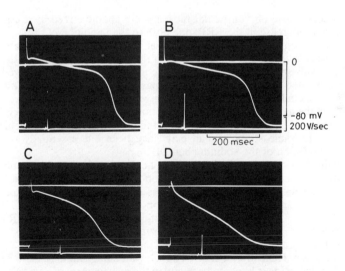

**FIGURE 5.** Effects of various concentrations of flecainide on the action potentials of the canine Purkinje fiber. The *upper trace* in each panel indicates zero potential, the *lower trace* the differentiated rate of rise of the phase 0 of the action potential ($dV/dt_{max}$ or $\dot{V}_{max}$). Vertical and horizontal calibrations are as indicated: **A** = control recording; **B** = changes after 0.1 $\mu$g/ml of flecainide (the main effects are the depression of $\dot{V}_{max}$ with shortening of the $APD_{50}$ and $APD_{90}$); **C** = changes after 1.0 $\mu$g/ml; **D** = effects of 10.0 $\mu$g/ml. Note the dose-related shortening of $APD_{50}$ and $APD_{90}$ and the reduction in $\dot{V}_{max}$. (From Ikeda *et al.*[34] Reproduced by permission.)

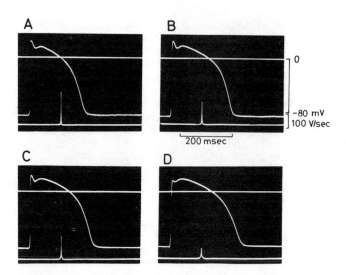

**FIGURE 6.** Effects of flecainide on several variables of transmembrane potential from canine ventricular muscle. Sequence as in FIGURE 1. The concentrations used were 0.1 $\mu$g/ml **(B)**, 1.0 $\mu$g/ml **(C)** and 10.0 $\mu$g/ml **(D)**. Note the dose-related *increase* in $APD_{50}$ and $APD_{90}$ and a decrease in $V_{max}$. (From Ikeda et al.[34] Reproduced by permission.)

Purkinje fibers, those on ventricular muscle were characterized by a concentration-dependent increase in the ERP, due both to the inhibition of the Na channel as well as to the lengthening of the $APD_{90}$ over a range of drug concentrations that were therapeutically and pharmacologically relevant. Although the lengthening of the $APD_{90}$ is still unexplained in terms of the ionic conductances involved, it has been demonstrated in man from the recordings of the right ventricular monophasic action potentials after flecainide was given intravenously.[42] However, the magnitude of the increase was small and did not influence the Q-Tc interval of the surface electrocardiogram, suggesting that the increases in the ventricular ERP observed in the same study in man may have been due essentially to a time-dependent inhibition of the sodium channel.

The clinical electrophysiologic effects of flecainide appear to be dominated by a profoundly depressant effect on conduction at nearly all levels in the myocardium, but the drug exerts a variable and less striking effect on refractoriness[2,43] after intravenous and oral drug administration. For example, when flecainide was given orally, in one study[44] there was a significant lengthening of the P-R interval (31%), QRS duration (47%), and Q-Tc interval (6%). The most extensive study delineating the electrophysiologic effects of intravenous flecainide have been reported recently by Hellestrandt et al.[2] The relevant data, summarized in TABLE 2, indicate that flecainide is likely to be useful in the management of a wide variety of cardiac arrhythmias. Preliminary experiences have tended to vindicate these expectations.[2,3,44–46]

### Control of Cardiac Arrhythmias by Flecainide

Human pharmacokinetic studies, even though incomplete as yet, suggest that flecainide has favorable kinetic features for both intravenous as well as oral use as an antiarrhythmic compound. The drug is almost completely absorbed after oral administration and undergoes minimal hepatic biotransformation, with a long plasma elimination half-life ranging from 11–22 hours.[47] These are highly desirable features for the long-term prophylactic use of antiarrhythmic agents. The protein binding of flecainide is moderate in serum, being between 37 and 58%; serum concentrations between 85 and 460 ng/ml have been considered within the therapeutic range.[48]

The most clearly documented antiarrhythmic effect of flecainide is in the control of ventricular arrhythmias,[3,44–46] especially premature ventricular contractions (PVCs). Although intravenous flecainide has been shown to suppress PVCs,[45] the effect of the oral drug is of greater therapeutic interest.[3,44–46] For example, in one study[49] in 8 patients with chronic PVCs, initially given 200 mg twice daily (plasma level 413–789 ng/ml) and then 50 mg twice daily, their was a >95% reduction in PVCs. At the lower dose (plasma level, 217–414 ng/ml) nearly complete PVC suppression was still evident, but levels <230 ng/ml tended to produce <70% PVC suppression. Therefore, the minimum therapeutic plasma concentrations of flecainide appear to be 200–400 ng/ml, which are associated with no significant side effects.[49]

The observations of Anderson *et al.*[3] on PVCs is of particular interest. In their study eleven patients were given incremental doses of flecainide, starting at 100 mg twice daily and increasing to 200, 250, and 300 mg twice daily every 3 days until complete PVC suppression was achieved as the maximum dose had been given; one patient was withdrawn because of intercurrent illness. Nine of the remaining ten patients attained near complete suppression of PVCs (average 99.2%; two on 100 mg, five on 200 mg, and two on 250 mg; one patient on 300 mg twice daily had only 68% suppression). Side effects included blurred vision in four patients, dizziness and light-headedness in three, abnormal taste, flushing, tinnitus and sleepiness in two, and paresthesias in one.

There were few comparative controlled data on the efficacy of flecainide until the results were reported of a recent multicenter study[50] comparing flecainide and

**TABLE 2.** Cardiac Electrophysiology of Flecainide in Man[a]

| Electrophysiologic Variable | n | Control (msec) | Flecainide (msec) | Statistical Significance (p) |
|---|---|---|---|---|
| Sinus cycle length | 47 | 745 ± 198 | 734 ± 18 | NS |
| P-A interval | 43 | 41 ± 13 | 50 ± 13 | <0.001 |
| A-H interval | 43 | 67 ± 21 | 81 ± 21 | <0.001 |
| H-V interval | 39 | 44 ± 9 | 61 ± 12 | <0.001 |
| QRS duration | 47 | 96 ± 21 | 118 ± 30 | <0.001 |
| Q-Tc interval[b] | 39 | 427 ± 34 | 446 ± 40 | <0.001 |
| WCL (AV) | 19 | 371 ± 153 | 410 ± 178 | <0.05 |
| WCL (VA) | 19 | 355 ± 91 | 496 ± 72 | <0.001 |
| ERP (atrial) | 47 | 213 ± 32 | 219 ± 28 | NS |
| ERP (AVN) | 10 | 314 ± 66 | 287 ± 21 | NS |
| ERP (ventricular) | 47 | 220 ± 22 | 229 ± 23 | <0.01 |
| ERP$_{AP}$ (antegrade) | 8 | 262 ± 47 | 361 ± 138 | <0.05 |
| ERP$_{AP}$ (retrograde) | 13 | 300 ± 49 | 453 ± 169 | <0.01 |

ABBREVIATIONS: WCL = Wenckebach cycle length; AV = atrioventricular; VA = ventriculoatrial; ERP = effective refractory period; AVN = atrioventricular node; AP = accessory pathway.

[a] Adapted from Hellestrandt *et al.*[2]

[b] Q-Tc lengthening was due entirely to the prolongation of the QRS duration.

quinidine. In this study of 280 patients, 80% suppression of PVCs was achieved in 85% of the patients taking flecainide versus 57% of those receiving quinidine sulfate ($p < 0.0001$). Of particular note was the finding that 65% of the patients taking flecainide not only had 80% suppression of PVCs but also had complete suppression of couplets and beats of ventricular tachycardia. The corresponding figure for quinidine was 33%.[50] While these data clearly document the striking potency of flecainide in suppressing and eliminating the frequent and complex PVCs, there are at present no systematic data that bear adequately on the effects of the drug on symptomatic ventricular tachycardias, whether spontaneously occurring or induced by programmed electrical stimulation (PES) of the heart. Such studies are in progress. However, it must be mentioned that in as yet undefined numbers of patients, especially those with marked depression of left ventricular ejection fraction, flecainide may aggravate ventricular tachycardia which may prove irreversible even to electroversion.[51] The reason for this is unclear, but it may be due to severe depression of conduction since the drug is known to be more depressant in tissues with preexisting disease than in the healthy myocardium. It is also conceivable that the differential effects of the drug on ventricular muscle and Purkinje fibers may aggravate the existing myocardial heterogeneity, augmenting the tendency to focal reexcitation, a possibility that might be a common feature of class 1C antiarrhythmic compounds.

The role of flecainide in treatment of the supraventricular tachyarrhythmias remains to be defined. It is of interest, however, that in one study all 13 patients with AV nodal reentrant tachycardia given flecainide intravenously reverted to sinus rhythm.[43] However, tachycardia could be reinitiated by PES in five after intravenous flecainide and in one after the oral drug. Flecainide markedly prolonged antegrade and retrograde conduction intervals at the AV node, with 5 of 13 patients developing complete retrograde block. Because flecainide also markedly prolongs the ERP (AV as well as VA) of the accessory pathways in the heart, it is likely to be of value in the management of all supraventricular tachyarrhythmias complicating the Wolff-Parkinson-White syndrome. Thus, the role of the drug in supraventricular tachyarrhythmias merits detailed study.

In summary, the available data from experimental observations and clinical studies indicate that the electrophysiologic effects of flecainide are complex and that its antiarrhythmic spectrum in man may be wider than that for many Class 1 agents. Moreover, its availability provides a new pharmacologic tool to study the nature of certain clinically occurring cardiac arrhythmias.

## AMIODARONE

Although the introduction of amiodarone as an antiarrhythmic drug has been gradual, the recognition of its unusual electropharmacologic properties[4] suggests a new departure in drug therapy of cardiac arrhythmias. Charlier et al.[52] were first to emphasize the broad pharmacologic profile of the drug, but more in relationship to the compound's potential for the control of myocardial ischemia. After the compound was seen to exert unique electrophysiologic effects in cardiac muscle, characterized by the slow onset of the propensity to homogeneously lengthen the action potential duration[53,54] in all cardiac tissues, interest in the drug's antiarrhythmic activity has burgeoned.[55-62] However, recent studies have only documented the extreme potency of the drug and its overall clinical toxicity profile. They have not provided newer insights into the fundamental mechanisms that might be involved in mediating the salutary therapeutic effects of the compound. In this paper, the known pharmacologic effects of the compound are discussed and its expanding clinical role in the control of cardiac dysrhythmias is summarized.

### Pharmacologic Considerations

When the action of amiodarone on cardiac muscle is considered, three features are of clinical significance. First, the drug is not soluble in physiologic media and, thus, superfusion studies in isolated tissues can reliably be undertaken only in homologous plasma or in blood containing amiodarone. The results of such studies have been conflicting (see References 4 and 63), but have to be reconciled with the observation that when the drug is given as a single intravenous bolus (in Tween 80 as the diluent), in experimental animals or man, the Q-T interval is not prolonged.[64,65] Second, the elimination half-life of amiodarone is exceedingly long and variable in different individuals.[66] Thus, it is impossible to standardize the

**TABLE 3.** Pharmacologic Properties of Amiodarone[a]

1. Electrophysiologic (chronic administration)
   (a) Lengthening of the action potential duration in all cardiac tissues
   (b) Depression of phase 4 (poorly defined)
2. Coronary arterial dilatation
3. Systemic vasodilatation
4. Noncompetitive alpha- and beta-catecholamine receptor antagonism
5. Probably no vagomimetic or vagolytic activity
6. Probably little or no intrinsic negative inotropic propensity
7. Complex interrelationships with thyroid hormone metabolism
8. Complex pharmacokinetics with long and variable elimination half-life
9. Pharmacodynamic and pharmacokinetic interactions with numerous cardioactive compounds

NOTE: The ionic translocation or other membrane and cellular processes involved in mediating the pharmacodynamic actions of amiodarone are poorly understood or not at all.
   [a] Modified from Singh.[4]

dosage regimen of the drug while determining the electrophysiologic and antiarrhythmic effects of the compound, and the reported electrophysiologic effects as well as efficacy and toxicity of the compound may therefore vary from center to center.[55-62] Third, it may also be significant that amiodarone is a benzofuran derivative with 37% of its weight due to iodine and that it shares structural similarities with triiodothyronine while producing a distinct pattern of changes in the levels of thyroid hormones without altering thyroid state.[67] Finally, it has an aggregate of associated pharmacologic properties which may all be relevant to its overall action in man. These are summaried in TABLE 3; the hemodynamic effects need emphasis.

The effects of intravenous amiodarone (the commercially available formulation containing Tween 80) on systemic and coronary hemodynamics have recently been reported by Coté *et al.*[68] in patients undergoing diagnostic cardiac catheterization. The drug decreased mean arterial pressure, left ventricular end-diastolic pressure, and systemic vascular resistance, while there was a mild but a significant increase in cardiac index. The coronary vascular resistance decreased, and coronary sinus flow, measured by thermodilution, increased significantly, thus confirming that amiodarone is a potent coronary and peripheral vasodilator. It is noteworthy, however, that despite the decrease in systemic vascular resistance, a reflex increase in heart rate did not occur, undoubtedly because of the drug's known nonspecific antiadrenergic actions.[69,70] There is still a paucity of data with respect to the hemodynamic effects of amiodarone when the compound is given by mouth orally. However, we found that doses of the drug that exert therapeutic effects in the control of cardiac arrhythmias do not depress ventricular ejection fraction measured by radionuclide ventriculography, even when the basal ejection fraction is severely reduced.[4] Possibly, the drug may exert a minor negative inotropic effect which is offset by its potent vasodilator properties[4]; this observation is in line with the knowledge that cardiac failure is rarely aggravated by amiodarone, even in patients with compromised ventricular farction.[57-59] However, the possibility remains that cardiac failure may be aggravated in patients in whom cardiac compensation is critically dependent on sympathetic drive, which may be influenced adversely by nonspecific adrenergic antagonism of amiodarone.

The general pharmacologic properties of amiodarone are of therapeutic significance. First, they provide the rational basis for the use of the drug for its original clinical indication—angina pectoris, in which reduction in the major determinants of $MVO_2$ may mediate the observed beneficial effect of the compound. The clinical relevance of the drug's coronary dilator properties has recently been suggested by its efficacy in Prinzmetal's angina.[71] Second, the presumed "antiischemic" and the recently demonstrated "cardioprotective" effects[72] may be significant in patients with ischemic heart disease complicated by the presence of recalcitrant cardiac arrhythmias and possibly in survivors of acute myocardial infarction. Third, because amiodarone possesses peripheral dilator actions, which result in impedance reduction, and because it lacks negative inotropic propensity, this drug is in a category distinct from that of most other antiarrhythmic agents, which aggravate existing myocardial dysfunction commonly present in patients needing antiarrhythmic therapy. For the delineation of the antiarrhythmic role of amiodarone, however, the drug's electrophysiologic effects are of direct relevance.

## Electrophysiologic and Antiarrhythmic Effects

The earliest electrophysiologic studies in rabbits chronically tested with amiodarone revealed no significant effect on $V_{max}$ on the action potential amplitude or the overshoot or resting membrane potential; by inference, the conduction velocity was not altered but the ERP was prolonged. The most consistent and striking finding was the lengthening of the overall action potential duration.[53,54] Thus, again by inference, the absolute as well as the effective refractory periods of cardiac muscle were lengthened. It was noteworthy that the effect of amiodarone on repolarization was discernible after 1 week of drug treatment and continued to increase for 6 weeks (FIG. 7), an observation that is directly relevant to the clinical observation of the gradual onset of antiarrhythmic effect of the drug[55-62] and the fact that significant differences exist between the overall changes induced by the acute intravenous formulations versus the chronic protracted oral therapy.[64,65] Also noteworthy is that the electrophysiologic changes in cardiac muscle produced by amiodarone pretreatment closely resembled those produced by thyroid gland ablation.[73] Moreover, it was found that iodine contained in the dose of amiodarone for the rabbit experiments did not lengthen the cardiac action potential if administered chronically. On the other hand, the effects of amiodarone on repolarization were all but prevented by the concomitant administration of $T_3$, suggesting the possibility that the fundamental action of amiodarone on cardiac muscle was due to the selective block of the $T_3$ effects on the myocardium.[54] If this were so, one might expect little or no effects on heart muscle after acute administration; the effect might be expected to be slow in onset and ubiqui-

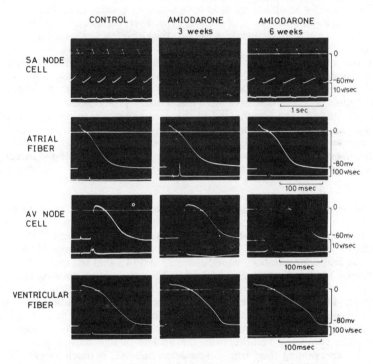

**FIGURE 7.** Changes in the action potentials of myocardial tissues obtained from the heart of rabbits that received chronic intraperitoneal administration of amiodarone (20 mg/kg) for 3 weeks and for 6 weeks compared to those from untreated animals. The *upper traces* of each panel show zero potential; the *middle traces* show transmembrane potential; and the *lower traces* represent the rate of rise of the action potential obtained by electronic differentiation. Amiodarone slows the spontaneous firing frequency of the SA node by retarding phase-4 depolarization. It also delays repolarization in atria, ventricle, and AV node without affecting the maximal rate of depolarization. (From Ikeda *et al.*[34] Reproduced by permission.)

tous in the heart and attained either by prolonged continuous intravenous infusion or by oral dosing. An alternative explanation might be that the delayed onset of amiodarone action is related to the slow formation of active metabolites.

The clinical electrophysiologic effects of amiodarone are in general agreement with those found in the experimental laboratory. Again, striking differences in the net effect after single intravenous doses of the drug and those that develop after chronic therapy are apparent (FIG. 8). The clinical effects are dominated by marked increases in the effective refractory periods of all cardiac tissues after chronic therapy, with the exception of the AV node, little or no effect being evident after single intravenous bolus injections (FIG. 7). Occasionally, unexpected increases in the atrial effective refractory period are found in a few patients, a change that may be due to an interaction with the autonomic nervous system and one that cannot be attributed to a fundamental alteration in either a voltage- or a time-dependent mechanism in ionic translocation mediating refractoriness in cardiac muscle. It is of interest that in the case of the AV node, the effect of the chronically administered drug is significantly greater than that found after the intravenous administration of the drug. However, the electrophysiologic basis for the increase in the intranodal conduction time or refractoriness in the AV node after intravenous amiodarone is not clear.

In contrast, the underlying mechanism of the change in the effective refractory period induced by chronically administered amiodarone is reasonably well defined.[58] It appears that the bulk of the observed changes are due to the lengthening of the action potential duration, with a secondary prolongation of the effective refractory period. The lengthening of the ventricular action potential duration after chronic amiodarone therapy is reflected in the consistent increases in the Q-Tc interval of the surface ECG[55,56,74] and, in the case of the atria, comparable lengthening of the time course of repolarization can be demonstrated directly by the use of intraatrial suction electrodes.[75]

### Antiarrhythmic-Pharmacokinetic Correlations and Drug Interactions

It has been apparent for some time that the "therapeutic half-life" of amiodarone is unusually long. After single oral doses of amiodarone (1400 to 1800 mg), peak drug concentrations were between 3 and 14 $\mu$g/ml and those of desethylamiodarone (metabolite) were much lower. The apparent elimination half-life of the drug after single doses was $7.2 \pm 5.0$ hours. Possibly, the decline in concentrations in the plasma after single doses might represent the distribution phase of the drug, with an extremely variable level being found in different patients given an identical dose. When amiodarone therapy is withdrawn after chronic maintenance dosage, the computed half-life from the decline of amiodarone serum levels, probably representing the "true" elimination half-life, is much longer: $29 \pm 19$ days (range 17–58). Even longer elimination half-life has been found in some patients, not uncommonly over 100 days (D. Holt, personal communication). On the other hand, the range of serum levels of amiodarone on chronic maintenance therapy is much narrower, about 0.5–4.0 $\mu$g/ml. However, the so-called "therapeutic range" as defined for conventional antiarrhythmic agents is not known at present. Furthermore, tentative data suggest that although serum levels of amiodarone and desethylamiodarone may increase as a function of dose, considerable overlap of values occurs between subjects for a given dose[76]; it remains uncertain whether a meaningful correlation between efficacy and side effects versus serum concentrations of the drug and its metabolite can be established for the purposes of clinical monitoring of drug effects. However, the clinical implications of the extremely variable and unusually long elimination half-life are clear. Thus, it is impossible to standardize a common dosage regimen of amiodarone for all patients and this may explain the variability in efficacy as well as toxicity noted by different investigators.[55-62] The variability in efficacy may be further complicated by the fact that numerous compounds such as quinidine, procainamide, disopyramide, and mexiletine, among others, interact with amiodarone.[77] Since amiodarone is used frequently in patients with cardiac decompensation, the interaction with digoxin[78,79] is particularly significant. Multiple pharmacokinetic mechanisms may mediate such an interaction.[77] It is of interest, however, that CNS and neuromuscular toxicity during combination therapy exceeds myocardial toxicity. Observations by Venkatesh *et al.*[80] from our laboratory suggest that this may be due to a differential tissue distribution of digoxin during the simultaneous administration of digoxin and amiodarone (FIG. 9).

### Clinical Efficacy and Concept of Amiodaronization

The overall antiarrhythmic effects of amiodarone in man are essentially predictable on the basis of the available experimental and clinical data; a significant

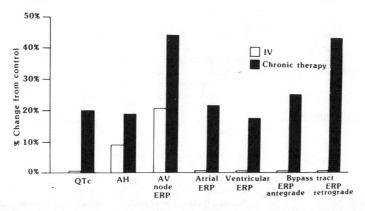

**FIGURE 8.** Percentage changes from control in various electrophysiologic parameters after intravenous amiodarone (5 mg/kg) and after chronic steady-state therapy with the drug. Note that the main effect of intravenous amiodarone is to slow atrioventricular (intranodal) conduction and to increase AV nodal refractoriness in patients with arrhythmias. In particular, the ventricular FRP is not affected. The chronically administered drug affects most variables, especially the lengthening of the ERP in all tissues. This also applies to accessory pathways, but the data are not shown. (From K. Nademanee, unpublished observations.)

difference might be expected between the effects of the acute intravenous single bolus injections and those evident after chronic drug administration. TABLES 4 and 5 summarize what appears to be the known spectrum of the antiarrhythmic actions of intravenous (single bolus) versus chronically administered amiodarone.

The wide spectrum of activity appears to be correlated with the increases in the ERP of the relevant cardiac tissue. Such an effect is accompanied by a potent suppressant action on ventricular and supraventricular ectopy by more than 90–98% and elimination of complex ectopy and runs of ventricular tachycardia.[57–59] Thus, it is possible that the removal of the "trigger" mechanism[58] in the form of ectopy may contribute importantly to the observed antiarrhythmic effects of amiodarone not only in ventricular tachyarrhythmias, but also in paroxysmal supraventricular tachycardia and paroxysmal atrial flutter and fibrillation with or without preexcitation. The increases in ERP of the relevant cardiac tissues must

**TABLE 4.** Antiarrhythmic Effects of Intravenously Administered Amiodarone

| Arrhythmia | Effect | Potential Mechanism(s) |
|---|---|---|
| 1. Sinus tachycardia | Variable but generally little effect; reduction in anesthetized patients | Antiadrenergic (?) |
| 2. Supraventricular ectopic beats | No systematic experience | — |
| 3. PSVT (narrow QRS) | (a) Conversion to sinus rhythm common (exact frequency of conversion not known)<br>(b) Enhanced difficulty in reinduction by PES | (a) AV nodal block and increase in ERP (antegrade)<br>(b) AV nodal block and increase in antegrade and retrograde ERP |
| 4. Ectopic PSVT | Unknown | Likely to produce AV block without effect on atrial rate |
| 5. PSVT (antidromic with wide QRS) | No effect | Intravenous amiodarone has no significant effect on antegrade conduction or ERP of bypass tracts |
| 6. Atrial flutter | (a) Atrial rate—unchanged or slowed little<br>(b) Ventricular response reduced<br>(c) Conversion to sinus rhythm in a small percentage of cases | Essentially by AV block |
| 7. Atrial fibrillation | (a) Ventricular response reduced<br>(b) Conversion to sinus rhythm in a small number of patients, especially with recent onset of the arrhythmia | Essentially by AV block |
| 8. Atrial flutter-fibrillation complicating Wolff-Parkinson-White syndrome | Either no effect or may aggravate the ventricular response | By AV block, ventricular response may be increased over the bypass tracts |
| 9. Multifocal atrial tachycardia | Effect not known | — |
| 10. Digitalis-induced arrhythmias (especially PAT with block) | Effect not known, but AV block likely to be aggravated | AV block |
| 11. Ventricular ectopic beats | Transiently reduced in many patients; effect not sustained even by intravenous infusion, except after 3–4 days | Mechanism not defined: antiadrenergic(?) diluent; ERP and Q-Tc not lengthened by intravenous bolus injections. |
| 12. Sustained VT | (a) Occasional terminations<br>(b) In occasional cases, cycle length of VT prolonged | As in No. 11 above. |
| 13. Inducible VT | No effect | |
| 14. Torsade de pointes | Effect not known | |
| 15. Ventricular parasystole | Effect not known | |

NOTE: The experience summarized herein is not based on controlled studies. It is an attempt to correlate the fragments of clinical experience with the known electrophysiologic effects of single intravenous doses of commercial preparations of amiodarone (usually 5 mg/kg).

**TABLE 5.** Antiarrhythmic Effects of Chronically Administered Oral Amiodarone

| Arrhythmia | Effect | Potential Mechanism(s) |
|---|---|---|
| 1. Sinus tachycardia | Reduced (modest effect) | Andiadrenergic; depression of phase-4 depolarization in the SA node |
| 2. Supraventricular ectopy | Reduced (marked effect) | Antiadrenergic; also exerts effect on the atrial muscle refractoriness |
| 3. PSVT (all forms) | (a) Prevents recurrences in most patients<br>(b) Prevents reinduction by PES or lengthens the cycle length of reinducible tachycardia | Lengthens ERP in all tissues involved in the reentrant circuit; also removes "trigger" mechanism (ectopy); in ectopic PSVT, depression of phase-4 depolarization of ectopic parameter probably involved |
| 4. Atrial flutter | (a) Atrial rate markedly reduced<br>(b) Ventricular response reduced<br>(c) Significant number convert to sinus rhythm and remain in sinus rhythm during chronic therapy | Probably due to the lengthening of the action potential duration and refractoriness |
| 5. Atrial fibrillation | (a) Ventricular response reduced<br>(b) Significant number convert to sinus rhythm and remain in sinus rhythm during chronic therapy<br>(c) Recurrences of paroxysmal atrial flutter-fibrillation (in patients with and without heart disease) nearly always prevented by amiodarone | As in No. 4. |
| 6. Atrial flutter-fibrillation complicating Wolff-Parkinson-White syndrome | (a) Recurrences prevented in most cases<br>(b) Inducibility obviated and the shortest R-R interval lengthened | As in No. 4; also lengthening of ERP over the bypass tract |
| 7. Multifocal atrial tachycardia | Unknown | — |
| 8. Digitalis-toxicity-induced arrhythmia | Unknown | Impractical to use because of the slow onset of action |
| 9. Ventricular ectopy | Reduced by more than 90% in most cases | By affecting automaticity (phase-4 depolarization) and re-entry (by lengthening ERP). |
| 10. Inducible VT/VF | (a) Variable suppression (possibly up to 50%)<br>(b) Lengthen cycle length of reinducible VT | By effect on ERP |

(TABLE 5 *Continued*)

| Arrhythmia | Effect | Potential Mechanism(s) |
|---|---|---|
| 11. Exercise induced VT (triggered automaticity[?]) | No systematic data | — |
| 12. Recurrent VT/VF | Highly effective in preventing recurrences (probably prolongs survival in survivors of cardiac arrest) | Probably affects reentry as well as trigger mechanism (ectopy) |
| 13. Long Q-T syndrome | Effect not known | May possibly be effective by reducing dispersion of refractoriness |
| 14. Ventricular parasystole | Effect not known | — |

NOTE: Again, efficacy of amiodarone on different dysrhythmias is a crude estimate from uncontrolled and controlled data in relation to our overall experience. It is subject to revision in light of the rapidly expanding clinical studies in various cardiac arrhythmias.

enhance the difficulty in the initiation of the tachycardia: in the case of ventricular tachycardia, the arrhythmia remains provokable (with a longer cycle length commensurate with the lengthened effective refractory period) in up to 50% of cases by appropriate electrical stimulation despite the abolition of the tendency for spontaneous recurrence of the arrhythmia. These observations may be interpreted as indicating the importance of PVCs in initiating sustained VT, thus providing a rational basis for the use of regimens that predictably suppress ventricular ectopy to manage recurrent cardiac arrhythmias in man. Whatever the relative importance of ectopy suppression and of lengthened refractoriness by amiodarone, the electrophysiologic data, when interpreted in light of the clinical experience, indicate a major role of the drug in the prophylactic control of: (1) recurrent life-threatening as well as other troublesome ventricular tachyarrhythmias; (2) recurrent atrial flutter and fibrillation occurring with and without

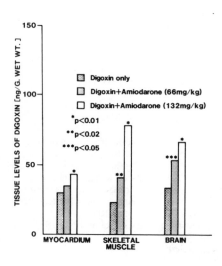

FIGURE 9. Effect of chronically administered amiodarone on steady-state tissue levels of digoxin in the myocardium, skeletal muscle and brain in rats. Two doses of amiodarone were given. Digoxin was given for five days (250 mg orally per day) followed by amiodarone (one of the two doses) with the digoxin for 21 days. In the control series (n = 6) digoxin alone was given for 3 weeks. In the group given 66 mg/kg of amiodarone orally, five rats were used; in the group given 132 mg/kg, 8 rats were used. Digoxin was measured by radioimmunoassay. Note the strikingly higher concentration of digoxin accumulating in skeletal muscle and in brain compared to that in the myocardium. (From Venkatesh *et al.*[80] Reproduced by permission.)

preexcitation syndromes; (3) all forms of paroxysmal supraventricular tachycardias; and (4) the ventricular response in atrial flutter and fibrillation in a number of cases in which conversion to sinus rhythm occurs on the drug (which then promotes the stability of normal rhythm if drug administration is continued).

As emphasized, the elimination half-life of the drug is unpredictable in an individual patient. However, the drug produces a number of measurable changes in the patient as a function not only of dose but also of duration of therapy. For the attainment of steady-state therapy, an individualized approach is always mandatory since the duration of therapy that might be necessary at a given dose in a given patient is difficult to determine except empirically. However, we have found that when Q-Tc interval of the ECG lengthens significantly, the ERP of the ventricle is prolonged by 30–50 msec, and the serum rT$_3$ levels[57] rise two to fourfold above baseline values, beneficial antiarrhythmic response is demonstrable in

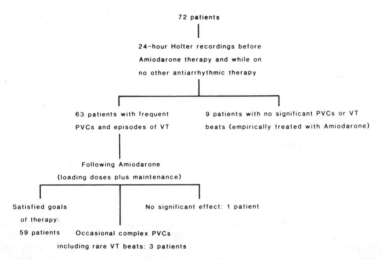

**FIGURE 10.** The effects of chronic amiodarone therapy on frequency of occurrence of premature ventricular contractions (PVCs) and ventricular tachycardia (VT) in patients with symptomatic and nonsymptomatic recurrent ventricular tachycardia and cardiac arrests. (From Nademanee *et al.*[81] Reproduced by permission.)

most patients. We believe that the magnitude of the changes in these variables indicates the degree of "amiodaronization." In the case of ventricular tachyarrhythmias, adequate amiodaronization is usually associated with more than 90% reduction in ventricular ectopy, with the elimination of runs of ventricular tachycardia, and with the long term that such a response is maintained.

It must be emphasized, however, that variables such as counts in ventricular ectopy, changes in the ERP and in the Q-Tc interval, as well as the overall antiarrhythmic response to chronically administered amiodarone for a given serum level of rT$_3$ (or, indeed, serum level of the drug or its metabolite) can be modified substantially by associated clinical features, such as drug interactions, as emphasized above. Under these circumstances, arrhythmogenic toxicity will not correlate with rT$_3$ levels. In our experience, the antiarrhythmic effects of amiodarone are particularly influenced by hypokalemia, a setting in which torsade de pointes may develop during chronic therapy with amiodarone. Indeed, we have not encountered torsade when amiodarone has been used as a single antiarrhythmic agent despite dramatic increases in the Q-Tc interval on the surface ECG. Torsade de pointes is particularly likely to occur in digitalized and hypokalemic patients taking combination therapy of amiodarone and Class 1 antiarrhythmic agents. The principle for the dosing schedule involved the use of a high initial loading dose of 1200–1600 mg/day for 1–2 weeks, followed by an intermediate dose of about 800 mg/day for 2–4 weeks, and then by a maintenance dose (generally 200–400 mg/day), which was the lowest dose that could produce the desired therapeutic response and did not lead to the development of limiting side effects. During long-term therapy, regular surveillance of patients is imperative since on the smallest doses of the drug the arrhythmia may recur, necessitating upward adjustment of dose. Conversely, at the higher maintenance doses (400–600 mg/day), a significant number of patients may develop side effects during

TABLE 6. Side Effects of Amiodarone Therapy in 96 Patients Treated Chronically

| Nature of Side Effects | No. of Patients with Side Effects |
|---|---|
| Gastrointestinal disturbances (constipation, anorexia, increases in SGPT) | 17 |
| Insomnia | 11 |
| Photosensitivity | 5 |
| CNS disturbances (uncoordination, tremor, ataxia, impaired memory) | 5 |
| Proximal muscle weakness | 2 |
| Interstitial pulmonary fibrosis | 3 |
| Halovision | 3 |
| Symptomatic bradycardia and sinus arrest | 3 |
| Weight loss | 1 |
| Hypothyroidism[a] | 1 |

[a] Confirmed by TSH measurements in the setting of a compatible clinical presentation. The frequency of development of hypothyroidism and hyperthyroidism during chronic amiodarone therapy is likely to be the same as in the general population in a particular geographical area given a particular iodine load. The complication is not specific for the drug (see text).

protracted therapy, thus requiring possible periodic reductions in dosage of amiodarone. These observations have been based on our experience in more than 300 patients in the last 5 years. The results for the first 96 patients treated for recalcitrant ventricular tachyarrhythmias and who were at high risk for sudden death were recently analyzed.[81]

All 96 patients (including 29 with recurrent cardiac arrest) had been treated previously by two or more conventional antiarrhythmic drugs; the arrhythmias either failed to respond to adequate doses of these compounds or the patients did not tolerate them. The dosage regimens utilized were those outlined above. On amiodarone, the patients were followed for 6–40 (mean 15) months. Seventy-five are alive and well. There have been five arrhythmic (three on apparently "adequate" and two on suboptimal therapy) and seven nonarrhythmic (six from heart and one from liver failure) deaths. Nonfatal arrhythmias recurred in four patients, one early and three late. The overall incidence of side effects was less than 10%

and the details are summarized in TABLE 6. In only five patients were the side effects deemed intolerable, necessitating withdrawal of the drug. Heart failure was not aggravated by the drug, and in 23 patients in whom the left ventricular ejection fraction could be measured by radiocuclide ventriculography before as well as during steady-state drug treatment, this variable was not reduced significantly by amiodarone. It is noteworthy that 24-hour Holter recordings made serially before and after treatment in 72 patients showed that amiodarone eliminated episodes of ventricular tachycardia and complex ectopy and reduced total ectopic beat count by more than 90% in all but 4 patients (FIG. 10). In contrast, ventricular tachycardia inducible by programmed electrical stimulation was suppressed in only 50% of patients, but failure of such suppression did not compromise an excellent clinical outcome in the long term. Thus, our data, which have been reported in detail elsewhere,[81] indicate that amiodarone is highly effective in the prophylaxis of recurrent refractory life-threatening ventricular arrhythmias. Particularly noteworthy is the observation that when used in an appropriate and individualized fashion, amiodarone, chronically administered, is associated with a low incidence of side effects, most of which develop as a function of dose as well as of duration of therapy. The advent of amiodarone is clearly an important advance in the pharmacologic control of a wide variety of cardiac arrhythmias.

## ACKNOWLEDGMENTS

We are grateful to Geetha Sritharan for typing this manuscript and to the Medical Media Department for help with the illustrations and photography.

## REFERENCES

1.  ELLRODT, G., C. Y. C. CHEW & B. N. SINGH. 1980. Therapeutic indications of slow-channel blockade in cardiocirculatory disorders. Circulation **62**: 669–679.
2.  HELLESTRANDT, K. J., R. S. BEXTON, A. W. NATHAN, R. A. J. SPURRELL & A. J. CAMM. 1982. Acute flecainide acetate on cardiac conduction and refractoriness in man. Brit. Heart J. **48**: 140–148.
3.  ANDERSON, J. L., J. R. STEWART & B. A. PERRY. 1981. Oral flecainide acetate for the treatment of ventricular arrhythmias. N. Engl. J. Med. **305**: 474–477.
4.  SINGH, B. N. 1983. Amiodarone: Historical development and pharmacologic profile. Am. Heart J. **106**: 788–797.
5.  SINGH, B. N. & E. M. VAUGHAN WILLIAMS. 1972. A fourth class of antidysrhythmic action? Effect of verapamil on ouabain toxicity, on atrial and ventricular intracellular potentials and on other features of cardiac function. Cardiovasc. Res. **6**: 109–114.
6.  CRANEFIELD, P. F., R. S. ARONSON & A. L. WIT. 1976. Effect of verapamil on the normal action potential and on a calcium-dependent slow response of canine cardiac Purkinje fibers. Circulation Res. **34**: 204–213.
7.  ROSEN, M. R., A. L. WIT & B. F. HOFFMAN. 1975. Appraisal and reappraisal of cardiac therapy: Electrophysiology and pharmacology of cardiac arrhythmias. VI. Cardiac effects of verapamil. Am. Heart J. **89**: 655–673.
8.  TRITTHART, H. A. 1980. Pharmacology and electrophysiology of calcium antagonists. Clin. Invest. Med. **3**: 1–7.
9.  HAEUSLER, G. 1972. Differential effect on verapamil on excitation-contraction coupling in smooth muscle and on excitation-secretion coupling in adrenergic terminals. J. Pharmacol. Exp. Ther. **180**: 672–679.
10. HARDER, D. R., L. BELARDINELLI, N. SPERELAKIS, R. RUBIO & R. M. BERNE. 1979.

Differential effects of adenosine and nitroglycerin on the action potentials of large and small coronary arteries. Circ. Res. **44:** 176–182.

11. SINGH, B. N., H. S. HECHT & K. NADEMANEE. 1982. Electrophysiologic and hemodynamic actions of slow-channel blocking compounds. Prog. Cardiovasc. Dis. **25:** 103–132.

12. CHEW, C. Y. C., H. S. HECHT, J. T. COLLET, R. G. MCALLISTER & B. N. SINGH. 1981. Influence of severity of ventricular dysfunction on hemodynamic responses to intravenously administered verapamil in ischemic heart disease. Am. J. Cardiol. **47:** 917–922.

13. CHEW, C. Y. C., G. B. BROWN, B. N. SINGH, M. M. WONG, C. PIERCE & R. PETERSEN. 1983. Effects of verapamil on coronary hemodynamic function and vasomobility relative to its mechanism of antianginal action. Am. J. Cardiol. **51:** 661–918.

14. BROWN, G. B., C. D. PIERCE, R. B. PETERSON, B. N. SINGH, E. L. BOLSON & H. T. DODGE. 1981. Verapamil, a mild coronary dilator, inhibits sympathetic and ergonovine-induced coronary constriction in humans (abstract). Circulation (Suppl. **IV–VI**): 150.

15. SPEAR, J. F., L. N. HOROWITZ, A. B. HODESS, H. MACVAUGH & E. N. MOORE. Cellular electrophysiology of human myocardial infarction. Abnormalities of cellular activation. Circulation **59:** 247–256.

16. WIT, A. L. & P. F. CRANEFIELD. 1981. Triggered activity in cardiac muscle fibers of the simian mitral valve. Circulation Res. **38:** 85–94.

17. KAWAI, C., T. KONISHI, E. MATSUYAMA & H. OKAZAKI. 1981. Comparative effects of three calcium antagonists, diltiazem, verapamil and nifedipine, on the sinoatrial and atrioventricular nodes. Experimental and clinical studies. Circulation **63:** 1035.

18. ZIPES, D. P. & J. C. FISCHER. 1974. Effects of agents which inhibit the slow channel automaticity and atrioventricular conduction in the dog. Circ. Res. **34:** 184–192.

19. OKADA, T. 1976. Effect of verapamil on electrical activities of SA node, ventricular muscle and Purkinje fibers in isolated rabbit hearts. Jpn. Circ. J. **40:** 329–341.

20. SINGH, B. N., G. ELLRODT & C. T. PETER. 1978. Verapamil: A review of its pharmacological properties and therapeutic uses. Drugs **15:** 169–197.

21. SINGH, B. N., K. NADEMANEE & S. H. BAKY. 1983. Calcium antagonists: Clinical use in the treatment of cardiac arrhythmias. Drugs **25:** 125–153.

22. SUNG, R., B. ELSER & R. G. MCALLISTER. 1980. Intravenous verapamil for termination of re-entrant supraventricular tachycardias. Intracardiac studies correlated with plasma verapamil concentrations. Ann. Intern. Med. **93:** 682–689.

23. RINKENBERGER, R. L., E. N. PRYSTOWSKY, J. J. HEGER, P. J. TROUP, W. M. JACKMAN & D. P. ZIPES. 1980. Effects of intravenous and oral verapamil administration in patients with supraventricular tachyarrhythmias. Circulation **62:** 996–1010.

24. STORSTEIN, O. & K. RASMUSSEN. 1974. Digitalis and atrial tachycardia with block. Br. Heart J. **36:** 171–176.

25. TONKIN, A. M., P. E. AYLWARD & S. E. JOEL. 1980. Verapamil in prophylaxis of paroxysmal atrioventricular nodal re-entrant tachycardia. J. Cardiovasc. Pharmacol. **2:** 473–480.

26. KLEIN, G. J., S. GULAMHUSSEIN & E. N. PRYSTOWSKY. 1981. Comparison of the electrophysiologic effects of intravenous and oral verapamil in patients with paroxysmal supraventricular tachycardia. Am. J. Cardiol. **49:** 117–124.

27. KLEIN, H. D., H. PAUZNER, E. D. SEGNI, D. DAVID & E. KAPLINSKY. 1979. The beneficial effects of verapamil in chronic atrial fibrillation. Arch. Intern. Med. **L39:** 747–749.

28. KLEIN, H. O., R. LANG, E. WEISS, E. DESEGNI, C. LIBHABER, J. GUERRERO & E. KAPLINSKY. 1982. The influence of verapamil on serum digoxin concentration. Circulation **65:** 998–1003.

29. GULAM HUSSEIN, S., P. KO, S. G. CARRUTHERS & G. J. KLEIN. 1982. Accleration of the ventricular response during atrial fibrillation in the Wolff-Parkinson-White syndrome after verapamil. Circulation **65:** 348–354.

30. LAZZARA, R. & B. SCHERLAG. 1980. The treatment of arrhythmias by blocking slow current. Ann. Intern. Med. **93:** 919–920.

31. SCHMID, J. F., B. D. SEEBACK, C. L. HENRIE, E. H. BANITT & D. C. KVAM. 1975. Some antiarrhythmic actions of a new compound, R-818, in dogs and mice. Fed. Proc. **34:** 775.
32. VERDOUW, P. D., W. D. JAAP & J. C. GORDON. 1979. Antiarrhythmic and hemodynamic actions of flecainide acetate (R-818) in the ischemic porcine heart. J. Cardiovasc. Pharmacol. **1:** 473–486.
33. HODESS, A. B., W. P. FOLLANSBEE, J. F. SPEAR & E. N. MOORE. 1979. Electrophysiological effects of a new antiarrhythmic agent, flecainide, on the intact canine heart. J. Cardiovasc. Pharmacol. **1:** 427–439.
34. IKEDA, N., B. N. SINGH, L. D. DAVIS & O. HAUSWIRTH. 1984. Effects of flecainide on the electrophysiologic properties of isolated canine and rabbit myocardial fibers. J. Am. Coll. Cardiol. Submitted for publication.
35. JOSEPHSON, M. A., N. IKEDA & B. N. SINGH. 1984. Effects of flecainide on ventricular function: clinical and experimental correlations. Am. J. Cardiol. **53:** 95B–100B.
36. COWAN, J. C. & E. M. VAUGHAN WILLIAMS. 1981. Characterization of a new oral antiarrhythmic drug, flecainide R-818. Eur. J. Pharmacol. **73:** 333–342.
37. BORCHARD, U. & M. BOISTEN. 1982. Effect of flecainide on action potentials and alternating current-induced arrhythmias in mammalian myocardium. J. Cardiovasc. Pharmacol. **4:** 205–212.
38. SCHULZE, J. J. & J. KNOPS. 1982. Effects of flecainide on contractile force and electrophysiological parameters in cardiac muscle. Arzneim. Forsch. **32:** 1025–1029.
39. HAUSWIRTH, O. & B. N. SINGH. 1978. Ionic mechanisms in heart muscle in relation to the genesis and pharmacological control of cardiac arrhythmias. Pharmacol. Rev. **30:** 5–63.
40. SINGH, B. N., J. R. COLLET & C. Y. C. CHEW. 1975. New perspectives in the pharmacologic therapy of cardiac arrhythmias. Prog. Cardiovasc. Dis. **22:** 243–301.
41. VAUGHAN WILLIAMS, E. M. 1975. Classification of antidysrhythmic drugs. Pharmacol. Ther. **B1:** 115–138.
42. OLSSON, S. B. & N. EDVARDSSON. 1981. Clinical electrophysical study of antiarrhythmic properties of flecainide: Acute intraventricular delayed conduction and prolonged repolarization in regular paced and premature beats using intracardiac monophasic action potentials with programmed stimulation. Am. Heart J. **102:** 864–871.
43. BEXTAN, R. S., K. J. HELLESTRANDT, A. W. NATHAN, R. A. J. SPURREL & A. J. CAMM. 1983. A comparison of the antiarrhythmic effects on AV junctional reentrant tachycardia of oral and intravenous flecainide acetate. Eur. Heart J. **4:** 92–102.
44. DURAN, D., E. V. PLATIA, L. S. C. GRIFFITH, G. ADHAR & P. R. REID. 1982. Suppression of complex ventricular arrhythmias by oral flecainide. Clin. Pharmacol. Ther. **32:** 554–561.
45. SOMANI, P. 1980. Antiarrhythmic effects of flecainide. Clin. Pharmacol. Ther. **27:** 464–470.
46. DUFF, H. J., D. M. RODEN, R. J. MAFFUCCI, B. S. VESPER, G. J. CONARD, S. B. HIGGINS, J. A. OATES, R. F. SMITH & R. J. WOOSLEY. 1981. Suppression of resistant ventricular arrhythmias by twice daily dosing with flecainide. Am. J. Cardiol. **48:** 1133–1140.
47. CONARD, G. J., G. L. CARLSON, J. W. FROST & R. E. OBER. 1979. Human plasma pharmacokinetics, a new antiarrhythmic, following single oral and intravenous doses (abstract). Clin. Pharmacol. Ther. **25:** 218.
48. MUHIDDIN, K. A., K. J. HELLESTRANDT, A. NATHAN, R. BEXTON & A. J. CAMM. 1982. The electrophysiologic effects of flecainide acetate (R-818) on the cardiac conducting system. Br. J. Clin. Pharmacol. **13** (2): 286P.
49. CONARD, G. J., G. E. CRANHEIM & H. W. KLEMPT. 1982. Relationship between plasma concentrations and suppression of ventricular extrasystoles by flecainide acetate (R-818) a new antiarrhythmic, in patients. Artzneim. Forsch. **32** (2): 155–160.
50. THE FLECAINIDE-QUINIDINE RESEARCH GROUP. 1983. Flecainide versus quinidine for treatment of chronic ventricular arrhythmias. A multicenter clinical trial. Circulation **67:** 1117–1123.

51. MUHIDDIN, K., A. W. NATHAN, K. J. HELLESTRANDT, S. O. BANIM & A. J. CAMM. 1982. Ventricular tachycardia associated with flecainide. Lancet 2: 1220–1221.
52. CHARLIER, R., G. DELTOUR, A. BAUDINE & F. CHAILLET. 1968. Pharmacology of amiodarone, an anti-anginal drug with a new biological profile. Artzneim. Forsch. 18: 1408–1417.
53. SINGH, B. N. 1971. A study of the pharmacological actions of certain drugs and hormones with a particular reference to cardiac muscle. D. Phil. thesis, University of Oxford, England.
54. SINGH, B. N. & E. M. VAUGHAN WILLIAMS. 1970. The effect of amiodarone, a new antianginal drug, on cardiac muscle. Br. J. Pharmacol. 39: 657–667.
55. ROSENBAUM, M. B., P. A. CHIALE, D. RYBA & M. V. ELIZARI. 1974. Control of tachyarrhythmias associated with Wolff-Parkinson-White syndrome by amiodarone hydrochloride. Am. J. Cardiol. 34: 215–223.
56. ROSENBAUM, M. B., P. A. CHIALE & M. S. HALPERN. 1976. Clinical efficacy of amiodarone as an antiarrhythmic agent. Am. J. Cardiol. 38: 934–944.
57. NADEMANEE, K., J. A. HENDRICKSON, D. S. CANNOM, B. N. GOLDREYER & B. N. SINGH. 1981. Control of refractory life-threatening ventricular arrhythmias by amiodarone. Am. Heart J. 101: 759–765.
58. NADEMANEE, K., J. A. HENDRICKSON, R. KANNAN & B. N. SINGH. 1982. Electrophysiological effects of amiodarone in patients with life-threatening ventricular arrhythmias: Modification of induced ventricular tachycardia versus suppression of spontaneously occurring tachyarrhythmias. Am. Heart J. 103: 950–959.
59. NADEMANEE, K., B. N. SINGH, J. A. HENDRICKSON, A. W. REED, S. MELMED & J. M. HERSHMAN. 1982. Pharmacokinetic significance of serum reverse T$_3$ levels during amiodarone treatment: A potential method for monitoring chronic drug therapy. Circulation 66: 202–211.
60. HEGER, J. J., E. PRYSTOWSKY, W. M. JACKMAN, G. V. NACARELLI, K. A. WARFEL, R. L. RINKENBERGER & D. P. ZIPES. 1981. Amiodarone: Clinical efficacy and electrophysiology during long-term therapy for recurrent ventricular tachycardia or ventricular fibrillation. New Engl. J. Med. 305: 539–545.
61. KASKI, J. C., L. A. FIROTTI, T. MESSUTI, B. RUBITZKY & M. B. ROSENBAUM. 1981. Long-term management of sustained recurrent symptomatic ventricular tachycardia with amiodarone. Circulation 64: 273–280.
62. PODRID, P. J. & B. LOWN. 1981. Amiodarone therapy in symptomatic, sustained, refractory, atrial and ventricular tachyarrhythmias. Am. Heart J. 101: 374–379.
63. IKEDA, N., K. NADEMANEE, R. KANNAN & B. N. SINGH. 1984. Electrophysiologic effects of amiodarone: experimental and clinical observations relative to serum and tissue drug concentrations. Am. Heart J. In press.
64. BRUGADA, P., D. ROY, F. W. BARR, B. HEDDLE, W. R. DASSEN & H. J. J. WELLENS. 1982. Electrophysiological effects of intravenous amiodarone (abstract). Am. J. Cardiol. 49: 1044.
65. NADEMANEE, K., G. FELD, J. A. HENDRICKSON, V. INTARACHOT, R. KANNAN & B. N. SINGH. 1983. Does intravenous amiodarone shorten the latency of the onset of antiarrhythmic action of oral amiodarone in ventricular arrhythmias? J. Am. Coll. Cardiol. 1: 360.
66. KANNAN, R., K. NADEMANEE, J. A. HENDRICKSON, H. J. ROSTAMI & B. N. SINGH. 1982. Amiodarone kinetics after oral doses. Clin. Pharmacol. Ther. 31: 438–444.
67. MELMED, S., K. NADEMANEE, A. W. REED, J. A. HENDRICKSON, B. N. SINGH & J. M. HERSHMAN. 1981. Hyperthyroxinemia with bradycardia and normal thyrotropin secretion following chronic amiodarone administration. J. Clin. Endoctrinol. Metab. 53: 997–1002.
68. COTE, P., M. G. BOURASSA, J. DELAYE, J. JANIN, R. FREMENT & P. DAVID. 1979. Effects of amiodarone on cardiac hemodynamics and/or myocardial metabolism in patients with coronary artery disease. Circulation 59: 1165–1172.
69. POLSTER, P. & J. BROEKHUYSEN. 1976. The adrenergic antagonism of amiodarone. Biochem. Pharmacol. 25: 131–136.
70. CHARLIER, R. 1970. Cardiac actions in the dog of a new antagonist of adrenergic

excitation which does not produce competitive blockade of adrenoceptors. Br. J. Pharmacol. **39:** 668–676.

71. RUTITZSKY, B., A. L. GIROTH & M. B. ROSENBAUM. 1982. Efficacy of chronic amiodarone therapy in patients with variant angina and inhibition of ergonovine coronary constriction. Am. Heart J. **103:** 38–44.
72. DEBOER, L. W. V., J. J. NOSTA, R. A. KLONER & E. BRAUNWALD. 1982. Studies of amiodarone during experimental myocardial infarction: Beneficial effects on hemodynamics and infarct size. Circulation **65:** 508–514.
73. FREEDBERG, A. S., J. G. PAPP & E. M. VAUGHAN WILLIAMS. 1970. The effect of altered thyroid state on atrial intracellular potentials. J. Physiol. **207:** 357–363.
74. PRITCHARD, D. A., B. N. SINGH & P. J. HURLEY. 1975. Effects of amiodarone on thyroid function in patients with ischemic heart disease. Br. Heart J. **37:** 856–861.
75. OLSSON, S. B., L. BRORSON & E. VARNAUSKAS. 1973. Class III antiarrhythmic action in man. Observations from monophasic action potential recordings and amiodarone treatment. Br. Heart J. **35:** 1255–1259.
76. BOPPANA, V. K., S. SHOSHANI, S. J. SPIELMAN, B. BELHASSEN & L. N. HOROWITZ. 1983. Steady state amiodarone and metabolite concentration—relationship to dosage and side effects. J. Am. Coll. Cardiol. **1:** 630.
77. MARCUS, F. I. 1983. Drug interactions with amiodarone. Am. Heart J. **106:** 924–930.
78. MOSEY, J. O., N. S. U. JAGGARAO, E. W. GRUNDY & D. A. CHAMBERLAIN. 1981. Amiodarone increases plasma digoxin concentrations. Br. Heart J. **282:** 272–273.
79. NADEMANEE, K., R. KANNAN, J. A. HENDRICKSON, M. BURNAM, I. KAY & B. N. SINGH. 1982. Amiodarone-digoxin interaction during treatment of resistant cardiac arrhythmias (abstract). Am. J. Cardiol. **49:** 1026.
80. VENKATESH, N., L. AL-SARRAF, R. KANNAN & B. N. SINGH. 1983. Tissue-serum correlates of digoxin-amiodarone interaction? Selective drug accumulation as a basis for neurotoxicity during combination therapy. J. Am. Coll. Cardiol. Submitted for publication.
81. NADEMANEE, K., B. N. SINGH, J. A. HENDRICKSON, V. INTARACHOT, V. LOPEZ, G. FELD, D. S. CANNOM & J. N. WEISS. 1983. Amiodarone in refractory life-threatening ventricular arrhythmias. Ann. Intern. Med. **98:** 577–584.

# Ventricular Premature Beats, Ventricular Tachycardia, and Sudden Cardiac Death: Identification of Patients and Drug Treatment

PHILIP R. REID

*Division of Cardiology*
*Sinai Hospital of Baltimore*
*Baltimore, Maryland 21215*

## INTRODUCTION

Sudden cardiac death (SCD) stands as one of our major health problems, claiming one life every 60–90 seconds.[1-2] Yet public awareness of this threat is appallingly low, and it appears that the majority of the nonmedical public is better informed on the problem of the sudden infant death syndrome, which frequently forms the basis for their understanding of what sudden cardiac death implies. Such a profound lack of medical understanding has only just begun to attract more scientific attention. Another example of this ignorance can be seen in some physicians' ascribing a patient's sudden death to a "massive heart attack." As we now know, it is only the minority[3] of patients who have evidence of acute myocardial infarction. Moreover, this kind of medical misunderstanding obscures the more important therapeutic goals of controlling cardiac electrical stability and the triggers of electrical instability rather than salvaging the myocardium. The former goal emphasizes prevention and reversibility, while the latter concern seeks to minimize damage that has already occurred.

Another factor that attends the retarded recognition of the problem of SCD has been the lack of effective therapy. However, recent years have been witness to an almost explosive development of such means of treatment as extremely potent antiarrhythmic agents,[4] antiarrhythmic surgery,[5,6] antitachycardia pacemakers,[7] and implantable cardioverter-defibrillators.[8-11] Whereas 15 years ago physicians bemoaned the lack of effective therapeutic alternatives, they are now faced with the opposite situation: Which of the many alternatives is most appropriate? Before this simple question can be effectively answered we must be able to assess accurately not only the risks of the therapy, but also the intrinsic risk of the patient.

The purpose of this discussion is to review the role of ventricular arrhythmias and clinical and physiologic measurements in identifying a patient at risk as well as to assess our ability to prospectively identify those initially (or recurrently) at risk; we will also review selected trials that were designed to determine whether or not therapy can make an impact on the problem of SCD. In the end, it appears that the most rational approach to the problem of sudden cardiac death is to provide a treatment strategy on the basis of individual risk stratification rather than to offer a single therapy to a group of patients with widely differing risks.

## VENTRICULAR PREMATURE BEATS, VENTRICULAR TACHYCARDIA, AND SUDDEN CARDIAC DEATH

Now, more than ever, we are able to obtain long-term electrocardiographic monitoring with highly accurate quantitation of ventricular ectopy and complexity. This has lead to the realization that some amount of ventricular ectopy is the rule, rather than the exception in apparently healthy[12] or asymptomatic[13] adults and that the amount of ectopy appears to increase with age. Thus, we are forced to deal with a continuum of ectopic frequency and complexity, rather than merely its presence or absence, in making therapeutic judgments. The need for some resolve becomes particularly apparent when the clinician is faced with the decision about whether to treat the asymptomatic patient who has frequent ventricular ectopy and nonsustained ventricular tachycardia. Unfortunately, there is no evidence that supports treatment as being effective in such a group, but there *are* compelling reasons to beware of the potential arrhythmogenic side effects of virtually any antiarrhythmic therapy that may be employed.[14]

Evidence for the associated risks of ventricular ectopy as a harbinger of SCD is best documented in patients after acute myocardial infarction[15-19] and in patients without myocardial infarction[20] who have had previous episodes related to ventricular tachyarrhythmias. While statistical controversy may exist as to the independent predictiveness of ventricular tachyarrhythmias, it is nevertheless abundantly clear that VT and VF are the overwhelming causes of sudden cardiac death. Although there may be general agreement that certain forms of ventricular ectopy place patients at increased risk, there is no agreement as to how much one must reduce frequency and/or complexity in order to lessen the risk.

The use of a classification system for ventricular ectopy is certainly an inviting approach to assess risk. However, the most widely used format[21] for risk assessment, that of Lown, was based on unquantitated clinical observations and its utility has been the subject of controversy and critical review[22] when applied to postinfarct patients. Although several deficiencies in this grading system are apparent with respect to quantitative data, the presence of repetitive forms (such as ventricular couplets and nonsustained ventricular tachycardia) was found to greatly increase risk. Despite the deficiencies of the Lown grading system, alternative systems based on more objective data are cumbersome for routine use.

## IDENTIFICATION OF PATIENTS AT RISK OF SUDDEN CARDIAC DEATH

### The Postmyocardial Infarction Patients

TABLE 1 lists by clinical diagnoses several patient groups considered to be at increased risk of sudden cardiac death from ventricular tachyarrhythmias. One of the largest groups is that of patients post myocardial infarction. In these patients many attempts have been made to assess prognosis[23] using clinical variables such as congestive heart failure,[19] infarct location,[24] laboratory measurements after the appearance of intraventricular conduction defects,[25] exercise testing,[26] Holter monitoring,[22] left ventricular ejection fraction,[27] and the coronary anatomy.[28] Only recently has an attempt been made to stratify by risk a large group of postinfarct patients. The Multicenter Postinfarction Research Group[19] prospectively examined 866 patients over a 3-year period and identified four independent

**TABLE 1.** Groups at Increased Risk of Sudden Cardiac Death from Ventricular Tachyarrhythmias

| |
|---|
| 1. Patients after acute myocardial infarction |
| 2. Survivors of sudden cardiac death |
| 3. Patients with ischemic cardiomyopathy |
| 4. Patients with nonischemic cardiomyopathy |
| 5. Patients with hypertrophic cardiomyopathy |
| 6. Patients with mitral valve prolapse |
| 7. Patients with prolonged Q-T syndrome(s) |
| 8. Patients with drug-induced tachyarrhythmias |

variables that greatly influenced survivorship: ejection fraction below 0.40, ventricular ectopy at a frequency of 10 or more per hour, advanced heart failure before infarction, and pulmonary rales in the early postinfarct period. These four factors identified five risk groups whose 2-year mortality rose from 3 to 60% as the number of risk factors increased. The importance of this study is the potential use of these variables to assess the individual patient and from this to develop a therapeutic plan that weighs the risks (and perhaps cost) of therapy against the probability of an undesirable outcome. For example, if the patient carried an intrinsic risk of 10% for death in 1 year and there was a therapy that provided 98% effectiveness in prevention, but a 15% chance of dying as a result of the treatment, the choice for the greatest therapeutic risk/benefit might well be another alternative or no treatment at all. Unfortunately, neither this nor any other study has controlled for treatment effects on outcome. Therefore, we must await additional information before being able to employ an idealized risk model in patient management. Nevertheless, it appears that studies such as this point to the prospect for enhancement of health care in a more rational and cost-effective manner.

## THE SURVIVOR OF SUDDEN CARDIAC DEATH

The typical patient who is a "survivor" of sudden cardiac death from symptomatic VT or VF differs from the postinfarct patient in at least one major respect: the lack of an acute myocardial infarction. However, detailed examination of this group reveals that it is distinctly unusual not to find some cardiovascular pathology. In our experience, only about 5% of these patients have no definable cardiovascular disease. TABLE 2 summarizes our results, based on clinical evaluation

**TABLE 2.** Clinical and Angiographic Findings in Survivors of Ventricular Tachycardia or Fibrillation

| Finding | No. and Percent of Patients |
|---|---|
| Coronary heart disease | 141 (67%) |
| Congestive cardiomyopathy | 32 (15%) |
| Mitral valve prolapse | 13 (6%) |
| Prolonged Q-T syndrome | 2 (1%) |
| Other | 11 (5%) |
| No structural heart disease | 11 (5%) |
| Total | 210 |

and cardiac angiography, in 210 patients who were survivors of VT and/or VF. Our findings are similar to those of other studies[5,29] with few exceptions[30] and typically demonstrate obstructive coronary artery disease in 65–75%; nonischemic cardiomyopathy (such as viral, rheumatic, alcoholic, and hypertrophic cardiomyopathy and mitral valve prolapse) in 20–25%; such events as prolonged Q-T syndrome or drug-aggravated arrhythmias in less than 5%; and no definable cardiovascular pathology in fewer than 5% of all survivors of sudden cardiac death. Mitral valve prolapse is included in our classification of nonischemic cardiomyopathy because those who have experienced SCD will usually be found to have segmental wall motion abnormalities (usually posterobasal) and electrocardiographic ST-T wave abnormalities (usually II, III, aVF and V5 or V6).

As a reflection of the relatively recent recognition of the importance of this rather large group of patients, within the last few years there has been a flurry of activity[5–11,14,29,30] to investigate the survivors of sudden cardiac death. Since the majority of these patients will not have acute myocardial infarction, the prognostic indices used for the postinfarct patient group may not be directly applicable. However, as would be expected, there are several similarities since both subgroups of patients have experienced sudden cardiac death and have been resuscitated. Although the number of studies made of these patients is relatively small, some have pinpointed important clinical variables such as a history of myocardial infarction, no infarction at the time of the SCD event, and complex arrhythmias on Holter monitoring.[31,32] The presence of all these variables placed the risk of recurrent SCD in excess of 70% within 1 year. In contradistinction, the presence of Q wave myocardial infarction with no previous myocardial infarction, no heart failure, and no complex arrhythmias would identify a patient whose chance of recurrent sudden cardiac death was less than 10%.[33]

The clinical advent of programmed electrical stimulation (PES) of the ventricle has provided a very sensitive and specific means for both identification of the patient at continued risk and assessment of the probability of prevention of VT or VF after therapeutic intervention.[31–39] Studies from many different institutions place the sensitivity at 85–95% for laboratory reproduction of VT or VF in the patient who has experienced sudden cardiac death. Furthermore, if a drug therapy is successful in suppression of induced tachyarrhythmias, a good clinical prognosis over the subsequent 12 months can be assumed for at least 85% of these patients. Equally important is the very low rate (less than 3%) of false-positive results, that is, the induction of tachyarrhythmias that are found to have no clinical significance. These results are based on the study of a wide variety of patients, most of whom have coronary artery disease. Closer examination of the results with PES clearly suggests that they are dependent on underlying cardiac pathology[30] in most, but not all,[40] studies where the prognostic sensitivity is in excess of 90% in patients with coronary artery disease, but drops to 65–70% in patients with nonischemic cardiomyopathy.

While PES is an invasive procedure and may require multiple studies, it provides one of the most accurate means available for assessing the patient who has been resuscitated from sudden cardiac death. Unfortunately, the requirement for repeat studies is more a reflection of our inability to provide adequate therapy than any limitation of the technique. However, several important aspects of this method remain poorly defined, such as standardization of the stimulation protocol and comparative studies with noninvasive techniques such as Holter monitoring.

While there has been impressive consistency of results, despite differing stimulation protocols, a recent report,[41] using increasing number of premature ventricular stimuli (such as $V_1$-$V_{2-4}$), suggests that there is an increase in the frequency of false-positive test results (that is, the induction of clinically irrelevant tachyarrhythmias). There is also lack of agreement on what constitutes a positive result; specifically, what is the significance of induced nonsustained VT and how many induced responses should be used to define a positive result? These issues of protocol, while solvable, currently hinder comparative evaluations of the same therapies between laboratories.

It appears that PES has a significantly higher predictive accuracy than has Holter monitoring in evaluation of the patient who has been resuscitated from SCD, but there are very few data. In a preliminary study,[42] we evaluated 44 patients with a history of VT/VF who underwent Holter monitoring (average = 62 hours), PES and clinical followup (average = 14 months) for recurrent syncope or SCD who were receiving the same antiarrhythmic therapy. These results demonstrated a predictive accuracy of 91% for PES and 55% for Holter monitoring (p < 0.001), but there was no consistent relationship of outcome on the basis of severity of the arrhythmias according to a modified Lown classification. The major weakness of Holter monitoring was the poor negative predictive value, that is, the suppression of nonsustained VT on the Holter recording correlated poorly with subsequent clinical outcome. Howver, we did find that persistence of nonsustained VT seen on the Holter recording was associated with a 70% chance of syncope or SCD during the followup period. Using these results, we have attempted to combine the use of Holter monitoring with PES by first making sure that all evidence of VT has been eliminated on the Holter recording (during 72 hours of monitoring) before subjecting the patient to repeat PES study. Despite the statistical significance obtained in this relatively small study, further investigation certainly seems warranted when taking into consideration the potential for cost savings (of repeat Holter compared to repeat PES) as well as patient morbidity.

The value of PES has been demonstrated for evaluation of several drugs such as quinidine, procainamide, disopyramide, and mexiletine.[31-39] However, it appears that PES cannot be assumed useful for all agents that may be clinically tested, the most notable of these being amiodarone,[43] where VT can be induced in the majority of patients taking this drug, but many fewer will go on to manifest clinical events during protracted followup study. The possibility of other such exceptions should be assumed, suggesting that new antiarrhythmic agents must go through a rather lengthy clinical trial before the utility of PES can be relied upon.

In contrast to the relatively large number of studies that examine risk stratification in postinfarct patients, relatively few studies have attempted risk stratification in the SCD survivor. In a recent retrospective analysis of 239 patients with a history of VT and/or VF, Swerdlow et al.[41] found that the two strongest predictors for both recurrent SCD and nonsudden cardiac death were the severity of congestive heart failure and the failure of response during PES. After 2 years of followup study, these investigators found that 85% of patients had a cardiac death if they were classified as NYHA Class IV (heart failure) and were also nonresponders to PES. In contrast, only 4% of patients were found to have a cardiac death at 2 years if they were in NYHA Class I and were PES responders. If we use these two variables, we can see that there were progressive gradations of risk, depending on the combination and severity of congestive heart failure with the response to PES.

There are no published comparative evaluations of clinical and laboratory variables that might be used to stratify the future risk of the SCD survivor. In our study of 67 patients, we initially examined more than 20 clinical variables in a univariate fashion and arrived at three that were used in a multivariate predictive equation which gave the probability of survival at 1 year: prior congestive heart failure, the presence of valvular heart disease (usually mitral regurgitation), and previous myocardial infarction. The overall accuracy for this equation was 77%; and it correctly classified 38 of 46 (82.6%) patients who were predicted to have an 80% or greater chance of survival at 1 year. Fifty-five of these patients underwent complete cardiac catheterization and the results were analyzed with respect to coronary artery and left ventricular segments according to AHA recommendations.[44] The univariate analysis selected three angiographic variables (the degree of obstruction in the left anterior descending coronary artery, posterobasal segmental dysfunction, and the anterior wall thickness) which were then fitted to a predictive equation in a manner analogous to that used for the clinical analysis. These results provided an overall predictive accuracy of 93% and correctly classified 10 of 14 (71%) patients predicted to have a 0% chance of survival at 1 year, 38 of 40 (95%) patients predicted to have ≥80% chance of survival at 1 year and 10 of 10 patients considered to have a 100% chance of survival at 1 year.

From studies in both the postinfarct patient and the SCD survivor, it thus becomes apparent that predictive equations can be developed to provide probability of survival for the individual patient. While clinical variables such as congestive heart failure and clinical evidence of coronary artery disease clearly provide important information in risk assessment, most studies demonstrate that greater accuracy can be achieved by use of more quantitative measurements such as the ejection fraction, degree of coronary artery disease, and response to programmed ventricular stimulation.

## ANTIARRHYTHMIC THERAPY TO PREVENT SUDDEN CARDIAC DEATH

Despite the appearance of newer modalities for management of ventricular tachyarrhythmias, antiarrhythmic drugs have been and remain the major therapeutic means in patients with ventricular arrhythmias. However, despite the many years of use of these drugs and the number of trials attempted, there has been no placebo-controlled evidence that (with the exception of beta-adrenergic blocking agents[45-49]) these drugs can decrease the frequency of SCD. These trials include attempts with agents such as procainamide,[50] phenytoin,[51] aprindine,[52] and mexiletine.[53] Furthermore, some studies that sought to evaluate therapy in "high"-risk patients showed not only an insignificant difference between the active drug and placebo groups, but also relatively low mortality rates within the placebo group. Thus, these studies also express inability to accurately identify the desired population.

An examination of these earlier trials furnishes important lessons in design. Frustrating flaws in these trials include underestimation of the sample size needed, "drop outs" because of the drug's side effects, lack of documentation of antiarrhythmic drug levels or compliance, failure to assess the potential for arrhythmogenic drug effects, and failure to control concurrent therapy (for example, digitalis and diuretics). One of the most difficult variables to control in study design is the effect of entering the study itself. The mere fact that a patient participates in a study, which probably guarantees greater attention given to his general health and more frequent hospital visits to satisfy the study protocol, may have a favorable influence on survival, but an unfavorable influence on accurate risk assessment in the placebo group.

While the fact that antiarrhythmic agents such as procainamide, phenytoin, aprindine, and mexiletine are unquestionably effective in reducing ventricular ectopy and, in our experience, more so than beta blockers, it is only the beta blockers that have been unequivocally demonstrated to reduce the incidence of SCD in the postinfarct population. Moreover, this group of drugs has also been shown to decrease total cardiac mortality and recurrent myocardial infarction.[45-49] However, the mechanism is unknown. Possibly the beta blockers do not particularly decrease ambient ectopy as much as they reduce the tendency to ischemia, which would have acted as a transient trigger for fatal ventricular arrhythmias. Furthermore, the success of the beta blockers is clearly in the lower-risk population. In fact, study designs tend to neglect patients with high-grade or symptomatic ventricular ectopy and depressed left ventricular function—two important factors that characterize a high-risk patient. Thus, we have evidence only to support a decrease in SCD in low-risk patients in an undefined manner.

In accepting the implications of the beta-blocker study—prophylactic use— one should consider the cost-effectiveness factor. If there are approximately 200,000 postinfarct patients who are annually eligible for beta-blocker therapy at an average daily cost of $0.40 for therapy, each patient would spend $146 per year for a total cost of $26,200,000! However, this cannot be considered money effectively spent since virtually 90% of the patients can be expected to live without beta blockers. Therefore, more than $26,000,000 could be saved annually if more accurate risk assessment were available to determine who, among the so-called "low-risk" group, was, in fact, destined for SCD.

If one does not demand placebo-controlled trials in order to be convinced that drug therapy can have an impact on the problem of sudden death the results of several other studies, most notably those using programmed electrical stimulation[31-39] or assessment of changes in ambient ectopy,[20] suggest that successful antiarrhythmic drug therapy results in an annual mortality rate of 4–15% compared to a mortality rate of 40–60% in patients who do not have their arrhythmias adequately controlled after therapy. It is also important to note that most of these studies deal with patients who have a history of symptoms related to ventricular tachyarrhythmias in contrast to the history of patients who entered the trials with beta-adrenergic blocking agents. Despite the inviting suggestion that therapy is truly effective in this group without placebo control, we must also consider the possibility that the test merely selected patients who were going to do well, independent of drug therapy. Conversely, one should also consider that therapy may have accelerated the death in certain patients.

In addition to pharmacologic means for the management of the patient at risk of SCD, newer treatment forms are now available, such as antitachycardia pacemakers,[7] antiarrhythmic surgery,[5,6] and implantable cardioverter-defibrillators.[8-11] Each of these modalities appears to offer effective therapy, but, as with drug therapy, there is no placebo control. Our experience[54] with the implantable cardioverter-defibrillator has demonstrated only 8% recurrent SCD over 12 months in a patient population that had survived an average of four cardiac arrests before implantation of the devices. This percentage seems much lower than expected. However, we did not employ controls (for example, sham implants) because of ethical restraints, which is one of the major reasons why other investigators have also refrained from using true placebo controls. However, the cardioverter-defibrillator may nevertheless give us the opportunity to examine the effectiveness of antiarrhythmic agents: If we provide all patients with a defibrillator to prevent SCD, we can then use a study drug in one-half of the population and a placebo in the other half while we measure the number of times the device discharges.

## SUMMARY

We now have a wide variety of potentially very effective means to approach the major health problem of SCD, but each carries its own intrinsic risk of worsening the problem. Consequently, it seems prudent to expend much greater effort in obtaining accurate risk assessment. The data from several investigators suggest that this is a real possibility and not something that must await future development. If we can attain accurate risk assessment, we should expect reduction in the study population size, improvement in the therapeutic risk/benefit to the individual patient who enters the study, and dramatic reduction in study costs, and we can also arrive at a quicker answer to the question of the effectiveness of the means of therapy under investigation.

It also appears likely that a more rational and cost-effective approach to the problem of the SCD will be by means of an entire treatment strategy or program of management rather than by a single therapy.

## REFERENCES

1. KULLER, L. 1969. Sudden death in arteriosclerotic heart disease: The case for preventive medicine. Am. J. Cardiol. **24:** 617–628.
2. INTER-SOCIETY COMMISSION FOR HEART DISEASE RESOURCES. 1970. Report on primary prevention of atherosclerotic diseases. Circulation **42:** A55–A95.
3. BAUM, R. S., H. ALVAREZ & L. A. COBB. 1974. Survival after resuscitation from out-of-hospital ventricular fibrillation. Circulation **50:** 1231–1235.
4. KEEFE, D. L., R. E. KATES & D. C. HARRISON. 1981. New antiarrhythmic drugs: Their place in therapy. Drugs **22:** 363–400.
5. HOROWITZ, L. N., A. H. HARKEN, J. A. KASTOR & M. A. JOSEPHSON. 1980. Ventricular resection guided by epicardial and endocardial mapping for treatment of recurrent ventricular tachycardia. N. Engl. J. Med. **302:** 589–593.
6. FONTAINE, G., G. GUIRAUDON, R. FRANK, F. FILLETTE, C. CABROL & Y. GROSGOGEAT. 1982. Surgical treatment of ventricular tachycardia unrelated to myocardial ischemia or infarction. Am. J. Cardiol. **49:** 397–410.
7. FISHER, J. D., G. K. SOO, S. FURMAN & J. A. MATOS. 1982. Role of implantable pacemakers in control of recurrent ventricular tachycardia. Am. J. Cardiol. **49:** 194–206.
8. MIROWSKI, M., P. R. REID, M. M. MOWER, L. WATKINS, V. L. GOTT, J. F. SHAUBLE, A. LANGER, M. S. HEILMAN, S. A. KOLENIK, R. E. FISCHELL & M. L. WEISFELDT. 1980. Termination of malignant ventricular arrhythmias with an implanted automatic defibrillator in human beings. N. Engl. J. Med. **303:** 322–324.
9. REID, P. R., M. MIROWSKI, M. M. MOWER, E. V. PLATIA, L. S. C. GRIFFITH, L. WATKINS, JR., S. M. BACH, JR., M. IMRAN & A. THOMAS. 1983. Clinical evaluation of the internal automatic cardioverter-defibrillator in survivors of sudden cardiac death. Am. J. Cardiol. **51:** 1068–1613.
10. ZIPES, D. P., W. M. JACKMAN, J. J. HEGER, D. A. CHILSON, K. F. BROWNE, G. V. NACCARELLI, G. T. RAHILLY, JR. & E. N. PRYSTOWSKY. 1982. Clinical transvenous cardioversion of recurrent life-threatening ventricular tachyarrhythmias: Low energy synchronized cardioversion of ventricular tachycardia and termination of ventricular fibrillation in patients using a catheter electrode. Am. Heart J. **103:** 789–794.
11. WASPE, L. E., S. G. KIM, J. A. MATOS & J. D. FISHER. 1983. Role of a catheter lead system for transvenous countershock and pacing during electrophysiologic tests: An assessment of the usefulness of catheter shocks for terminating ventricular tachyarrhythmias. Am. J. Cardiol. **52:** 477–484.
12. BRODSKY, M., W. DELON, P. DENES, C. KANAKES & K. ROSEN. 1977. Arrhythmias

documented by 24-hour continuous electrocardiographic monitoring in 50 male medical students without apparent heart disease. Am. J. Cardiol. **39:** 390–395.

13. HINKLE, L. E., JR., S. CARVER & M. STEVENS. 1969. The frequency of asymptomatic disturbances of cardiac rhythm and conduction in middle-aged men. Am. J. Cardiol. **24:** 629–650.

14. VELEBIT, V., P. PODRID, B. LOWN, B. COHEN & S. GRABOYS. 1982. Aggravation and provocation of ventricular arrhythmias by antiarrhythmic drugs. Circulation **65:** 886–894.

15. THE CORONARY DRUG PATIENT RESEARCH GROUP. 1972. The prognostic importance of the electrocardiogram after myocardial infarction: Experience in the coronary drug project. Ann. Intern. Med. **77:** 677–689.

16. SHULZE, R. A., JR., J. ROULEAU, P. RIGO, S. BOWERS, H. W. STRAUSS & B. PITT. 1975. Ventricular arrhythmias in the late hospital phase of acute myocardial infarction: Relation to left ventricular function detected by gated cardiac blood pool scanning. Circulation **52:** 1006–1011.

17. RUBERMAN, W., E. WEINBLATT, J. D. GOLDBERG, C. W. FRANK & S. SHAPIRO. 1977. Ventricular premature beats and mortality after myocardial infarction. N. Engl. J. Med. **297:** 750–757.

18. BIGGER, J. T., JR., F. M. WELD & L. M. ROLNITZKY. 1981. Prevalence, characteristics and significance of ventricular tachycardia (three or more complexes) detected with ambulatory electrocardiographic recording in the later hospital phase of acute myocardial infarction. Am. J. Cardiol. **48:** 815–823.

19. THE MULTICENTER POSTINFARCTION RESEARCH GROUP. 1983. Risk stratification and survival after myocardial infarction. N. Engl. J. Med. **309:** 331–336.

20. GRABOYS, T. B., B. LOWN, P. J. PODRID & R. DeSILVA. 1982. Long-term survival of patients with malignant ventricular arrhythmias treated with antiarrhythmic drugs. Am. J. Cardiol. **50:** 437–443.

21. LOWN, B. & M. WOLF. 1971. Approaches to sudden death from coronary heart disease. Circulation **44:** 130–142.

22. BIGGER, J. T., JR. & F. M. WELD. 1981. Analysis of prognostic significance of ventricular arrhythmias after myocardial arrhythmias after myocardial infarction: Shortcomings of the Lown grading system. B. Heart J. **45:** 717–724.

23. PEEL, A. A. F., T. TAMPLE, I. WANG, W. M. LANCASTER & J. L. G. DALL. 1962. A coronary prognostic index for grading the severity of infarction. Br. Heart J. **24:** 745–760.

24. LURIA, M. H., J. D. KNOKE & J. S. WACHS. 1979. Survival after recovery from acute myocardial infarction: Two- and five-year prognostic indices. Am. J. Med. **67:** 7–14.

25. LIE, K. I., H. J. J. WELLENS, E. DOWNAR & D. DURRER. 1975. Observations on patients with primary ventricular fibrillation complicating acute myocardial infarction. Circulation **52:** 755–759.

26. THEROUX, P., D. D. WATERS, C. HALPHEN, J.-C. DEBAISIEUX & H. F. MIZALA. 1979. Prognostic value of exercise testing soon after myocardial infarction. N. Engl. J. Med. **301:** 341–345.

27. SCHULZE, R. A., H. W. STRAUSS & B. PITT. 1977. Sudden death in the year following myocardial infarction: Relation to ventricular premature contractions in the late hospital phase and left ventricular ejection fraction. Am. J. Med. **62:** 192–199.

28. TAYLOR, G. J., J. O. HUMPHRIES, E. D. MELLITS, B. PITT, R. A. SCHULZE, L. S. C. GRIFFITH & S. C. ACHUFF. 1980. Predictors of clinical course, coronary anatomy and left ventricular function after recovery from acute myocardial infarction. Circulation **62:** 960–970.

29. SWERDLOW, C. D., R. A. WINKLE & J. W. MASON. 1983. Determinants of survival in patients with ventricular tachyarrhythmias. N. Engl. J. Med. **308:** 1436–1442.

30. NACCARELLI, G. V., E. N. PRYSTOWSKY, W. M. JACKMAN, J. J. HEGER, G. T. RAHILLY & D. P. ZIPES. 1982. Role of electrophysiologic testing in managing patients who have ventricular tachycardia unrelated to coronary artery disease. Am. J. Cardiol. **50:** 165–171.

31. COBB, L. A., J. A. WERNER & G. B. TROBAUGH. 1980. Sudden cardiac death. I. A

decade's experience with out-of-hospital resuscitation. Mod. Concepts Cardiovasc. Dis. **49:** 31–36.

32. COBB, L. A., J. A. WERNER & G. B. TROBAUGH. 1980. Sudden cardiac death. II. Outcome of resuscitation: Management and future directions. Mod. Concepts Cardiovasc. Dis. **49:** 37–42.

33. COBB, L. A., A. P. HALLSTROM, W. D. WEAVER, M. K. COPASS & R. E. HAYNES. 1978. Clinical predictors and characteristics of the sudden cardiac death syndrome. The Proceedings of the USA/USSR. First Joint Symposium on Sudden Death.: 99–116. DHEW Publication O. (NIH) 78-1470.

34. WELLENS, H. J., D. R. DURRER & K. L. LIE. 1976. Observations on mechanisms of ventricular tachycardia in man. Circulation **54:** 237–244.

35. FISHER, J. D., H. L. COHEN, R. MEHRA, H. ALTSCHULER, D. J. W. ESCHER & S. FURMAN. 1977. Cardiac pacing and pacemakers. II. Serial electrophysiologic-pharmacologic testing for control of recurrent ventricular tachycardia. Am. Heart J. **93:** 658–668.

36. HOROWITZ, L. N., M. E. JOSEPHSON, A. FARSHIDI, S. R. SPIELMAN, E. L. MICHELSON & A. M. GREENSPAN. 1978. Recurrent sustained ventricular tachycardia. 3. Role of the electrophysiologic study in selection of antiarrhythmic regimens. Circulation **58:** 986–997.

37. MASON, J. W. & R. A. WINKLE. 1980. Accuracy of the ventricular tachycardia-induction study for predicting long-term efficacy and inefficacy of antiarrhythmic drugs. N. Engl. J. Med. **303:** 1073–1077.

38. RUSKIN, J. N., J. P. DiMARCO & H. GARAN. 1980. Out-of-hospital observations and selection of long-term antiarrhythmic therapy. N. Engl. J. Med. **303:** 607–613.

39. PLATIA, E. V., H. L. GREEN, S. C. VLAY, J. A. WERNER, B. GROSS & P. R. REID. 1983. Sensitivity of various extrastimulus techniques in patients with serious ventricular arrhythmias. Am. Heart J. **106:** 698–703.

40. LIVELLI, F. D., JR., J. T. BIGGER, JR., J. A. REIFFEL, E. S. GANG, J. N. PATTON, P. M. NOETHLING, L. M. ROLNITZKY & J. I. GLIKLICH. 1982. Response to programmed ventricular stimulation: Sensitivity, specificity and relation to heart disease. Am. J. Cardiol. **50:** 452–458.

41. SWERDLOW, C. D., J. BLUM, R. A. WINKLE, J. C. GRIFFIN, D. L. ROSS & J. W. MASON. 1982. Decreased incidence of antiarrhythmic drug efficacy at electrophysiologic study associated with use of a third extrastimulus. Am. Heart J. **104:** 1004–1011.

42. PLATIA, E. V., S. C. VLAY & P. R. REID. 1982. A comparison of the predictive value of programmed electrical stimulation and Holter monitoring in patients with malignant ventricular arrhythmias. Am. J. Cardiol. **49:** 928.

43. HEGER, J. J., E. N. PRYSTOWSKY, W. M. JACKMAN, G. V. NACCARELLI, K. A. WARFEL, R. L. RINKENBERGER & D. P. ZIPES. 1981. Amiodarone. Clinical efficacy and electrophysiology during long-term therapy for recurrent ventricular tachycardia or ventricular fibrillation. N. Engl. J. Med. **305:** 539–545.

44. AUSTEN, W. G., J. E. EDWARDS, R. L. FYE, G. G. GENSINI, V. L. GOTT, L. S. C. GRIFFITH, D. C. McGOON, M. L. MURPHY & B. B. ROWE. 1975. A reporting system in patients evaluated for coronary artery disease. Circulation **51:** 5–40.

45. WILHELMSSON, C., J. A. VEDIN, L. WILHELMSEN, G. TIBBLIN & L. WERKS. 1974. Reduction of sudden deaths after myocardial infarction by treatment with alprenolol: Preliminary results. Lancet **2:** 1157–1160.

46. MULTICENTRE INTERNATIONAL STUDY. 1975. Improvement in prognosis of myocardial infarction by long-term beta adrenoreceptor blockade using practolol: A multicentre international study. Br. Med. J. **3:** 735–740.

47. THE NORWEGIAN MULTICENTER STUDY GROUP. 1981. Timolol-induced reduction in mortality and reinfarction in patients surviving acute myocardial infarction. N. Engl. J. Med. **304:** 801–807.

48. HJALMARSON, A., D. ELMFELDT, J. HERLITZ, S. HOLMBERG, I. MALEK, G. NYBERG, L. RYDEN, K. SWEDBERG, A. VEDIN, F. WAAGSTEIN, A. WALDENSTROM, J. WALDENSTROM, H. WEDEL, L. WILHELMSEN & C. WILHELMSSON. 1981. Effect on

mortality of metoprolol in acute myocardial infarction: A double-blind randomized trial. Lancet **2:** 823–827.

49. BETA-BLOCKER HEART ATTACK TRIAL RESEARCH GROUP. 1974. A randomized trial of propranolol in patients with acute myocardial infarction. I. Mortality results. JAMA **247:** 1707–1714.

50. KOSOWSKY, B. D., J. TAYLOR, B. LOWN & R. RITCHIE. 1973. Long-term use of procainamide following acute myocardial infarction. Circulation **97:** 1204–1210.

51. COLLABORATIVE GROUP. 1971. Phenytoin after recovery from myocardial infarction: Controlled trial in 568 patients. Lancet **2:** 1055–1057.

52. WINKLE, R. A. 1982. Clinical efficacy of antiarrhythmic drugs in prevention of sudden coronary death. *In* Sudden Coronary Death. H. M. Greenberg & E. M. Dwyer, Eds. Ann. N. Y. Acad. Sci. **382:** 247–257.

53. CHAMBERLAIN, D. A., D. E. JEWITT, D. G. JULIAN, R. W. F. CAMPBELL, D. MC BOYLE & R. G. SHANKS. 1980. Oral mexiletine in high-risk patients after myocardial infarction. Lancet **2:** 1324–1327.

54. MIROWSKI, M., P. R. REID, R. A. WINKLE, M. M. MOWER, L. WATKINS, E. B. STINSON, L. S. C. GRIFFITH, H. KALLMAN & M. L. WEISFELDT. 1983. Mortality in patients with implanted automatic defibrillator. Ann. Intern. Med. **98:** 585–588.

# Considerations in the Long-Term Management of Survivors of Cardiac Arrest[a]

LEONARD A. COBB,[b] ALFRED P. HALLSTROM,
W. DOUGLAS WEAVER, GENE B. TROBAUGH, AND
H. LEON GREENE

*Departments of Medicine (Cardiology) and Biostatistics*
*University of Washington*
*Seattle, Washington 98195*

*Harborview Medical Center*
*Seattle, Washington 98104*

Nearly 15 years' experience in following patients resuscitated from out-of-hospital cardiac arrest has helped us to gain insight into certain aspects of sudden cardiac death. In spite of the value of this experience, there remain a number of uncertainties as to how such patients should be managed. Approximately 80% of the victims of sudden cardiac death have coronary heart disease, and in this paper our observations and discussion will be focused on the management of that group.

It is widely held that most episodes of sudden cardiac death are due to ventricular fibrillation (VF), and indeed this has been recorded by paramedics in 78–95% of victims after a witnessed cardiac arrest.[1] Additionally, the overwhelming majority of patients with exertionally related cardiac arrest have been reported to show VF.[2] Although most episodes of VF are probably initiated by a few cycles of ventricular flutter or polymorphous ventricular tachycardia,[3–5] very few resuscitated patients have had histories consistent with symptomatic, recurrent ventricular tachycardia prior to cardiac arrest. Furthermore, in our experience, such histories are also distinctly uncommon after resuscitation from VF. This is in accord with findings on ambulatory electrocardiographic recording; in 144 ambulatory patients previously resuscitated from VF, ventricular tachycardia (more than three repetitive complexes) was recorded in only 9% of patients during 24-hour monitoring.[6] Thus, recurrent ventricular tachycardia and sudden cardiac death are by no means synonymous, and the therapeutic strategies for these disorders may well be quite dissimilar.

## RECURRENT CARDIAC ARREST AND RISK STRATIFICATION

Although the numbers of patients resuscitated from out-of-hospital VF are relatively modest, the natural history of these survivors has helped to extend our

[a] This work was supported by Grant HL-18805 from the National Heart, Lung and Blood Institute of the National Institutes of Health and by a grant from Ayerst Laboratories.

[b] Address for correspondence: Leonard A. Cobb, M.D., Division of Cardiology, Harborview Medical Center, 325 Ninth Avenue, Seattle, Washington 98104.

**TABLE 1.** Univariate Predictors of Recurrent Cardiac Arrest in Previously Resuscitated Patients

---

    1. Abnormal left ventricular function[9-11]
        History of remote myocardial infarction prior to VF
        History of congestive heart failure prior to VF
        Segmental left ventricular dysfunction and reduced ejection fraction
    2. Extensive coronary artery obstruction[12]
    3. VF *not* precipitated by acute infarction[11]
    4. Complex or high frequency of ventricular ectopic activity[6,10]
    5. Age[13]
    6. Exercise-evoked hypotension or angina[14]

---

understanding of sudden cardiac death. Overall there is a high incidence of recurrent cardiac arrest, particularly in the first 1 to 2 years after resuscitation,[7-9] and several factors have been recognized as predictors of recurrence. Of most significance in our experience is impairment of left ventricular function, as reflected by the systolic ejection fraction.[10] Ventricular ectopy, particularly complex forms, was also significant, but in our patients did not have the impact of ventricular dysfunction in predicting individuals likely to develop recurrent cardiac arrest.[10] TABLE 1 shows the major univariate predictors of recurrences of the sudden cardiac death syndrome in patients with coronary heart disease.

A very practical aspect of recognizing predictors for recurrent cardiac arrest is that of risk stratification. Although the overall likelihood of a patient's developing recurrent cardiac arrest within a year after resuscitation approximates 20%,[11] that risk is remarkably variable from one subgroup to another. Accordingly, the need for intervention ought to be related to the anticipated natural history. For instance, of 45 resuscitated patients with left ventricular ejection fractions above 0.50, only two died during an observational period of at least 2.5 years. In contrast, 52 of 109 patients with ejection fraction of 0.50 or less died during the same follow-up period.[10]

Although sudden cardiac death (SCD) is usually a consequence of VF, the pathophysiologic derangements underlying the emergence of that arrhythmia are undoubtedly variable and highly complex. In this regard it is important to emphasize that the sudden cardiac death syndrome occurs in a markedly heterogenous group of patients. At one extreme are persons whose first manifestation of coronary heart disease is acute infarction with VF; on the other end of the spectrum are patients with advanced disease who have left ventricular scars or aneurysms and who develop VF without evidence of acute myocardial ischemia. Also within this spectrum is a group in whom sudden cardiac arrest develops apparently because of transient myocardial ischemia.

Whereas sudden cardiac death in industrialized nations is usually a manifestation of coronary heart disease, it is precipitated by acute myocardial infarction in only a minority of cases.[7] At autopsy, coronary thrombosis is usually absent[15]; furthermore, in resuscitated patients diagnostic electrocardiographic and enzymatic findings of acute infarction were present in only 19% and 38% of cases, respectively.[16] Since most episodes of SCD are not initiated by acute infarction, the possibility of preventing SCD by measures influencing "primary" arrhythmic events seems at least plausible. To this end, antiarrhythmic agents, beta blocking drugs, antifibrillatory agents, and coronary artery bypass grafting have all been proposed as possible and logical therapies.

## USE OF CLASS I ANTIARRHYTHMIC AGENTS

To our knowledge, no controlled trials of Class I, membrane-active antiarrhythmic agents have been reported in survivors of out-of-hospital ventricular fibrillation. Nevertheless, some relevant data are available and will be reviewed here.

### *Uncontrolled Community Experience.*

One hundred forty-four resuscitated patients with coronary heart disease were followed for an average of 32 months after 24-hour ambulatory monitoring.[6] Fifty-one patients died, 32 from recurrent cardiac arrest. Although the patients were followed in a research clinic for VF survivors, their medical care was the responsibility of many physicians in the community. Antiarrhythmic therapy was usually prescribed empirically, and plasma levels of the drugs were not regularly monitored in these years (1972–1978). The presence of any complex ventricular ectopy (defined here as bigeminy, trigeminy, repetitive forms, or frequent multiforms) during a 24-hour recording was a relatively sensitive predictor (84% sensitivity), of patients who were to develop recurrent sudden cardiac arrest, but its specificity was only 40%.

We recognized five treatment groups in these 144 patients; their outcomes and ambulatory arrhythmias are shown in TABLE 2.

Patients chronically treated with quinidine as well as those receiving no antiarrhythmic therapy had mortality rates significantly lower then that of the patients who received procainamide (p < .05). However, the clinical characteristics of patients in these treatment groups were not uniformly distributed. As shown in FIGURE 1, there was substantial variation among the drug groups in the proportion

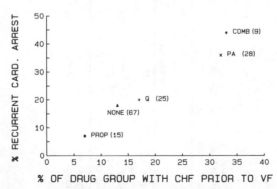

VF SURVIVORS
ANTIARRHYTHMICS, PRIOR CHF, AND SURVIVAL

**FIGURE 1.** The relationship between recurrent cardiac arrest and history of congestive heart failure prior to the initial episode of ventricular fibrillation. One hundred forty-four resuscitated patients comprise five groups according to the type of chronic antiarrhythmic therapy prescribed. PROP = propranolol, Q = quinidine, PA = procainamide, COMB = combination of these drugs. Figures in parentheses represent the number of patients in each group. (Adapted from Weaver *et al.*[6])

**TABLE 2.** Antiarrhythmic Drugs, Ambulatory Arrhythmias, and Survival in 144 Survivors of Out-of-Hospital Ventricular Fibrillation[a]

| | Drug Groups | | | | |
| | Procainamide | Quinidine | Propranolol | Combination | No Antiarrhythmic Agents |
|---|---|---|---|---|---|
| Number of patients | 28 | 25 | 15 | 9 | 67 |
| Patients with complex ventricular ectopy | 22 (79%) | 15 (60%) | 6 (40%)[b] | 7 (78%) | 45 (67%) |
| Recurrent cardiac arrest | 10 (36%)[b] | 5 (20%) | 1 (7%) | 4 (44%) | 12 (18%) |
| Total number of deaths | 16 (57%) | 7 (28%) | 2 (13%)[b] | 6 (67%)[b] | 20 (30%) |

[a] Adapted from Weaver et al.[6]
[b] $p < 0.05$ comparing a drug group with those who received no antiarrhythmic therapy ($\chi^2$ analysis).

of patients who had experienced congestive heart failure prior to VF, and this measure of morbidity was closely related to the proportion who later developed recurrent cardiac arrest. Although the high mortality in patients taking procainamide was likely related to the severity of underlying heart disease, it has been suggested that protection from sudden cardiac death may be less with procainamide than with quinidine.[17]

In an analysis of 70 men previously resuscitated from out-of-hospital VF not associated with acute infarction, we tested in a multivariate model[18] the influence of chronic treatment with quinidine and/or procainamide, complex arrhythmias, and a history of prior myocardial infarction in predicting survival.[19] There was no evidence that chronic antiarrhythmic therapy benefited the 37 patients who received procainamide or quinidine compared to 33 patients who were not treated with antiarrhythmic agents.

There are, of course, major limitations to the above retrospective observations. Nevertheless, when Class I antiarrhythmic agents were administered in an empirical and uncontrolled manner, we were unable to demonstrate obvious protection from recurrences of the sudden cardiac death syndrome.

### Antifibrillatory Effects

Myerburg and coworkers reported on the use of quinidine or procainimide in 32 patients who had been resuscitated from out-of-hospital cardiac arrest.[20] These investigators found no correlation between the incidence of recurrent cardiac arrest and suppression of ventricular ectopy. Rather, the salient observation in that report was that the maintenance of relatively stable plasma drug levels in a "therapeutic range" seemed to afford protection from sudden death. This is a provocative observation, suggesting an "antifibrillatory" effect of these agents separate from their suppression of ventricular ectopy. These findings, of course, are limited by the small number of patients, and the authors' hypothesis requires a larger prospective evaluation.

### Adverse Effects

An important consideration in evaluating the use of quinidine as well as other antiarrhythmic agents is the possibility that in some patients these agents may render the myocardium more electrically unstable and actually facilitate the emergence of ventricular arrhythmias.[21,22] This is potentially very serious, particularly in an unmonitored situation, where the adverse effects of antiarrhythmic agents may not be recognized. Therefore, even if antiarrhythmic agents could actually protect some patients from SCD, others might well be victims of such therapy. An additional limitation to the use of presently available antiarrhythmic agents is their well-recognized propensity to evoke disturbing noncardiac side effects.

## PREVENTION OF SCD BY BETA-ADRENERGIC BLOCKERS

Clinical trials of beta-adrenergic blocking drugs administered for 1 to 4 years after acute myocardial infarction have shown that total mortality and deaths from sudden cardiac arrest are reduced in patients who receive beta blockers compared to those on placebo.[23–27] In spite of these important and conclusive findings, these interventions will not have a major impact on the community incidence of sudden cardiac death, primarily because the reduction in first-year mortality affects only a small proportion (2–4%) of eligible patients discharged after a recent myocardial infarction. Additionally, half or more of the patients who die suddenly because of coronary heart disease do not have a history of ever having had a previously recognized myocardial infarction.[28,29] Finally, an inspection of the approximate numbers of events shows that an intervention that affects the first-year mortality of 2 to 4% of 600,000 patients hospitalized for acute myocardial infarction cannot be expected to have a major impact on the estimated 400,000 victims of sudden cardiac death each year in the United States.

The mechanisms underlying the protection afforded by beta blocking drugs after myocardial infarction are not known. It is possible that mortality might be reduced through antiarrhythmic effects of by decreased myocardial oxygen requirements. However, it seems to us that the observed reduction in sudden cardiac deaths should be considered in light of the fact that beta blocking drugs are also associated with a reduced incidence of recurrent, nonfatal myocardial infarction.[27] Since a proportion of sudden cardiac deaths are secondary to acute myocardial infarction, it is reasonable to consider that the protection from sudden death with beta blockers is at least in part a reflection of the lowered incidence of reinfarction.

### Propranolol in VF Survivors

Impressed by the early reports of beta blockers in patients who recovered from recent myocardial infarction, we carried out a small trial of propranolol in ambulatory patients who had been resuscitated from out-of-hospital ventricular fibrillation.[30] In that study, 52 patients were randomly assigned, after risk stratification, to a regimen of receiving either propranolol or no propranolol; other therapy, including antiarrhythmic agents, was continued as already prescribed. The study was not blinded, and both patients and physicians were aware of the therapy. We excluded from the study patients who had angina and thus who were likely to require beta blockers as well as patients who had sustained a recent myocardial infarction. Twenty-three patients were allocated to receive propranolol and twenty-nine no propranolol. The daily dosage of propranolol after titration ranged from 90 to 640 (median 165) mg, and the goal was to achieve a trough plasma level of 40 to 50 ng/ml. Although the trial was small, there was a total of 16 fatal events (30%) during an average follow-up period of 36 months. The mortality rates in the two treatment groups were approximately equal, although there were retrospectively defined subjects who had a lower incidence of sudden death than did others. The major findings in this pilot study are summarized in TABLE 3.

These findings, which did not show protection by beta blockers, are, of course, limited by the relatively small number of patients and the possibility of a type II error. However, these results are consistent with those of Taylor and colleagues,[31] who reported a large trial of oxprenolol in 1103 men with stable coronary heart disease enrolled an average of 13 months after myocardial infarction. These investigators also found no overall "protective" effect of oxprenolol on mortality and suggested that beta blockers may prevent sudden cardiac death only in a select group, that is, those who have sustained a recent myocardial infarction.[31]

## MYOCARDIAL ISCHEMIA

Although the association between sudden cardiac death and coronary heart disease is well established, the role of myocardial ischemia per se in this interaction is not well defined. However, there are cases in which there is circumstantial evidence pointing to an association between transient myocardial ischemia and sudden cardiac death: first, the recognized temporal association between strenuous exertion and cardiac arrest,[14,32,33] and, second, the fact that some victims have evidence of neither myocardial dysfunction nor infarction in spite of extensive coronary atherosclerosis. In following a large number of patients resuscitated from out-of-hospital cardiac arrest, we estimated that up to one-third of these patients could have had cardiac arrest due to transient myocardial ischemia.[11,14]

**TABLE 3.** Propranolol in Survivors of Out-of-Hospital Cardiac Arrest

| | Group A (Propranolol) | Group B (No Propranolol) |
|---|---|---|
| No. of patients | 23 | 29 |
| Average age ± S.D. | 62 ± 8 | 59 ± 8 |
| Percent with histories of: | | |
| Angina | 45% | 41% |
| Remote MI | 48% | 45% |
| CHF before cardiac arrest | 30% | 7% |
| Drug therapy at entry | | |
| Digitalis | 30% | 31% |
| Beta blockers | 13% | 24%[a] |
| Diuretics | 30% | 41% |
| Antiarrhythmics | 74% | 62% |
| Average percent ± S.D. of half-hour intervals with complex ventricular arrhythmia[b] at baseline | 17 ± 28 | 21 ± 27 |
| Average LV ejection fraction ± S.D. at baseline | .44 ± 16 | .39 ± 17 |
| Mortality[c] 1 yr after randomization | | |
| Total deaths | .17 ± .08 (n = 4) | .21 ± .08 (n = 6) |
| Recurrent cardiac arrest | .09 ± .06 (n = 3) | .18 ± .07 (n = 5) |
| Mortality 2 yr after randomization | | |
| Total deaths | .23 ± .09 (n = 5) | .24 ± .08 (n = 7) |
| Recurrent cardiac arrest | .13 ± .06 (n = 3) | .22 ± .08 (n = 6) |

ABBREVIATIONS: MI = myocardial infarction; CHF = signs and symptoms thought to represent congestive heart failure; LV = left ventricular.

[a] Propranolol was stopped on the day of randomization in six patients previously taking this drug.

[b] During 24-hr ambulatory ECG recording.

[c] Mortality rates were determined by life-table analysis.[18] The observational time varied from 1 to 4 years.

This estimate was based on the circumstances and symptoms surrounding cardiac arrest as well as the responses to exercise testing.

### Coronary Revascularization

The use of propranolol in survivors of out-of-hospital ventricular fibrillation in one small study has been discussed earlier. A second, and more direct, attack on transient myocardial ischemia is to improve coronary perfusion, particularly by coronary artery bypass grafting. The data on prevention of sudden cardiac death and reduction of arrhythmias after bypass surgery are seemingly inconsistent. There appears to be no reduction in exercise-induced ventricular ectopy in patients who have had coronary artery bypass grafting.[34] Nonetheless, in the European Coronary Surgery Study, an impressive case was made for preventing sudden cardiac death by coronary artery bypass grafting in patients who had stable angina pectoris, relatively preserved left ventricular function, and triple-vessel coronary artery disease. In that study there was a significant reduction in total as well as sudden deaths in patients who were randomly assigned to surgical treatment compared to those treated medically.[35] On the other hand, the multicenter Coronary Artery Surgery Study[36] in the United States did not demonstrate such an improvement. It should be emphasized that in the latter study the patients were either asymptomatic or only mildly symptomatic and that the mortality in the control patients was sufficiently small so that the effect of any form of life-extending therapy, regardless of its magnitude, would have been most difficult to demonstrate.

In managing patients who have been resuscitated from out-of-hospital ventricular fibrillation, surgery is clearly a consideration. We recently compared the

TABLE 4. Variables Used to Select a Matched Medically Treated VF Survivor for Each Surgically Treated Patient

| | |
|---|---|
| 1. Age | (average, 56 yrs) |
| 2. Sex | (all males) |
| 3. History of remote myocardial infarction | (26%) |
| 4. History of congestive heart failure | (8%) |
| 5. History of angina | (46%) |
| 6. Left ventricular ejection fraction (in 34 of 39 patients) | (average, 0.52) |
| 7. Complex arrhythmias during ambulatory monitoring | |

follow-up of 39 VF survivors treated by coronary bypass grafting with the same number of patients treated medically: each surgically treated patient was matched to a medically managed patient. With the assistance of a computer, the characteristics shown in TABLE 4 were utilized to match the patients. The matching process also required that each medically treated patient must have survived at least as long after cardiac arrest as the time from cardiac arrest to the surgery of the matched patient.

In these 39 paired survivors of cardiac arrest, recurrent sudden cardiac arrests were significantly reduced in those who underwent surgery compared to the medically treated patients.[37] During follow-up study, there was a total of 24 deaths or recurrent cardiac arrests—16 in the medical group and 8 in those who had surgery (including one operative death). At 2 years of follow-up, the total mortality rates were 22% and 13% in the medical and surgical groups, respectively (p = 0.11), and the rates of recurrent unexpected cardiac arrest were 17% and 3% in the two groups (p = 0.02).

Clearly, this retrospective analysis has shortcomings. There is the question of why some patients were operated upon and others not and also whether their characteristics were truly "matched." However, it is our belief that the decision to proceed with surgery was primarily a physician-biased action and was not determined by the status of the patient. Although a randomized prospective trial is necessary to test the hypothesis in VF survivors, our observations are in accord with those of the European Coronary Surgery Study cited earlier: relief of myocardial ischemia in selected patients is one measure to prevent sudden cardiac death.

### Ischemia from Coronary Artery Spasm

Temporary restriction and restoration of coronary blood flow, apparently mediated through coronary artery spasm, can result in cardiac arrhythmias, including ventricular tachycardia and fibrillation.[38-40] If the vast numbers of victims of sudden cardiac death are considered, those deaths attributed to coronary artery spasm in persons with otherwise normal hearts represent but a very small proportion of episodes. On the other hand, coronary spasm in patients with fixed coronary atherosclerosis can potentiate the degree of myocardial ischemia and conceivably could be of major importance in initiating ventricular fibrillation in large numbers of patients. At this time we are unaware of studies that provide an estimate of the significance of coronary vasomotion in sudden cardiac death in the setting of coronary heart disease, and techniques adequate for the direct study of this problem are probably not available. Clinical trials of drugs known to inhibit coronary artery spasm could help to clarify this potentially important issue.

### SUMMARY AND CONCLUSIONS

The heterogeneity of resuscitated patients at risk of recurrent cardiac arrest serves to make their management difficult and complex. It is logical that therapy should be tailored to each patient and certainly to the mechanism whereby sudden cardiac death occurred. It is important, also, to recognize that *not* all resuscitated victims are at high risk for recurrence and that aggressive interventions are not necessarily mandatory. In the patient with cardiac arrest related to transient myocardial ischemia, a direct approach toward relieving ischemia seems appropriate. Antiarrhythmic agents may have a role in the treatment of some patients, but to this date the efficacy of such therapy is speculative, at best. The development and testing of agents that have "antifibrillatory" properties seems a logical approach at this time.

Clearly, efforts to lessen the mortality of patients who have been resuscitated from out-of-hospital cardiac arrest are important, not only for the particular patients themselves, but also in an effort to develop rational, prophylactic interventions for the large numbers of patients with coronary heart disease who are at risk for the development of sudden cardiac death.

### REFERENCES

1. HALLSTROM, A. P., M. S. EISENBERG & L. BERGNER. 1983. Emerg. Health Services Q. **1:** 41–49.
2. HOSSACK, K. F. & R. HARTWIG. 1982. J. Cardiac Rehab. **2:** 402–408.
3. HINKLE, L. E., JR., D. C. ARGYROS, J. C. HAYNES, T. ROBINSON & D. R. ALONSO. 1977. Am. J. Cardiol. **39:** 873–879.

4. AXELROD, P. J., R. L. VERRIER & B. LAUN. 1976. Am. J. Cardiol. **36:** 776–781.
5. NIKOLIC, G., R. L. BISHOP & J. B. SINGH. 1982. Circulation **66:** 218–225.
6. WEAVER, W. D., L. A. COBB & A. P. HALLSTROM. 1982. Circulation **66:** 212–218.
7. COBB, L. A., R. S. BAUM, H. ALVAREZ & W. A. SCHAFFER. 1975. Circulation **51 & 52** (Suppl. III): 223–228.
8. LIBERTHSON, R. R., E. L. NAGEL, J. C. HIRSCHMAN & S. R. NUSSENFIELD. 1974. N. Engl. J. Med. **291:** 317–321.
9. GOLDSTEIN, S., J. R. LANDIS, R. LEIGHTON, G. RITTER, M. VASU, A. LANTIS & R. SEROKMAN. 1981. Circulation **64:** 977–984.
10. RITCHIE, J. L., A. P. HALLSTROM, G. B. TROBAUGH, J. H. CALDWELL & L. A. COBB. 1985. Am. J. Cardiol. In press.
11. COBB, L. A., J. A. WERNER & G. B. TROBAUGH. 1980. Mod. Concepts Cardiovasc. Dis. **49:** 37–42.
12. WEAVER, W. D., G. S. LORCH, H. A. ALVEREZ & L. A. COBB. 1976. Circulation **54:** 895–900.
13. EISENBERG, M. S., A. P. HALLSTROM & L. BERGNER. 1982. N. Engl. J. Med. **306:** 1340–1343.
14. WEAVER, W. D., L. A. COBB & A. P. HALLSTROM. 1982. Am. J. Cardiol. **50:** 671–676.
15. REICHENBACH, D. D., N. S. MOSS & E. MEYER. 1977. Am. J. Cardiol. **39:** 865–872.
16. COBB, L. A., J. A. WERNER & G. B. TROBAUGH. 1980. Mod. Concepts Cardiovasc. Dis. **49:** 31–36.
17. KLETZKIN, M. 1980. Circulation **61:** 214.
18. COX, D. R. 1972. J. Royal Stat. Soc. (B) **34:** 187–220.
19. COBB, L. A. & A. P. HALLSTROM. 1980. *In* Current Controversies in Cardiovascular Disease. E. Rapaport, Ed.: 359–364. W. B. Saunders. Philadelphia, PA.
20. MYERBURG, R. J., K. M. KESSLER, L. ZALMAN, C. A. CONDE & A. CASTELLANOS. 1982. JAMA **247:** 1485–1490.
21. VELEBIT, V., P. PODRID, B. LOWN, B. H. COHEN & T. B. GRABOYS. 1982. Circulation **65:** 886–894.
22. RUSKIN, J. N., B. McGOVERN, H. GARAN, J. P. DiMARCO & E. KELLY. 1983. N. Engl. J. Med. **309:** 1302–1306.
23. WILHELMSSON, C., J. A. VEDIN, L. WILHELMSEN, G. TIBBLIN & L. WERKO. 1974. Lancet **2:** 1157–1160.
24. — 1977. Reduction in mortality after myocardial infarction with long-term beta-adrenoceptor blockade: Multicentre International Study. Supplementary report. Br. Med. J. **2:** 419–421.
25. NORWEGIAN MULTICENTER STUDY GROUP. 1981. N. Engl. J. Med. **304:** 801–807.
26. BETA-BLOCKER HEART ATTACK TRIAL RESEARCH GROUP. 1982. JAMA **247:** 1707–1714.
27. FRISHMAN, W. H., C. D. FURBERG & W. T. FRIEDEWALD. 1984. N. Engl. J. Med. **310:** 830–837.
28. FRIEDMAN, G. D., A. L. KLATSKY & A. B. SIEGELAUB. 1975. Circulation **51 & 52** (Suppl. III): 164–169.
29. COBB, L. A. & J. A. WERNER. 1982. Predictors and prevention of sudden cardiac death. *In* The Heart, 5th ed. J. W. Hurst, Ed.: 599–610. McGraw-Hill. New York, NY.
30. COBB, L. A., T. L. CHINN, A. P. HALLSTROM, M. J. SWAIN, G. B. TROBAUGH, J. A. WERNER & H. L. GREENE. 1981. Circulation **64** (Suppl. IV): 35 (abstract).
31. TAYLOR, S. H., B. SILKE, A. EBUTT, G. C. SUTTON, B. J. PROUT & D. M. BURLEY. 1982. N. Engl. J. Med. **307:** 1293–1300.
32. FRIEDMAN, M., J. H. MANWARING, R. H. ROSENMAN, G. DONION & P. ORGEGA. 1973. JAMA **225:** 1319–1328.
33. THOMPSON, P. D., M. P. STERN, P. WILLIAMS, K. DUNCAN, W. L. HASKELL & P. D. WOOD. 1979. JAMA **242:** 1265–1267.
34. TILKIAN, A. G., J. F. PFEIFFER, W. J. BARRY, M. J. LIPTON & H. N. HULTGREN. 1976. Am. Heart J. **92:** 707–714.
35. EUROPEAN CORONARY SURGERY STUDY GROUP. 1982. Lancet **2:** 1173–1180.

36. CASS PRINCIPLE INVESTIGATORS. 1983. Circulation **68:** 939–950.
37. COBB, L. A., A. P. HALLSTROM, M. ZIA, G. B. TROBAUGH, H. L. GREENE & W. D. WEAVER. 1983. J. Am. Coll. Cardiol. (abstract) **1:** 688.
38. KERIN, N. Z., M. RUBENFIRE, M. NAINI, W. J. WAJSZCZUK, A. PAMATMAT & P. N. CASCADE. 1979. Circulation **60:** 1343–1350.
39. LEVI, G. F. & C. PROTO. 1973. Br. Heart J. **35:** 601–606.
40. MURDOCK, D. K., J. M. LOEB, D. E. EULER, W. C. RANDALL. 1980. Circulation **61:** 175–182.

# Atrial Flutter and Atrial Fibrillation: Drug Therapy and Recent Observations[a]

ALBERT L. WALDO,[b] RICHARD W. HENTHORN, AND
VANCE J. PLUMB

*Department of Medicine and the*
*Cardiovascular Research and Training Center*
*University of Alabama in Birmingham*
*School of Medicine*
*Birmingham, Alabama 35294*

## INTRODUCTION

Atrial flutter and atrial fibrillation are arrhythmias that have long been recognized in patients, yet surprisingly little is understood about their mechanism. In addition, despite our having recognized these clinical entities for so very long, their management has changed little over the years. Thus, therapy classically has been to use digitalis to slow and control the ventricular response rate to either of these atrial arrhythmias, and, should the arrhythmia persist, to convert it to sinus rhythm using quinidine or procainamide.[1] In most instances, therapy to prevent recurrence of either atrial flutter or atrial fibrillation has employed these same Type I antiarrhythmic agents, along with digitalis to control the ventricular response rate, should either recur.[1]

The last two decades have witnessed small, but significant improvements in therapy of both atrial flutter and atrial fibrillation beginning with the advent of DC cardioversion in the 1960s.[2] The most recent decade has seen the addition of the beta blocking agents, primarily propranolol, as an adjunct to digitalis therapy (but, on occasion, in lieu of it) in an effort to control ventricular response rate in the presence of either of these supraventricular tachyarrhythmias.[1] The last few years have seen the advent of the use of the so-called calcium channel blockers, verapamil and, recently, diltiazem, also primarily as an adjunct to digitalis therapy in the control of ventricular response rate in the presence in either of these arrhythmias, or occasionally in lieu of digitalis therapy.[1,3] And finally, there has been a growing experience, primarily in Europe and South America, with the use of amiodarone in the successful treatment of recurrent atrial flutter and atrial fibrillation.[4]

[a] This work was supported in part by Grant 1R01HL29381-01A1 and SCOR in Ischemic Heart Disease Grant 5P50HL17,667 from the National Heart, Lung and Blood Institute of the National Institutes of Health.
[b] Address for correspondence: Albert L. Waldo, M.D., UAB Medical Center, Room 336LHR, University Station, Birmingham, Alabama 35294.

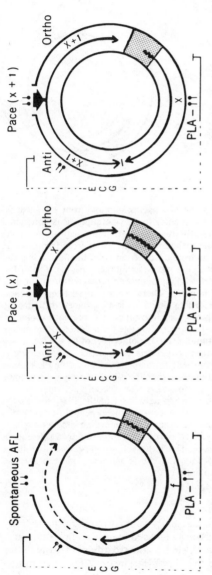

**FIGURE 1.** (*Left*): The reentry loop during spontaneous, Type I atrial flutter (AFL). In this and subsequent diagrams of transient entrainment and interruption of classical atrial flutter, the **f** represents the orthodromic wavefront, the **arrow** indicates the direction of spread of the impulse, the **serpentine line** indicates slow conduction through an area of slow connection (**stippled region**) in the reentry loop, the **ECG electrodes** represent the recording of a body surface electrocardiogram, and the **black dots with tails** indicate bipolar electrodes at an atrial pacing site, at a posterior-inferior left atrial (PLA) site and another atrial site. The **dashed lines** indicate the direction of continued spread of the orthodromic atrial flutter impulse in the reentry loop. Note that there is a gap of excitability in the reentry loop. (*Middle*): The introduction of the first pacing impulse (×) during rapid pacing from a site high in the right atrium during the spontaneous atrial flutter. The **large arrow** indicates the entry of the pacing impulse into the excitable gap of the reentry loop, whereupon it is conducted orthodromically (**Ortho**) and antidromically (**Anti**). The antidromic wavefront (×) collides with the orthodromic wavefront of the previous spontaneous atrial flutter beat (**f**), resulting in atrial fusion. This, in effect, terminates the tachycardia. However, the orthodromic wavefront from the pacing impulse (×) continues the tachycardia, resetting it to the rapid pacing rate. (*Right*): The introduction of the second pacing impulse (× + 1) during rapid pacing from the high right atrium during the atrial flutter. The **large arrow** again indicates the entry of the pacing impulse into the excitable gap of the reentry loop, whereupon it is conducted orthodromically and antidromically. Once again, the antidromic wavefront (× + 1) collides with the orthodromic wavefront of the previous paced beat (×), resulting in atrial fusion, and, once again, the orthodromic wavefront (× + 1) resets the tachycardia to the rapid pacing rate. Subsequent paced beats at this same pacing rate behave similarly. Thus, as illustrated in these diagrams, transient entrainment results from repeated early entrance of the wavefront from the pacing impulse into the reentry loop. This results in continuous resetting of the tachycardia, causing an increase of the tachycardia to the rapid pacing rate. (Modified from Plumb *et al.*[14])

LAST PACED BEAT (Entrained, but not fused)

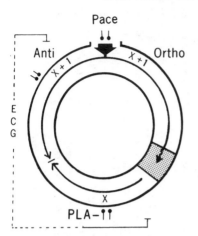
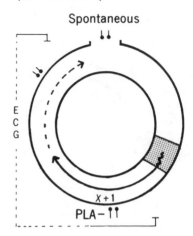

**FIGURE 2.** (*Left*): The **large arrow** indicates the last pacing impulse from a high atrial pacing site entering into the excitable gap of the reentry loop, whereupon it is conducted orthodromically (**Ortho**) and antidromically (**Anti**). Just as diagrammed in FIGURE 1, the antidromic wavefront ($\times$ + 1) collides with the orthodromic wavefront from the previous beat ($\times$), resulting in atrial fusion, and the orthodromic wavefront from the pacing impulse ($\times$ + 1) continues the tachycardia, resetting it to the rapid pacing rate. (*Right*): The orthodromic wavefront of the last pacing impulse ($\times$ + 1) is unopposed by an antidromic wavefront because there is no subsequent pacing impulse. Therefore, no atrial fusion occurs, despite treatment entrainment of the PLA recording site. This last entrained orthodromic wavefront continues the tachycardia (**dashed lines**), which resumes at its previous spontaneous rate. This diagram also illustrates why the PLA recording site is entrained at the pacing cycle length one beat beyond the last pacing stimulus, but the other recording site is not (see FIGURE 3). Note in the *left panel* and in FIGURE 1 that this other atrial recording site is activated antidromically during the period of transient entrainment, whereas the PLA site is activated orthodromically. However, note further that when the other recording site is being activated by the antidromic wavefront ($\times$ + 1), the PLA site is being activated by the previous orthodromic wavefront ($\times$). Therefore, when activation of the PLA site by the orthodromic wavefront of the last paced beat ($\times$ + 1) occurs at the expected time, there is no subsequent antidromic wavefront to activate the other atrial recording site. As a result, the orthodromic wavefront of the last paced beat ($\times$ + 1), now unopposed by a subsequent beat, proceeds to activate the other recording site. This latter activation necessarily follows activation of the PLA site. This explains why the PLA site is entrained one beat beyond entrainment of the other site. (Modified from Plumb *et al.*[12])

Thus, in a brief introduction, one can succinctly summarize the drug therapy of atrial flutter and atrial fibrillation. Necessarily glossed over in such a summary, of course, are many nuances to drug therapy, such as the treatment of atrial flutter and atrial fibrillation in the presence of the Wolff-Parkinson-White syndrome.[5] Nevertheless, it seems clear that as more is learned about these arrhythmias, additional advances in their therapy will be forthcoming. In this spirit, we present some of our recent observations concerning atrial flutter and atrial fibrillation, two arrhythmias in which we have been particularly interested.

## TRANSIENT ENTRAINMENT AND INTERRUPTION OF
## ATRIAL FLUTTER

Transient entrainment of a tachycardia may occur during cardiac pacing at a rate faster than the intrinsic rate of the tachycardia. It is an increase to the pacing rate of all tissue responsible for sustaining the tachycardia, with resumption of the intrinsic rate of the tachycardia upon either abrupt cessation of pacing or slowing of the pacing rate below the intrinsic rate of the tachycardia.[6-9] We have now been able to demonstrate transient entrainment of a tachyarrhythmia during rapid pacing in five different arrhythmias: atrial flutter, ventricular tachycardia, atrioventricular (AV) bypass pathway type of paroxysmal atrial tachycardia, ectopic atrial tachycardia, and AV nodal reentrant tachycardia.[6-14] On the basis of studies done during rapid pacing of these arrhythmias, we have suggested that the demonstration of transient entrainment and subsequent interruption of an arrhythmia necessarily mean that the arrhythmia results from reentry, and, moreover, that it is reentry with an excitable gap.[9-14]

Transient entrainment of a tachyarrhythmia was first recognized and described during rapid pacing of atrial flutter,[6] and then of ventricular tachycardia,[7] but the

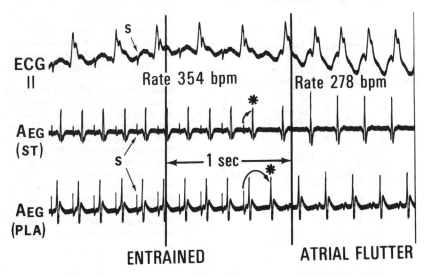

**FIGURE 3.** ECG lead II recorded simultaneously with bipolar atrial electrograms ($A_{EG}$) from the sulcus terminalis (**ST**) and from the posterior-inferior left atrium (PLA) at the termination of rapid pacing from Bachmann's bundle during a classical (Type I) atrial flutter. Pacing was performed at a rate of 354 beats/min. Note that immediately after termination of pacing, the spontaneous atrial flutter (rate of 278 beats/min) recurs. The **asterisks** denote the last beat entrained at each recording site, and the arrows point from the last stimulus artifact to the resulting atrial electrogram at each recording site. Note that the last entrained beat at the sulcus terminalis site is associated with a fused, positive atrial complex, but the last entrained beat at the posterior-inferior left atrial recording site is associated with an unfused atrial flutter complex. See FIGURE 2 for a diagrammatic explanation of these events. Time lines are at 1-sec intervals. **S** = stimulus artifact. (Modified from Plumb *et al.*[12])

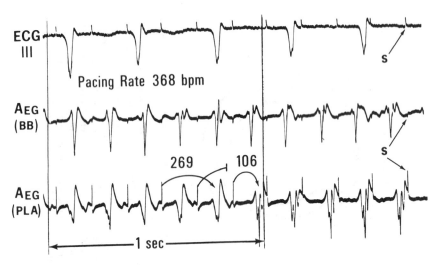

**FIGURE 6.** ECG lead III recorded simultaneously with bipolar atrial electrograms ($A_{EG}$) recorded from Bachmann's bundle (**BB**) and the posterior-inferior left atrium (**PLA**) during rapid pacing of atrial flutter (spontaneous rate, 273 beats/min) from a mid-sulcus terminalis pacing site. In the PLA electrogram recording, the **arrows** connect each stimulus with the resulting atrial electrogram and the **numbers** indicate the conduction time from the stimulus artifact to each recording site. During pacing at a rate of 368 beats/min, localized conduction block to the posterior-inferior left atrial recording site of one pacing impulse develops, followed by activation of that site from a different direction (note the change in the atrial electrogram morphology), and with a shorter conduction time (note the decrease in conduction time from 269 msec to 206 msec). These observations are diagrammatically explained in FIGURE 7. Subsequently, after termination of pacing, sinus rhythm was present. **S** = stimulus artifact. Time lines are at 1-sec intervals. (Modified from Plumb et al.[12])

fusion beats at each pacing rate, which fails to interrupt the arrhythmia, but different degrees of fusion at each of the pacing rates (progressive fusion) (FIGS. 4 and 5). Similarly, interrupting a tachyarrhythmia with pacing at a rate faster than the spontaneous rate does not permit one to establish the presence of reentry. Rather, associated with interruption of a tachyarrhythmia, localized conduction block of one beat to a site must be shown, followed by activation of that site by the subsequent pacing impulse from a different direction and with a shorter conduction time than that before the localized block (FIGS. 6 and 7).[8-14]

During rapid pacing of a tachyarrhythmia whose underlying mechanism is reentry with an excitable gap, transient entrainment may occur without demonstrating any of the aforementioned criteria.[8] Should this occur, it is most likely due to inadequacies in recording technique. These inadequacies may be simple, such as not recording from the coronary sinus during rapid pacing from the high right atrium of a paroxysmal atrial tachycardia associated with a left-sided AV bypass pathway; or complex, such as the practical inability to record from appropriate sites close to or within the reentry loop of a ventricular tachycardia during rapid ventricular pacing. Nevertheless, if transient entrainment occurs, but cannot be clearly established, one then cannot distinguish reentry from other possibilities. These possibilities include the presence of (1) overdrive suppression of an automatic focus or of a parasystolic focus, (2) termination followed by reinitiation of a reentrant tachycardia, and (3) failure to interrupt a triggered rhythm.[8,9,12-23] Similarly, if interruption of a tachyarrhythmia occurs during rapid pacing, but localized conduction block is not demonstrated, a reentry rhythm may not be distinguished from a triggered rhythm.[8,9,12,20,21]

In sum, our studies which demonstrated transient entrainment and subsequent interruption of atrial flutter indicate that classical atrial flutter is a reentrant rhythm with an excitable gap. This knowledge plus the use of the rapid pacing techniques to achieve transient entrainment and interruption of atrial flutter (and of other apparent reentrant arrhythmias) provide both a new opportunity and a new tool to investigate further and in more detail the various components of the

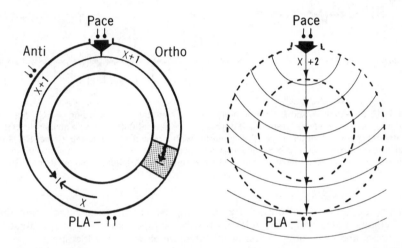

**FIGURE 7.** Diagrammatic explanation of the events illustrated in FIGURE 6. (*Left*): The **large arrow** indicates the pacing impulse from an atrial site entering into the excitable gap of the reentry loop, whereupon it is conducted orthodromically (**Ortho**) and antidromically (**Anti**). The antidromic wavefront ($\times + 1$) collides with the orthodromic wavefront from the previous beat ($\times$), resulting in atrial fusion. The orthodromic wavefront ($\times + 1$) also blocks during the same beat, presumably in the area of slow conduction, so that the tachycardia is no longer reset. In fact, because the orthodromic and antidromic wavefronts of the same pacing impulse have blocked during the same beat, the tachycardia has been interrupted. Note that block of both the antidromic and orthodromic wavefronts of the same pacing impulse is associated with absence of conduction of one pacing impulse to the posterior-inferior left atrial recording site (**PLA**). (*Right*): The **large arrow** indicates the next pacing impulse ($\times + 2$) from the same atrial pacing site as in the *left* diagram. The **dashed circle** indicates the reentry loop present during both the previous periods of spontaneous atrial flutter and of transient entrainment of the atrial flutter during rapid pacing. Because the atrial flutter has been interrupted by the previous pacing impulse ($\times + 1$), the sequence of atrial activation of the next pacing impulse ($\times + 2$) is, as one would expect, during overdrive pacing of a sinus rhythm. Therefore, the PLA recording site is activated from a different direction and with a shorter conduction time than during previous periods of transient entrainment of atrial flutter during pacing from the same site. The isochromes are drawn to indicate the general direction of spread of the impulse, and are not meant to imply that the sequence of activation from the pacing site to the PLA recording site is radial. (Modified from Plumb *et al.*[12])

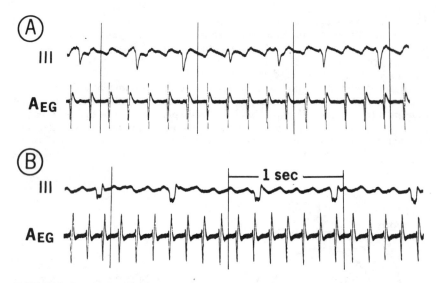

**FIGURE 8.** Panels **A** and **B** both demonstrate the simultaneous recording of ECG lead **III** and a bipolar atrial electrogram ($A_{EG}$) during a Type I atrial flutter with an atrial rate of 296 beats/min (panel A), and a Type II atrial flutter with a rate of 420 beats/min (panel B). Note that in each instance there is an irregular ventricular rate in response to the atrial flutter. Time lines are at 1-sec intervals. See text for discussion. (Modified from Wells *et al.*[24])

reentry circuit in atrial flutter. By so doing, we should learn more about this arrhythmia and, particularly relevant for this symposium, more about effective treatment and even suppression of this arrhythmia with drug therapy.

## TYPES OF ATRIAL FLUTTER

We recently have provided evidence that there are two types of atrial flutter: Type I (classical) and Type II (very rapid) (FIG. 8).[24] This classification is independent of the morphology or polarity of the atrial flutter waves in the ECG. Type I atrial flutter can always be influenced by rapid atrial pacing from sites high in the right atrium, whereas Type II atrial flutter cannot.[24] This major difference served as the initial distinction between these two types of atrial flutter. The reason for the inability to interrupt Type II atrial flutter with rapid atrial pacing from high right atrial sites is unknown. However, it may be that the atrial refractoriness and prolonged atrial conduction time preclude the interruption of Type II atrial flutter when pacing from this site because the site is too far from the atrial flutter focus, or the mechanism of this type of atrial flutter may not be reentry with an excitable gap.[25] Nevertheless, if the only difference between Type I and Type II atrial flutter was the response to rapid atrial pacing from high right atrial sites, there might be insufficient reason to separate atrial flutter into a slower and faster type.

Two observations have provided additional reasons to suggest that a separation of atrial flutter into two types is valid. First, Type II atrial flutter was observed to convert spontaneously to Type I atrial flutter in a stepwise fashion in several patients.[24] Second, on several occasions, when rapid atrial pacing from a high right atrial site was utilized to treat Type I atrial flutter, Type II atrial flutter was present after termination of the rapid pacing.[24] Thus, it would appear that Type I and Type II atrial flutter are not really part of a continuum of atrial flutter, but rather are separate entities, although perhaps quite closely related.

The foregoing observations permitted further differentiation between two types of atrial flutter in terms of range of rates. Type I atrial flutter is characterized by a range of rates from 240–340 beats/min and Type II atrial flutter is characterized by a range of rates from 340–433 beats/min.[24] There probably is some overlap in the upper range of rates for Type I atrial flutter and the lower range of rates for Type II atrial flutter, as well as some flexibility in the upper and lower range of rates of each of these types of atrial flutter in any event. Additional

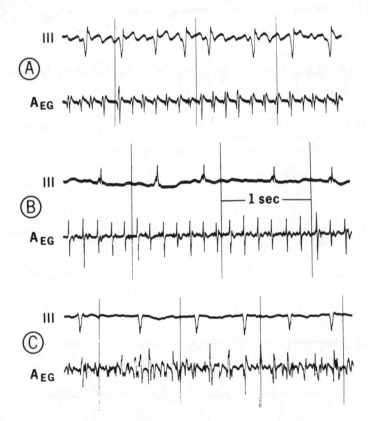

**FIGURE 9.** In each of the three panels in this figure, ECG lead **III** has been recorded simultaneously with a bipolar atrial electrogram ($A_{EG}$). Panel **A** demonstrates the characteristic atrial electrogram for Type I atrial fibrillation, panel **B** for Type II atrial fibrillation, and panel **C** for Type III atrial fibrillation. Time lines are 1-sec intervals. (Modified from Wells *et al.*[26])

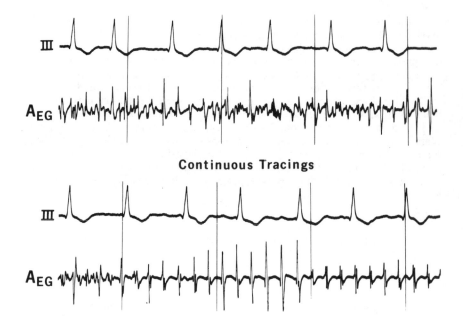

**Continuous Tracings**

**FIGURE 10.** ECG lead **III** recorded simultaneously with a bipolar atrial electrogram ($A_{EG}$) demonstrating the atrial electrogram characteristic of Type IV atrial fibrillation. Time lines are at 1-sec intervals. (From Wells *et al.*[26] Reproduced by permission.)

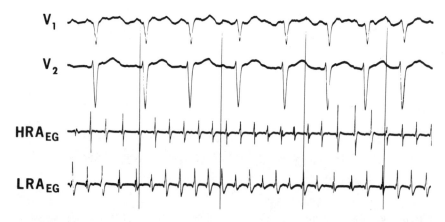

**FIGURE 11.** ECG leads $V_1$ and $V_2$ recorded simultaneously with bipolar atrial electrograms from the high right atrium ($HRA_{EG}$) and from the low right atrium ($LRA_{EG}$) during Type I atrial fibrillation. $V_1$ shows a course atrial fibrillation pattern. See text for discussion. (From Wells *et al.*[26] Reproduced by permission.)

insights into these rhythms, their interrelationships, and their mechanisms should be most useful as a guide to effective drug therapy.

## TYPES OF ATRIAL FIBRILLATION

Recent studies of atrial fibrillation showed that there was a characteristic variation in the beat-to-beat polarity, morphology, amplitude, and cycle length of the recorded bipolar atrial electrogram. On the basis of these characteristics, four descriptive types of atrial fibrillation were identified.[26] Type I atrial fibrillation was characterized by discrete atrial electrograms separated by discrete isoelectric

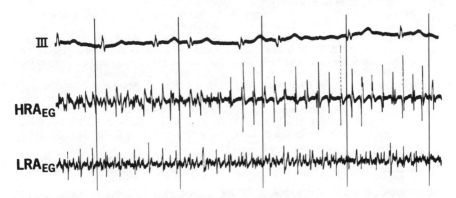

**FIGURE 12.** ECG lead **III** recorded simultaneously with bipolar atrial electrogram from the high right atrium (**HRA$_{EG}$**) and the low right atrium (**LRA$_{EG}$**) during Type IV atrial fibrillation. Initially, both electrogram recordings show a Type III pattern. Note that when the HRA$_{EG}$ pattern changes, the LRA$_{EG}$ pattern does not. This is one of the characteristics of atrial fibrillation and does not represent dissimilar atrial rhythms. See text for discussion. (From Wells *et al.*[26] Reproduced by permission.)

intervals (FIG. 9). Type II atrial fibrillation was characterized by discrete atrial electrograms that were not separated by isoelectric intervals (FIG. 9). Type III atrial fibrillation was characterized by the absence of discrete atrial electrograms (they were chaotic in appearance) and the absence of isoelectric intervals of any sort (FIG. 9). Type IV atrial fibrillation was an amalgam of Types I, II, and III, that is, the recorded atrial electrogram varied between Type III and Types I and II (FIG. 10). Presently, the importance of recognizing these different types is largely limited to preventing confusion with other rhythms such as atrial flutter (FIG. 11) or dissimilar atrial rhythms (FIG. 12). However, it is not unreasonable to suggest that as we learn more about these different types of atrial fibrillation, we may find important implications for therapy. Whether or not there will be clinical significance in differentiating these four types, however, remains to be proven.

## REFERENCES

1. BIGGER, J. T., JR. 1980. Management of arrhythmias. *In* Heart Disease—A Textbook of Cardiovascular Medicine. E. Braunwald, Ed.: 691. W. B. Saunders. Philadelphia, PA.
2. SELTZER, A., J. J. KELLY, R. B. JOHNSON & L. J. KEITH. 1966. Immediate and long term results of electrical conversion of arrhythmias. Prog. Cardiovasc. Dis. **9:** 90.
3. TALANO, J. V. & C. TOMMASO. 1982. Slow channel calcium antagonists in the treatment of supraventricular tachycardia. Prog. Cardiovasc. Dis. **5:** 141.
4. GRABOYS, T. B., P. J. PODRID & B. LOWN. 1983. Efficacy of amiodarone for refractory supraventricular tachyarrhythmias. Am. Heart J. **106:** 870.
5. SELLERS, T. D., JR., T. M. BASHORE & J. J. GALLAGHER. 1977. Digitalis in the preexcitation syndrome. Analysis during atrial fibrillation. Circulation **56:** 260.
6. WALDO, A. L., W. A. H. MACLEAN, R. B. KARP, N. T. KOUCHOUKOS & T. N. JAMES. 1978. Entrainment and interruption of atrial flutter with atrial pacing: Studies in man following open heart surgery. Circulation **56:** 737.
7. MACLEAN, W. A. H., V. J. PLUMB & A. L. WALDO. 1981. Transient entrainment and interruption of ventricular tachycardia. PACE **4:** 358.
8. WALDO, A. L., V. J. PLUMB, J. G. ARCINIEGAS, W. A. H. MACLEAN, T. B. COOPER, M. F. PRIEST & T. N. JAMES. 1983. Transient entrainment and interruption of the atrioventricular bypass pathway type of paroxysmal atrial tachycardia. A model for understanding and identifying reentrant arrhythmias. Circulation **67:** 73.
9. WALDO, A. L., R. W. HENTHORN, V. J. PLUMB & W. A. H. MACLEAN. 1984. Demonstration of the mechanism of transient entrainment and interruption of ventricular tachycardia with rapid atrial pacing. J. Am. Coll. Cardiol. **3:** 422–430.
10. PLUMB, V. J., W. A. H. MACLEAN, T. B. COOPER, T. N. JAMES & A. L. WALDO. 1979. Atrial events during entrainment and interruption of atrial flutter by rapid atrial pacing (abstract). Circulation **60** (Suppl. II): II-64.
11. PLUMB, V. J., T. N. JAMES & A. L. WALDO. 1980. Evidence that atrial flutter is due to circus movement with an excitable gap (abstract). Circulation **62:** (Suppl. III): III-46.
12. WALDO, A. L., V. J. PLUMB & R. W. HENTHORN. 1984. Observations on the mechanism of atrial flutter. *In* Tachycardias. B. Surawicz, Ed.: 213. Martinus Nijhoff. The Hague.
13. HENTHORN, R. W., V. J. PLUMB, J. G. ARCINIEGAS & A. L. WALDO. 1982. Entrainment of "ectopic atrial tachycardia:" Evidence for reentry (abstract). Am. J. Cardiol. **39:** 920.
14. BRUGADA, P., A. L. WALDO & H. J. J. WELLENS. 1984. Transient entrainment and interruption of AV nodal reentrant tachycardia (abstract). J. Am. Coll. Cardiol. **3:** 537.
15. VASSALLE, M. 1977. The relationship among cardiac pacemakers. Overdrive suppression. Circ. Res. **41:** 269.
16. WELLENS, H. J. J. 1978. Value and limitations of programmed electrical stimulation of the heart in the study and treatment of tachycardias. Circulation **57:** 845.
17. CRANEFIELD, P. F. 1975. The Conduction of the Cardiac Impulse.: 207, 263, 272. Futura. Mt. Kisco, NY.
18. WIT, A. L. & P. F. CRANEFIELD. 1977. Triggered and automatic activity in the canine coronary sinus. Circ. Res. **41:** 435.
19. CRANEFIELD, P. F. 1977. Action potentials, after potentials and arrhythmia. Circ. Res. **41:** 415.
20. WIT, A. L., P. F. CRANEFIELD & D. C. GADSBY. 1981. Electrogenic sodium extrusion can stop triggered activity in the canine coronary sinus. Circ. Res. **49:** 1029.
21. ROSEN, M. R. & R. F. REDER. 1981. Does triggered activity have a role in the genesis of cardiac arrhythmias? Ann. Intern. Med. **94:** 794.
22. JALIFE, J. & G. K. MOE. 1979. A biologic model of parasystole. Am. J. Cardiol. **43:** 761.
23. FURESE, A., G. SHINDO, H. MAKUNCH, M. SAIGUSA, H. MATRSUO, K. TAKAANAGI &

H. INOUE. 1979. Apparent suppression of ventricular parasystole by cardiac pacing. Jpn. Heart J. **29:** 843.

24. WELLS, J. L., JR., W. A. H. MacLEAN, T. N. JAMES & A. L. WALDO. 1979. Characterization of atrial flutter. Studies in man after open heart surgery using fixed atrial electrodes. Circulation **6:** 665.

25. ALLESSIE, M. A., F. I. M. BONKE & F. J. G. SCHOPMAN. 1977. Circus movement in rabbit atrial muscle as a mechanism of tachycardia. III. The "leading circle" concept: A new model of circus movement in cardiac tissue without involvement of an anatomical obstacle. Circ. Res. **41:** 9.

26. WELLS, J. L., JR., R. B. KARP, N. T. KOUCHOUKOS, W. A. H. MacLEAN, T. N. JAMES & A. L. WALDO. 1978. Characterization of atrial fibrillation in man. Studies following open heart surgery. PACE **1:** 426.

# Drug Therapy of Patients with Arrhythmias Associated with Bypass Tracts

HEIN J. J. WELLENS,[a] PEDRO BRUGADA, AND
HOSHIAR ABDOLLAH

*Department of Cardiology*
*University of Limburg*
*Annadal Hospital*
*Maastricht, The Netherlands*

In the Wolff-Parkinson-White syndrome there is a second pathway, in addition to the AV nodal His-Purkinje pathway, that is able to conduct impulses from the atrium to the ventricle. This second atrioventricular connection is usually able not only to conduct from the atrium to the ventricle, but also from ventricle to atrium.

The presence of such an accessory atrioventricular pathway may lead to two arrhythmic complications: Firstly, a circus movement tachycardia may develop, during which an impulse circulates in a pathway from atrium → AV node → ventricle → accessory atrioventricular pathway → atrium. Usually, during such a circus movement tachycardia, atrioventricular conduction occurs over the AV node–His pathway, and ventriculoatrial conduction occurs by way of the accessory connection (the orthodromic circus movement tachycardia). A circus movement tachycardia in the reverse direction (antidromic circus movement tachycardia) is much rarer. Second, in patients with anterograde conduction over an accessory pathway, life-threatening high ventricular rates may occur in case of atrial fibrillation if the atrioventricular pathway has a short anterograde refractory period.

In recent years it has become clear that in a significant number of patients suffering from supraventricular tachycardia, an accessory atrioventricular pathway is able to conduct from ventricle to atrium only (the so-called "concealed" accessory pathway). In these patients, during supraventricular tachycardia, an orthodromic circus movement tachycardia is present.

The introduction of programmed stimulation of the heart allows the study of the effect of different drugs on the components of the circuit involved in circus movement tachycardia and on the anterograde refractory period of the accessory pathway in patients suffering from atrial fibrillation.

## PROGRAMMED STIMULATION IN PATIENTS WITH ACCESSORY ATRIOVENTRICULAR PATHWAYS

TABLE 1 lists the reasons for performing programmed stimulation of the heart in patients with accessory atrioventricular pathways.

To adequately study the effect of drugs, the site of the accessory pathway

---

[a] To whom correspondence should be addressed.

should be determined to allow positioning of the catheter as closely as possible to this structure. This minimizes the role of drug-induced changes in electrophysiological properties of the tissue in between the site of stimulation and the accessory atrioventricular pathway. To obtain information of the effect of drug on the different components of the reentry circuit in patients with circus movement tachycardia, several catheters are positioned as closely as possible to the circuit. Usually a minimum of four catheters is required: one in the right atrium, one in the coronary sinus, one at the site of the bundle of His, and one in the right ventricle.

Basic measurements before drug administration include determination of the refractory period of the right atrium, the coronary sinus, the atrioventricular node, the accessory atrioventricular pathway in anterograde and retrograde direction, the right ventricle, the A-H and H-V interval and the modes of initiation and termination and rate of tachycardia. These measurements are made using single-test stimulation at different cycle lengths of pacing. Also the ventricular rate after induction of atrial fibrillation is determined. After drug administration, these measurements are repeated using the same stimulation sites and pacing intervals. When the effect of intravenous drug administration is studied, repeated measurements are required to obtain information about the time course and maximal effect of the drug. Drug administration should preferably be done through one of the intracardiac catheters to minimize the chance of extravasation and phlebitis. While drug levels are frequently routinely determined after intravenous drug ad-

TABLE 1. Value of Programmed Stimulation of the Heart in Patients with the Wolff-Parkinson-White Syndrome

| |
|---|
| 1. To study mechanisms and pathways of tachycardias. |
| 2. To localize accessory pathways and study their electrophysiologic properties. |
| 3. To study the effect of drugs on accessory pathways. |
| 4. To select patients for surgery or for pacemaker implantation. |
| 5. To evaluate the success of surgery. |

ministration, their value, in our opinion, is questionable in the absence of information on correlation between rapidly changing blood levels and cardiac drug concentration.

During chronic oral drug administration, which results in less important changes in blood levels and therefore cardiac concentration, a better correlation between these two values can be expected. To study the effect of a drug on the ventricular rate during atrial fibrillation, this arrhythmia should again be provoked after the drug has been given. Also, since the electrophysiologic properties of the different parts of the heart are affected by sympathetic tone, it is important to know whether the patient was sedated before the study.

## ELECTROPHYSIOLOGIC EFFECTS OF DIFFERENT DRUGS

TABLES 2 and 3 list the electrophysiologic effects of different conventional and investigational drugs. These results are based upon data reported by numerous investigators.[1-20] Unfortunately, few systematic analyses have been made of the effect of the different drugs on retrograde conduction over the accessory pathway, and so the data on the accessory pathway given in TABLES 2 and 3 applies to anterograde conduction only.

**TABLE 2.** Effect of Conventional Drugs on the Duration of the Refractory Period of Different Parts of the Heart

| Drug | Atrium | AV Node | His-Purkinje | Ventricle | Accessory AV Pathway |
|------|--------|---------|--------------|-----------|----------------------|
| Digitalis | ± | + | ? | ± | − |
| Procainamide | + | 0 | + | + | + |
| Quinidine | + | ± | + | + | + |
| Ajmaline | + | 0 | + | + | + |
| Disopyramide | + | ± | + | + | + |
| Diphenylhydantoin | ± | − | − | ± | ± |
| Propranolol | ± | + | ? | ± | 0 |
| Lidocaine | ± | 0 | + | + | + |
| Verapamil | ± | + | ? | ± | ± |
| Atropine | 0 | − | ? | 0 | 0 |
| Isoproterenol | ± | − | ? | ± | − |

NOTE: + = lengthens; − = shortens; 0 = no change; ± = variable; ? = unknown.

It is well known[21] that the electrophysiologic properties of accessory pathways may differ with respect to anterograde and retrograde direction. It is of interest that some investigational drugs, such as encainide,[12] flecainide,[13] and propafenon,[20] seem to lengthen the retrograde refractory period of the accessory pathway more than the anterograde one.

Our group has previously commented upon the relation between the initial value of the duration of the anterograde effective refractory period of the accessory pathway and the effect of different drugs such as quinidine, procainamide, ajmaline, and amiodarone.[21] It is not clear at the present time whether this relationship holds for all drugs. In our experience, drugs that lengthen the H-V

**TABLE 3.** Effect of Investigational Drugs on the Duration of the Refractory Period of Different Parts of the Heart

| Drug | Atrium | AV Node | His-Purkinje | Ventricle | Accessory AV Pathway |
|------|--------|---------|--------------|-----------|----------------------|
| Amiodarone (oral) | + | + | + | + | + |
| Amiodarone (intravenous) | 0 | + | 0 | 0 | + |
| Encainide | 0 | 0 | + | + | + |
| Flecainide | + | ± | + | + | + |
| Sotalol | + | + | ± | + | + |
| Lorcainide | 0 | 0 | + | + | + |
| Mexiletine | 0 | 0 | + | + | ± |
| Tocainide | 0 | 0 | + | + | ± |
| Bepridil | 0 | + | 0 | 0 | ± |
| Aprindine | 0 | ± | + | + | + |
| Moxaprindine | 0 | ± | + | + | + |
| Propafenone | + | 0 | + | 0 | + |
| Ethmozin | ? | ? | + | + | + |
| Diltiazem | 0 | + | 0 | 0 | + |

NOTE: + = lengthens; − = shortens; 0 = no change; ± = variable; ? = unknown.

conduction time also lengthen the anterograde refractory period of the accessory atrioventricular pathway. Therefore, if an investigational drug is found to lengthen the H-V interval, a lengthening effect can also be expected on the anterograde refractory period of the accessory atrioventricular pathway.

When interpreting the data presented in TABLES 2 and 3, one should realize that frequently the relation between dose and electrophysiologic effects, cumulative effects, especially after oral drug administration, and the role of degradation products are not known. Also, there may be individual differences in the effect of different drugs. Again, we want to stress that drugs may not have the same effect on anterograde and retrograde conduction over the AV node and the accessory atrioventricular pathway. And, last, sympathetic stimulation may counteract drug-induced lengthening of the refractory period of the accessory pathway.[8]

## THE PRACTICAL APPROACH

### Circus Movement Tachycardia

As pointed out elsewhere,[22] several mechanisms may lead to the initiation of a circus movement tachycardia. The most common mechanism is by a premature beat which creates unidirectional block in either the atrioventricular pathway or the AV node in the anatomically determined circuit consisting of atrium → AV node → ventricle → accessory pathway → atrium. For persistence of circus movement tachycardia a delicate interplay is required between conduction velocity of the circulating impulse and the duration of the refractory period within the circuit. The purpose of drug therapy is therefore to prevent the initiating event or to disrupt the balance between conduction velocity and refractoriness within the circuit. Drug therapy is always a trade-off between efficacy, dosing requirements, and side effects. If circus movement tachycardia occurs rarely and is well tolerated, we advise the patient to try vagal maneuvers and, if these are unsuccessful, to take one tablet of 200 mg of quinidine sulfate or 80 mg of verapamil at 20-minute intervals for a maximum of three times. For intravenous termination of circus movement tachycardia, 10 mg of verapamil given over a 3-minute period is the therapy of choice. If circus movement tachycardia occurs frequently or is poorly tolerated, continuous drug therapy is required. Amiodarone has the distinct advantage of requiring only one dose per day or even on alternate days. Usually only 1000 mg per week is needed, making the incidence of side effects small.[22] If amiodarone is not available, sotalol or long-acting quinidine alone or in combination with a beta blocking agent are acceptable alternatives. Our present approach in the patient with circus movement tachycardia is summarized in TABLE 4.

### Atrial Fibrillation

The danger of this arrhythmia is related to the duration of the anterograde refractory period of the accessory atrioventricular pathway.[23] Therefore the primary objective of drug therapy is to increase this value. Unfortunately, we have observed that the effect of drugs is disappointing in the presence of a short refractory period of the accessory pathway.[21] In reporting on the effect of drugs in patients with the Wolff-Parkinson-White Syndrome it is important therefore to

**TABLE 4.** Treatment of Circus Movement Tachycardia in Patients with the Wolff-Parkinson-White Syndrome

| |
|---|
| *Treatment during the Attack of Circus Movement Tachycardia* |
| Vagal maneuvers |
| Verapamil, 10 mg, intravenously |
| Propranolol, 5–10 mg, intravenously |
| Ajmaline, 50 mg, intravenously |
| Procainamide, up to 10 mg/kg body weight, intravenously |
| Pacing |
| Direct-current shock |
| |
| *Prophylaxis of Circus Movement Tachycardia* |
| Amiodarone |
| Sotalol |
| Long-acting quinidine |
| Long-acting quinidine + propranolol |

stress the necessity of distinguishing patients with a short (<270 msec) from those with a longer refractory period of the accessory pathway.

Some reports suggest that such a relation between the effect of the drug and the initial value of the duration of the refractory period of the accessory pathway does not exist with some of the investigational agents. Unfortunately, for most of these drugs the follow-up period is insufficiently long to establish their practical value for long-term oral treatment. In Europe, orally taken amiodarone is the drug of choice for treatment of patients with the Wolff-Parkinson-White Syndrome and atrial fibrillation. The dosage varies between 1000 to 2000 mg per week. Amiodarone not only lengthens the refractory period of the accessory pathway, but also markedly reduces the incidence of paroxysms of atrial fibrillation. When amiodarone is not available, long-acting quinidine should be given. In case of a recurrence of atrial fibrillation with a high ventricular rate, the patient should be considered a candidate for surgical interruption of the accessory pathway.[24] TABLE 5 gives our present views on the treatment of atrial fibrillation in the patient with the Wolff-Parkinson-White syndrome.

**TABLE 5.** Treatment of Atrial Fibrillation in Patients with the Wolff-Parkinson-White Syndrome

| |
|---|
| *Treatment during the Attack* |
| Hemodynamically not tolerated: |
| Direct-current shock |
| Hemodynamically tolerated: |
| Procainamide |
| Ajmaline |
| Disopyramide |
| |
| *Prophylaxis of Atrial Fibrillation* |
| Amiodarone |
| Long-acting quinidine |
| Long-acting quinidine + propranolol |
| Sotalol |

## REFERENCES

1. WELLENS, H. J. J. & D. DURRER. 1973. Effect of digitalis on atrioventricular conduction and circus movement tachycardias in patients. Circulation **47:** 1229–1237.
2. WELLENS, H. J. J. & D. DURRER. 1979. Effect of procainamide, quinidine, and ajmaline in the Wolff-Parkinson-White syndrome. Circulation **50:** 114–120.
3. SPURRELL, R. A. J., C. W. THORBURN, E. SOWTON & D. C. DEUCHAR. 1978. Effects of disopyramide on electrophysiological properties of specialized conduction system in man and on accessory atrioventricular pathway in Wolff-Parkinson-White syndrome. Br. Heart J. **37:** 861–867.
4. BENNETT, D. H. 1978. Disopyramide in patients with the Wolff-Parkinson-White syndrome and atrial fibrillation. Chest **74:** 624–628.
5. ROSS, D., J. VOHRA, P. COLO, D. HUNT & G. SLOMAN. 1980. Electrophysiology of disopyramide in man. Aust. N. Zeal. J. Med. **8:** 922–923.
6. ROSEN, K. N., C. BÄRWOLF, A. ELSANI & S. H. RAHIMTOOLA. 1982. Effects of lidocaine and propranolol on the normal and anomalous pathways with pre-excitation. Am. J. Cardiol. **50:** 180–184.
7. SPURRELL, R. A. J., D. M. KRIKLER & E. SOWTON. 1974. Effect of verapamil on electrophysiological properties of the anomalous atrioventricular connection in Wolff-Parkinson-White syndrome. Br. Heart J. **36:** 256–264.
8. Wellens, H. J. J., P. Brugada, D. Roy, J. Weiss & F. W. Bär. 1982. Effect of 150 proterenol on the anterograde refractory period of the accessory pathway in patients with the Wolff-Parkinson-White syndrome. Am. J. Cardiol. **50:** 180–184.
9. ROSENBAUM, M. B., P. A. CHIALE, D. RYBA & M. V. ELIZARI. 1974. Control of tachyarrhythmias associated with Wolff-Parkinson-White syndrome by amiodarone hydrochloride. Am. J. Cardiol. **34:** 215–223.
10. WELLENS, H. J. J., K. I. LIE, F. W. BÄR, J. C. WESDORP, H. J. DOHMEN, D. R. DUREN & D. DURRER. 1976. Effect of amiodarone in the Wolff-Parkinson-White syndrome. Am. J. Cardiol. **38:** 189–194.
11. WELLENS, H. J. J., P. BRUGADA & H. ABDOLLAH. Effect of amiodarone in patients with supraventricular tachycardia. Am. Heart J. In press.
12. JACKMAN, W. M., D. P. ZIPES, G. V. NACCARELLI, R. L. RINKENBERGER, J. J. HEGER & E. N. PRYSTOWSKY. 1982. Electrophysiology of oral encainide. Am. J. Cardiol. **49:** 1270–1278.
13. HELLESTRAND, K. J., R. S. BEXTON, A. W. NATHAN, R. A. J. SPURRELL & A. J. CAMM. 1982. Acute electrophysiological effects of flecainide acetate on cardiac conduction and refractoriness in man. Br. Heart J. **48:** 140–148.
14. KASPER, W., T. MEINERTZ, F. KERSTING, H. LOLLGEN, K. LANG & H. JUST. 1979. Electrophysiologic actions of lorcainide in coronary artery disease. J. Cardiovasc. Pharmacol. **1:** 343–352.
15. BÄR, F. W., J. FARRÉ, D. ROSS & H. J. J. WELLENS. 1981. Electrophysiological effects of lorcainide, a new antiarrhythmic drug. Br. Heart J. **65:** 292–298.
16. WALEFFE, A., P. BRUINIX, L. MARY-RABINE & H. E. KULBERTUS. 1979. Effects of tocainide studied with programmed stimulation of the heart in patients with reentrant tachyarrhythmias. Am. J. Cardiol. **43:** 292–299.
17. Zipes, D. P., W. E. Gaum, P. R. Foster, K. M. Rosen, D. Wu, F. Amat-y-leon & R. J. Noble. 1977. Aprindine for treatment of supraventricular tachycardias. Am. J. Cardiol. **40:** 586–596.
18. REID, P. R., L. GREENE & P. J. VARGHESE. 1977. Suppression of refractory arrhythmias by aprindine in patients with the Wolff-Parkinson-White syndrome. Br. Heart J. **39:** 1353–1360.
19. WALEFFE, A., L. MARY-RABINE & H. E. KULBERTUS. 1972. Study of moxaprindine with programmed electrical stimulation of the heart in patients with re-entrant tachyarrhythmias. Am. J. Cardiol. **45:** 297–303.
20. WALEFFE, A. & H. E. KULBERTUS. 1983. Electrophysiologic effects and antiarrhythmic efficacy of Rytmonorm, evaluated with programmed electrical stimulation of

the heart in patients with reentrant supraventricular tachycardia. *In* Cardiac Arrhythmics. M. Schlepper & B. Olsson, Eds.: 191–198. Springer Verlag. Berlin.

21. WELLENS, H. J. J., F. W. BÄR, W. R. DASSEN, P. BRUGADA, E. VANAGT & J. FARRÉ. 1980. Effect of drugs in the Wolff-Parkinson-White syndrome. Importance of initial length of effective refractory period of the accessory pathway. Am. J. Cardiol. **46:** 665–671.

22. WELLENS, H. J. J. 1977. Modes of initiation of circus movement tachycardia in 139 patients with the Wolff-Parkinson-White syndrome studied by programmed electrical stimulation. *In* Re-entrant Arrhythmias. H. Kulbertus, Ed.: 153. M.T.P. Lancaster.

23. WELLENS, H. J. J., P. BRUGADA, H. ABDOLLAH & W. R. DASSEN. A comparison of the electrophysiologic effects of intravenous and oral amiodarone in the same patient. Circulation. In press.

24. SEALY, W. C., E. L. C. PRITCHETT, J. J. GALLAGHER & J. KASELL. 1979. The surgical problems with the identification and interruption of the bundle of Kent. *In* Cardiac Arrhythmias. O. Narula, Ed.: 636. Williams and Wilkins. Baltimore, MD.

# Drug Development: Risks
# and Problems

DANIEL L. AZARNOFF AND ROBERT L. HERTING

*Searle Research and Development*
*G. D. Searle and Company*
*Skokie, Illinois 60077*

Drug discoveries originate from many sources, both inside and outside the pharmaceutical industry. Drug development, on the other hand, takes place almost exclusively as a result of the investment and skills of the pharmaceutical industry.

Although this symposium is concerned with antiarrhythmic drugs in particular, development of this class of drugs undergoes a process which is similar to that of most of the other drugs conceived and synthesized by the medicinal chemist. Therefore, we will examine several general factors that influence drug development in today's regulatory, economic, and social climate.

Many United States pharmaceutical companies now make a significant portion of their sales outside of this country.[1-2] Thus, drug development is most economical if the process utilized satisfies the requirements of the developed countries of the world, even for drugs whose greatest use may be in less-developed countries.

## THE ROLE OF PATENTS

It is currently estimated that the development of a new drug in the United States costs about $70,000,000 and takes an average of 8 years from discovery to FDA approval.[4] Although the rate is increasing, only about 1 of every 10 new chemical entities studied in human beings for the first time will ever become a product. The others will fail for a variety of reasons, primarily related to toxicity, lack of efficacy, or inability to provide advantages over competitive products.[5,6] A patent, which protects the product from competition for 17 years in the United States and for variable but similar durations in other countries, is usually the basis on which a company is willing to invest in the quite risky development of a new drug.[4,7]

Many discussions about patents have taken place over the past 2–3 years in the United States Congress. The Senate passed a patent extension bill in the 97th Congress, only to have it die in the House in the final hectic minutes of a special session.[8] Now again congressional committees are considering legislation to extend the patent life of an invention for which the development phase is prolonged due primarily to government regulatory agency review time. For the most part this problem applies to new drugs, although other regulated articles, such as pesticides, may also be affected.[9] Concern over the erosion of patent life by lengthy government procedures has also surfaced in the United Kingdom.

The fundamental socioeconomic issue under debate is whether or not patent protection is a stimulus to encourage research and development, a process of recognized value to society. If so, the corollary question to be asked is whether or not the shortening of patent life caused by FDA requirements and lengthy review processes negatively affects the incentive of the pharmaceutical industry to invest in R&D. We believe that it does. One need only look at the lack of new drug development in Canada, where compulsory outlicensing is required as a means of bypassing a valid patent, to find evidence that patents are important.[10-12] In fact, a study recently issued by the National Academy of Engineering recommends that the patent protection of drugs be extended to include the time spent testing the compound to meet health and safety requirements.[13]

The size of a company's investment for the future is determined by what they can afford on the basis of their current flow of profit. Even a company with annual sales greater than 1 billion dollars has limited R&D resources and probably can successfully search for new drugs in only four to six major therapeutic areas. A publicly owned corporation has to provide from its income a return to its stockholders as well as the resources needed to maintain the flow of sales dollars and the production and distribution of products. The cost of marketing drugs has increased significantly in the past few years.[14,15] Finally, what is left is considered for investment in R&D.

Because of their marketing and manufacturing start-up costs, many drugs may not make a profit until the second or third year on the market. Thus, remaining patent life when the product is marketed becomes especially important for long-term projects since the projected investments in such projects require a longer pay-back period to recoup the costs incurred. Yet it is these same projects that erode remaining patent life the most. Extended patent protection can go a long way toward giving a greater potential return to such projects and make them a significantly more attractive investment risk.

Today we take for granted a large number of effective drugs for treating a wide variety of human illnesses. Undeniably, there are many additional medical problems which still need more effective therapy. However, those disorders for which the major advances in therapy have already been made are also the disorders for which the greatest background of scientific knowledge is available. Consequently, many research programs tend to focus on previously worked areas of disease because the science base for new drug discovery and development is best and the chances of finding an effective drug are increased. As a result, new drugs in an area where therapy is already available need not only be effective, but must also offer at the least a perceived advantage over available agents. Currently, many new chemical entities which show satisfactory activity on screening tests in animals are being discarded because they fail to meet the higher standards of offering significant improvement over existing therapy. Ten years ago these discarded molecules might have been a "breakthrough" in therapy. This problem is only partially offset by the modern techniques of computer-assisted drug design, which has permitted a structural lead to be assessed by the synthesis of far fewer well-planned molecules.[16]

The advantage of a new drug for a disease for which effective therapy exists must now frequently be found in its prevention of progression of the disease and/or mortality. For example, a question of the efficacy of an antiarrhythmic agent is now framed in terms of whether or not only a reduction in cardiac premature beats is a medically significant estimate of efficacy. Drugs with this effect are available, but their long-term effect on death from arrhythmia is not known. Prophylactic agents demand expensive, long-term clinical trials as well as a higher level of safety to prove the benefit of the new agent. The resources and risk to carry out the appropriate studies may be unacceptably large to a company, even if the potential return from a successful product appears quite large.

So far, the considerations discussed have stressed the need for a large high-risk investment of resources. At the same time, the economic forces working against such an investment are strengthening. More and more pressure has developed to substitute generic drugs for those marketed by the innovator, thus transferring the cash flow and profit margins to companies who make little or no contribution to the discovery and development of new drugs.

## EFFECT OF GOVERNMENTAL ACTIONS

The rising cost of medical care is increasingly carried by governments whose own budgets are far out of balance. Their efforts to reduce medical-care costs often focus on drug costs since they are controllable. Many countries have price controls on the sale of drugs, only some of which have profit margins large enough to justify continued research investment.

The decrease in support provided by the government for basic research is another factor which increases the cost of new drug development. As a consequence investigators turn to the private sector for funds to support their research. The result is an increase in the cost to the pharmaceutical company of conducting clinical research since some academic clinicians inflate their grant requests for clinical trials of new drugs to obtain support for their fundamental research interests.

## PAPER NDAs AND ABBREVIATED NDAs

The FDA has a procedure that allows a company to market generic dosage forms of an innovator's product by establishing the safety and efficacy of the drug with evidence from the published literature. The data from these published clinical trials, although "peer-reviewed" in the aggregate, certainly do not get the intense case-by-case review of a new chemical entity in a New Drug Application (NDA) by the Medical Reviewing Officer at the FDA.[17,23] The paper NDA process has several consequences that may not have been considered. To minimize the ability of another company to obtain an NDA, the innovating company will not publish key pieces of information. In addition, the innovator is no longer motivated to obtain new claims. Why spend significant resources on a new claim if when you are finished, the generic manufacturer will be allowed the same claim? It certainly would make no sense to have the same drug on the market with different claims and labelling.

## BENEFIT-TO-RISK RATIO

Everyone agrees that the benefit of a new therapy has to outweigh the associated risk. Although "benefit-to-risk ratio" has a distinctly mathematical ring, rarely do we have the data available to make this judgment in any quantitative sense, especially at the time a new drug is proposed for marketing.

It is difficult to produce numerator and denominator data in the same units. However, an antiarrhythmic drug would appear to overcome this difficulty in the case of a life-threatening cardiac arrhythmia, where both benefit and risk could be measured in terms of mortality. But mortality alone does not account for all the risk: We must also consider other adverse reactions which can alter the quality of life. Suppose that the mortality ratio significantly favors the person receiving the drug but that a large proportion of patients receiving the drug are drowsy much of the time or have an excess number of hospitalizations for congestive heart failure or other disorders thought to be attributable to the new drug. How then does one evaluate the benefit-to-risk ratio where the denominator is in units different from that of the numerator? Only by means of experienced medical judgment can a reasonable evaluation be made.

The ultimate question regarding efficacy of a drug for many disorders is whether or not the drug therapy reduces progression of the disease and/or mortality. But can we afford to wait until evidence of efficacy of the latter type is available? Or should we accept other variables that are based on well-founded, yet less convincing endpoints? Are reductions in number of hospitalizations and their inherent costs or improvements in the quality of life sufficient benefits to expose patients to the risk of the drug, even tentatively pending the outcome of more definitive long-term trials? If it is required that a reduction in these long-term outcomes is the measure of efficacy, can the individual pharmaceutical company afford such studies? They will be very expensive and their duration will undoubtedly reduce the available patent life once the drug is marketed. Assume that the goal of development of an antiarrhythmic agent is to find a well-tolerated drug that will prevent death from ventricular fibrillation in apparently healthy persons as well as in those with coronary artery disease. The financial investment needed to demonstrate the value of such a drug will be extremely large if it is to address the issues of long-term safety and efficacy.

## GOVERNMENTAL CONTROLS

The standards for proof of efficacy required by drug regulatory agencies vary widely, even among the developed countries of the world. At present, the FDA's standards are the highest in the world, in our opinion. For example, the requirement for a placebo treatment varies from agency to agency. FDA guidelines generally require a placebo treatment group in any controlled trial. Although the well-controlled trial has its greatest power when a placebo group is included, in more and more instances investigators are refusing to do placebo-controlled trials when they believe there is an already established therapy. This creates a dilemma for the pharmaceutical company.

The requirements for preclinical safety assessment also vary widely among regulatory agencies throughout the world. The differences, however, are diminishing in favor of the model of the FDA, which is still the most demanding in most instances. In other words, increasingly more effort and resources are required to produce sufficient data to register a new drug in all developed countries. On the other hand, the United States is perhaps one of the most rational countries in the world with respect to the duration of treatment allowed in a clinical trial relative to the duration in available animal safety studies. Also, the FDA does not use regulations as an artificial trade barrier, as do some countries.

The suggestion that expensive animal carcinogenicity studies be required prior to exposing any human being to a new drug, despite the fact that no data suggest that our current standards are inadequate to protect the public health, has raised new concerns.[25,26] Since efficacy of a new drug can only be determined from careful trials in human beings, unreasonable preclinical requirements have a serious and hampering effect on research investments. It certainly would be hard to convince the management of a pharmaceutical company to support long and expensive animal carcinogenicity studies before it is known whether or not a drug candidate is effective in man. Again, consider what effect this would have on the remaining patent life of this product.

Another source of increasing cost, not only in dollars but also in use of human resources, is the trend by regulatory agencies to require more testing in human subjects of old, established drugs to validate a change in manufacturing site or to re-prove that a new dosage form reliably producing plasma levels in an established therapeutic range is still clinically effective.

On balance, although unwarranted requirements are imposed from time to time, most governmental agency requirements at present do not exceed the standards a reputable company would apply to assure themselves of having a safe and effective new drug. The greatest problem with the FDA is the slow rate at which the agency carries out its reviews. There appears to be no sense of urgency and little appreciation of the economic loss to the company of even one day's delay in the approval process. In general, other countries have a more rapid review process. In addition, in many countries, an outside group of experts, rather than civil servants, makes the final scientific and medical judgments for approval of a new chemical entity.

## FINDING CLINICAL INVESTIGATORS

Problems do not exist only with the FDA. The clinical investigator is a key person in the process of developing a new drug. Appropriate design and other aspects of the controlled clinical trial are done by groups that include clinical pharmacologists, biostatisticians, medical subspecialists, and so forth. With a detailed protocol, a good clinician, although inexperienced in clinical trials, can now participate competently in developing a new drug. As a result, larger numbers of trials of higher quality are being conducted today than ever before. The availability of appropriate patients, not investigators, is rate-limiting. In this regard, in many instances investigators still enter into a trial patients who do not meet the admission criteria.

There was a short period when clinical investigators complained about the increasing complexity of protocols, procedures for obtaining informed consent, institutional review boards, and the dictation of trial design by the pharmaceutical company monitor. The last is essential if a sufficient number of subjects is to be evaluated to obtain a definitive answer from the trial. Most clinicians have become used to these procedures and now deal with them in a more or less routine manner. A significant delay in carrying out trials is caused by institutional review boards, for they do not seem to realize the importance and economic consequences of not carrying out their reviews expeditiously.

If several drugs of the same type are under study at the same time, the competition for investigators and scarce patients becomes a significant problem. For example, it appears that there are at least 23 antiarrhythmic agents currently under clinical investigation. Most multinational companies have minimized this problem by having organizations capable of conducting clinical research on a worldwide scale.

## CONCLUSION

Significant problems are associated with new drug development in today's environment. We need to reduce the risk attending long-term investment by finding innovative ways to predict success from short-term trials.

The pharmaceutical industry has an obligation to discover and develop new treatments for man's ailments. This industry has a further obligation to prove or disprove the safety and efficacy of new drugs by using money and persons as efficiently as possible and by conducting trials that truly answer the necessary and relevant questions. Such a venture is, however, a cooperative effort. The public, clinical investigators, and regulatory agencies also have an obligation. They must be aware of the benefits and risks associated with new drug development and not hinder the process by inappropriate legislation, undue delays in carrying out their part in the investigation, the conduction of poor quality trials, or unwarranted regulatory constraints.

## REFERENCES

1. ANON. 1983. U.S. slipping in world market. Standard and Poor's Industry Surveys Sept. 1, Sec 2: H22–23.
2. ANON. 1983. Good prognosis for pharmaceutical industry. Scrip 803: 10.
3. DE HAEN, P. 1983. A new look at pharmaceutical operations. Drug & Cosmetic Industry May: 32.
4. SEITZER, R. J. 1983. Drop in U.S. share of drug R & D endangers world position. Chem. & Eng. News Aug 8: 16.
5. ANON. 1983. Patterns of the U.S. NCE development. Scrip 814: 4–5.
6. WARDELL, W. M. 1982. New drug development by United States pharmaceutical firms. Clin. Pharm. Ther. 32: 410–417.
7. EISMAN, M. M. & W. M. WARDELL. 1981. The decline in effective patent life of new drugs. Res. Management Jan: 18–21.
8. ANON. 1983. Patent restoration may need new sponsor in 1983: House roadblocks seen. F-D-C Reports (The Pink Sheet) 45(1): 4.
9. HUTT, P. B. 1982. The case for drug patent life extension. Med. Marketing & Media May: 10–20.
10. ANON. 1983. Canadian IND seriously affected. Scrip 799 & 800: 22.
11. ANON. 1983. Canada: New moves on patents. Scrip 773: 12.
12. ANON. 1983. Canada: Pressure over patents. Scrip 780: 11.
13. 1983. The Competitive Status of the U.S. Pharmaceutical Industry: A Study of the Influences of Technology in Determining International Industrial Competitive Advantage (ISBN 0309 033969). National Academy Press. Washington, DC.
14. PORTMAN, R. 1983. A new strategy for promotional spending. Pharmaceut. Exec. April: 42–45.
15. ANON. 1981. The U.S. pharmaceutical industry faces rising foreign competition, market concentration and other factors encouraging a complete restructure. Marketing News 11/31: 7 & 14.
16. OLSON, E. C. & R. E. CHRISTOFFERSEN, Eds. 1979. Computer Assisted Drug Design, Vol. 112. ACS Symposium Series. Washington, DC.
17. ANON. 1983. Generix Case Challenges the ANDA System. Med. Marketing & Media Jan: 48.
18. ANON. 1983. FDA sued over post '62 ANDAs. Scrip 811: 12.
19. ANON. 1983. Waxman presses generics bill. Scrip 817: 9.
20. ANON. 1983. ANDA drug labelling bills marked up. Scrip 821: 9.

21. ANON. 1983. Post-1962 ANDA: 15-year delay is not legally permissible. F-D-C Reports (The Pink Sheet) Vol 45 (27), July 4: T&G–1.
22. ANON. 1981. Publication of paper NDA memorandum. Fed. Reg. 46(96): 27396–27397.
23. ANON. 1983. New bill to aid generic producers. Standard and Poor's Industry Surveys. Sec 2, Sept 1: H–21.
24. ANON. 1978. OSHA ongoing carcinogenic risk hearings: Animal test results—two opposing views. F-D-C Reports (The Pink Sheet) 40(29): 11.

# Antiarrhythmic Therapy: The Issue of Patient Compliance

CAROLYN SOMELOFSKI

*Department of Medicine, Cardiology Division*
*University of California, San Francisco, and*
*San Francisco General Hospital*
*San Francisco, California 94110*

ROBERT W. PETERS

*Department of Medicine, Division of Cardiology*
*Veterans Administration Medical Center, and the*
*University of Maryland School of Medicine*
*Baltimore, Maryland 21218*

The recent development of a variety of antiarrhythmic medications has ushered in a new era in the treatment of cardiac arrhythmias. Interest in the therapy of arrhythmias has been heightened by the recent demonstration that certain antiarrhythmic drugs may actually prolong life in some clinical situations.[1] Generally ignored in the midst of all this excitement is the question of compliance: medications can be maximally effective only if the patient is taking them as prescribed. Unfortunately, there is a paucity of information about compliance with antiarrhythmic regimens, especially those involving new drugs. As a group, antiarrhythmic agents tend to have many side effects, making compliance rather difficult. This difficulty is reinforced by the fact that arrhythmias may be intermittent, with long asymptomatic periods between attacks. Because the therapeutic goal is often suppression of ventricular arrhythmias and ultimately prevention of sudden death, the problem of persuading a patient to take a toxic drug or group of drugs regularly is considerable, especially without the reinforcement of symptoms. Studies of commonly used medications such as digoxin and propranolol suggest that compliance is generally in the range of only 50–60%.[2,3] These studies have profound implications for our present perception of the efficacy of medication. They suggest that the expenditure of huge amounts of money to develop new medications might be inappropriate; we might be better off devoting some of our time and energy to ascertaining that the drugs that are already commercially available are actually being taken as prescribed. Recently, several multicenter clinical trials of beta blocking drugs provided a unique opportunity to examine drug compliance in a systematic and controlled fashion. The results of these trials with respect to long-term compliance with antiarrhythmic regimens are discussed herein. Although the subject is discussed from the perspective of an outpatient clinic, the conclusions are also applicable for the most part to patients seen in private practice.

## DEFINITION OF COMPLIANCE

What constitutes compliance? The best definition may involve some type of quantitative assessment of the frequency with which a patient follows a given regimen.

However, there is no universal agreement as to the desired goal. Does taking 75% of the prescribed medication constitute good compliance or is greater than 90% necessary? The answer seems to vary with the type of medication, its margin of safety, the amount and frequency of dosing, the type of disease process, characteristics of the individual patients, and the methods used to assess compliance.[4] Before a therapeutic plan is put into effect, either with an individual patient or in a clinical trial, a means of assessing compliance and an acceptable level of compliance should be determined. For example, acceptable compliance for a relatively long-acting drug such as digoxin by a patient with mildly symptomatic supraventricular tachycardia may be very different than the level of compliance required in a patient with life-threatening ventricular tachycardia whose dose of procainamide has been carefully titrated by means of serial electrophysiologic studies.

## METHODS OF ASSESSING COMPLIANCE (TABLE 1)

Direct biologic determinations such as measurement of blood concentrations of drug[2,5] and the detection of metabolites[6,7] in body fluids are useful and commonly

TABLE 1. Methods of Assessing Compliance

| |
|---|
| *Direct:* |
|     Measurement of drug concentrations in body fluids |
| *Indirect:* |
|     Clinic attendance |
|     Pill counts |
|     Interviews |
|     Self-monitoring (diary or drug dispenser, for example) |
|     Clinician's evaluation |
|     Biologic markers (such as pulse, blood pressure) |
|     Surprise home visits |

employed methods for measuring compliance. Serum concentrations of drug may be misleading if blood samples are obtained only at regular clinic visits because the patient may only take the drug several days preceding each visit. Additional limitations of this method are that the timing of the determination may be critical to its interpretation, particularly in medications with short half-lives, and that marked intra- and interindividual variations in absorption and metabolism occur. However, when performed at random times and coordinated with other methods of assessing compliance, direct biologic determinations (those involving pulse or blood pressure measurements, for example) may be extremely useful in providing objective data.[8] Addition of a pharmacologic marker such as riboflavin to a drug can also be employed to assess compliance. However, the marker itself can cause difficulties. For example, riboflavin is rapidly excreted so that only recent drug ingestion can be assessed. Also, riboflavin may be detected if the patient is taking vitamin pills.[9] Markers must be demonstrated to be harmless and require approval from the Food and Drug Administration before they can be added to a medication.

Among the various indirect methods of assessing compliance, keeping records of attendance in the outpatient clinic is probably the simplest. Keeping appointments is objective, easy to tabulate, and identifies the most severe form of non-

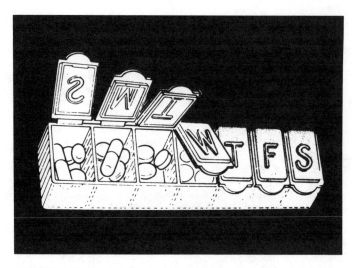

**FIGURE 1.** Medication dispenser to aid self-monitoring of drug-taking.

compliance, that of dropping out of care. However, the fact that a patient faithfully attends a clinic does not necessarily mean that he or she is faithful in taking his or her medication. Several studies have shown a relatively poor correlation between clinic attendance and medication compliance, so that this method, by itself, provides an incomplete measure of compliance.[10–12]

Pill counts have the advantage of providing a quantitative assessment of compliance over a period of time. However, pill counts do not identify the pattern of noncompliance (that is, whether a patient randomly skips medication or does so with a particular pattern) and can fail to show if a patient is simply discarding the medication merely to indicate medication compliance. In addition, pill counts are time-consuming and necessitate careful control of the number of pills dispensed. It has been shown that pill counts generally indicate a higher degree of compliance than measurements of serum concentrations of drug, but a lower degree of compliance than the patient indicates in an interview.[13–15]

Patient interviews are another commonly employed means of assessing compliance. Although deliberate misrepresentation during an interview appears to be uncommon, interviews correlate poorly with other measures of compliance. Not surprisingly, patients tend not to report poor compliance fully,[15,16] and major deviations from the prescribed regimen are more likely to be reported than minor ones.[17,18] Interviews are also relatively subjective and there is the possibility of misunderstanding between the examiner and the patient.

In contrast, self-monitoring techniques may provide a more objective assessment of a patient's compliance. Such self-reporting has an advantage over reliance on memory in that it encourages the patient to record information on behavior at the time that it occurs. In particular, self-reporting may document patterns of variation in compliance that may be essential in planning the intervention strategy and in evaluating therapeutic efficacy (for example, by correlating the onset of palpitations with failure to take the evening dose of medication). However, it must be kept in mind that in some cases the placebo effect may leave the patient asymptomatic. Various types of medication dispensers (FIG. 1) provide another method of self-monitoring and have the advantage of reminding patients to take their medication.

The physician's assessment is probably the poorest method of evaluating compliance. Studies indicate that physicians consistently overestimate compliance, often by as much as 50%, and that their judgement is not improved by experience or increased contact with the patient.[17,19,20]

Biologic markers such as pulse rate, blood pressure, or suppression of extrasystoles are a particularly attractive means of assessing compliance because the patient can be taught to measure them, thus increasing his or her involvement in the therapeutic process. Unfortunately, the response to a medication can vary considerably from patient to patient and also from day to day in a given patient, possibly causing disappointment and loss of confidence in the therapeutic regimen. Thus, when patients and their physicians were asked to determine whether they were taking propranolol or placebo at the conclusion of the double-blind Beta Blocker Heart Attack Trial (BHAT), 30–50% incorrectly identified their medical regimen.[21]

Surprise home visits can also be a useful method of assessing compliance, especially if serum samples for determination of drug concentrations and urine samples for measurement of biologic markers can be obtained and unobtrusive pill counts carried out at that time. However, this method is extremely time-consuming and expensive, and requires a trusting relationship between the patient and the health-care team.

Ideally, compliance assessment should provide reliable information and should be easy and inexpensive to carry out. No single method is invariably effective. In clinical trials, an antiarrhythmic effect can be compared between the placebo and experimental groups; however, this is impossible in clinical practice and so other methods must be employed.

First, clinic attendance should be monitored in all patients. If a satisfactory therapeutic response is not achieved, an interview should be arranged and followed or supplemented by determination of drug concentration, pill count and other means of assessment, depending on the patient, type of medication, and the disease process. In particular, compliance with the regimen of medication should have priority and be the subject of frequent specific discussions between the patient and the health-care team.

## FACTORS INFLUENCING COMPLIANCE

A major misconception prevalent in the medical profession is that poor compliance is the fault of the patient. Although this is sometimes the case, there are a variety of factors that affect compliance, and the health-care provider must understand them to achieve a therapeutic goal. Factors that affect compliance have traditionally been divided into five areas[22] (TABLE 2). The patient's sociodemo-

TABLE 2. Factors Influencing Compliance

| |
|---|
| Patient characteristics |
| Health-care providers' characteristics |
| Health-care provider–patient relationship |
| Medical regimen characteristics |
| Illness characteristics |

graphic characteristics can have a major influence on compliance. For example, the elderly and the poorly educated tend to be more forgetful and may have a fear of physicians and hospitals and are thus more likely to develop problems with compliance. Similarly, ethnic factors may play a role, especially if a language barrier exists. Various personality traits have also been shown to adversely affect compliance. Patients experiencing social isolation tend to be poorly compliant,[23] as do patients with type A personalities, possibly because they fear dependency and loss of control.[24] Finally, a significant factor affecting compliance behavior is cost: a medication regimen that is a financial burden to the patient may be the cause for therapeutic failure and noncompliance.

It must be remembered that the health-care providers may have a major influence on compliance. In a recent study involving antihypertensive medication, physicians were carefully educated about the problem of noncompliance.[25] This education was reflected by an increase in the amount of time that they spent educating patients about their illnesses and therapeutic regimens, and a corresponding increase in their comments in the medical record relating to the patient's understanding. The results of the study revealed a significant increase in the number of patients taking at least 75% of their prescribed medications and achieving satisfactory control of blood pressure. There is also evidence that the nature of the doctor-patient relationship, especially in regard to initial contact, continuity of care, and patient satisfaction, may influence compliance. Brevity in giving instructions is of the utmost importance because it has been shown that after the first 5 minutes, patients forget approximately half of what is told to them and remember best the information in the first third of the presentation.[26,27] It is also advisable to inquire about the patient's "hidden agenda" for an outpatient visit: that is, what complaints he or she feels are most important, what therapy and outcome he or she expects, and what his or her understanding is of "obeying doctor's orders." In this way, some peculiar preconceived ideas about taking medications may surface, for example the notions that "you need to give your body some rest from the medication occasionally" or "your body might become immune to it."[28-31]

The medical regimen itself is known to have a particularly strong effect on compliance.[23,32-35] Among factors that are especially important are the type and severity of side effects of a given medication, the frequency of dosing, the degree to which a medical regimen interferes with a patient's life-style (for example, taking a few pills each day that have no side effects is considerably easier than losing weight, stopping smoking, or taking a medication that causes fatigue and impotence) and the length of time that a patient is expected to follow this regimen. Thus, patients who have been following a regimen for a long time tend to be less compliant, especially if the condition for which they are receiving the medication is not life-threatening. It also must be kept in mind that a medication schedule that is unusually complicated or lengthy is unlikely to be followed closely: consider, for example, the inconvenience of applying nitroglycerin ointment while at work. TABLE 3 shows a sample medication schedule given to us by one of our clinic patients with angina pectoris and hypertension. The impossibility of following such a regimen can easily be appreciated. This list also reveals that it is possible for a patient to unwittingly be taking an excess of drug by taking the same medication more than once because it can be prescribed by both generic and one or more trade names.

Factors relating to the patient's disease process may also affect compliance. A previous illness or a family-related illness tends to improve compliance, perhaps because of the patient's belief that therapy can have positive effects. However, excessive use of fear motivation—"take your medicine or your will die"—may lead to denial of the illness and ultimately a decrease in compliance. In dealing with long-term follow-up, it must be kept in mind that the more symptomatic and recent the illness, the greater the compliance. As the acuteness of the illness fades in the patient's memory, symptom reinforcement must be replaced by staff intervention and support.

## BETA BLOCKER HEART ATTACK TRIAL

The BHAT was a clinical study that evaluated the efficacy of propranolol in reducing mortality, sudden death, and reinfarction in a population of almost 4000 patients who had recently had a myocardial infarction. The study was randomized, double-blind, placebo-controlled, and involved an extended (25-month mean) follow-up period. Careful monitoring of compliance was especially crucial in this study because prevention, rather than treatment, was the primary goal and because low-risk patients, many of whom had few or no symptoms after their

**TABLE 3.** Medication Schedule

| Drug | Schedule |
| --- | --- |
| Nitropaste | 1" q.4h. and 2" q.h.s. |
| Isordil | 20 mg q.i.d. and 40 mg q.h.s. |
| HCTZ | 50 mg b.i.d. |
| KCl | 20 mEq in juice t.i.d. |
| Propranolol | 60 mg q.i.d. |
| Nifedipine | 20 mg t.i.d. |
| Hydralazine | 25 mg q.i.d. |
| Procainamide | 500 mg q.i.d. |
| Pronestyl | 500 mg q.i.d. |
| Digoxin | 0.25 mg q.a.m. |
| Lanoxin | 0.25 mg daily |

myocardial infarction, were selected to participate. San Francisco General Hospital Medical Center was one of 31 clinical centers involved in the BHAT study. The interventions that we developed at our center to improve compliance followed the general principles outlined earlier and also evolved to meet the specific needs of our patient population, many of whom were indigent and non-English-speaking with relatively low levels of education. Self-monitoring techniques were particularly important in our clinic and included the use of weekly medication dispensers, diaries, and medication charts, especially in patients with complicated medical regimens. Every effort was made to keep the medical regimen simple, stressing medications that could be administered in single daily doses whenever possible, especially when therapy was being initiated, so that the patient would not be overwhelmed by his or her regimen. Patients were taught how to take their own pulses and to correlate a slow pulse rate with medication compliance. We also found that compliance was improved when patients were educated about their disease and therapy and particularly when they were forewarned about side effects of the medication. The physiology of beta blockers was stressed as much as possible, particularly the dangers of sudden cessation of therapy. Instructions were reinforced verbally before the patient's departure from the clinic, provided in written form for them to take home, and further reinforced by telephone calls in between clinic visits. Frequent telephone contact had the additional advantage of minimizing social isolation. In addition, patients were sent birthday cards, Christmas cards, appointment reminder cards, and educational booklets. When patients arrived at the clinic for outpatient visits, a friendly and professional atmosphere was provided and patients were carefully informed about their health status. After each visit, patients were notified of the results of their laboratory tests by telephone. In addition, they were provided with an identification card (FIG. 2) with the names of the staff and a telephone number that was manned 24 hours a day. We found that this approach was helpful with regard to answering questions, clarifying misunderstandings, and identifying early symptoms. We also initiated a weekly cardiac group therapy session in which health-care team members would lead discussions of common problems such as fear of dying and medication toxicities. Groups were extremely well received and attended and seemed to help keep potential dropouts within the system. In summary, our approach was aimed at providing comprehensive care and a regimen tailored to the needs of the individual patient with emphasis upon patient education and maximum contact between the patient and the health-care team.

In TABLE 4, follow-up data from our first 96 BHAT patients are compared with data from the remainder of the outpatient cardiac clinic over the same period of time. There were significantly fewer missed clinic visits and patients lost to follow-up among the BHAT patients. Compliance in the BHAT group was 80% when assessed by random measurements of serum propranolol concentrations and 94% when assessed by pill counts. The number of patients who were poorly compliant was so small that a statistical comparison between them and the remainder of the BHAT group would not be meaningful. However, it is noteworthy that almost all

**BETA-BLOCKER HEART ATTACK TRIAL**

*This is to certify that*

*M* _____

*Drug No.* _____

*is a participant in the Beta-Blocker Heart Attack Trial at*

San Francisco General Hospital

*WEEKDAYS:*

    *Robert Peters, M.D. or*
    *Carolyn Somelofski, R.N.*
    *(415) 821-8315*

*In case of EMERGENCY*
*NIGHTS OR WEEKENDS:*

    *Coronary Care Unit (CCU)*
    *Head Nurse*
    *(415) 821-8311*

**FIGURE 2.** Patient's identification card.

TABLE 4. Compliance in BHAT Patients Compared with That in the Remainder of the Clinic Population (Clinic)

| | BHAT (%) | Clinic (%) | p Value |
|---|---|---|---|
| Missed visits | 44/419 (11) | 499/1656 (30) | <0.005 |
| Lost to follow-up | 3/96 (3) | 106/248 (43) | <0.005 |

of the patients who were poorly compliant had a history of heavy alcohol intake. Exact figures are not available for the remainder of the regular clinic population. We estimate that in contrast to compliance of the BHAT patients, compliance in the other clinic patients was no better than 50%. We believe that our approach to compliance outlined herein was responsible for the difference.

## CONCLUSION

In conclusion, a systematic approach provides the opportunity to markedly enhance patient compliance. As newer and more effective antiarrhythmic drugs become available, it is hoped that this improvement will be translated into an improvement in the quality of life and a decrease in the incidence of sudden death. Most of the data available in the medical literature on antiarrhythmic drugs deals primarily with efficacy; the issue of compliance is either examined only superficially or ignored altogether. On the basis of current estimates, it is conceivable that in many studies of antiarrhythmic drugs, only 50% of patients were taking the medication as prescribed. Further clinical trials are urgently needed, utilizing more enlightened methods to improve compliance in order to provide a more realistic assessment of the clinical efficacy of antiarrhythmic drugs.

## REFERENCES

1. BETA BLOCKER HEART ATTACK TRIAL RESEARCH GROUP. 1982. A randomized trial of propranolol in patients with acute myocardial infarction. I. Mortality results. JAMA 247: 1707–1714.
2. JOHNSTON, G. D., J. G. KELLY & D. G. McDEVITT. 1978. Do patients take digoxin? Br. Heart J. 40: 1–7.
3. INUI, T. S., W. B. CARTER, R. E. PECORARO, R. A. PEARLMAN & J. J. DOHAN. 1980. Variations in patient compliance with common long-term drug. Med. Care 15: 986–993.
4. EVANS L. & M. SPELMAN. 1983. The problem of noncompliance with drug therapy. Drugs 25: 63–76.
5. REDDY, C. P., J. DOMINIC & B. SURAWICZ. 1980. Monitoring blood levels of cardioactive drugs. Cardiovasc. Clin. 11: 267–290.
6. FITZLOFF, J. & F. ESHELMAN. 1976. Quantitative urine analysis for measuring compliance. Am. J. Hosp. Pharmacol. 33: 990–992.
7. GORDIS, E. & K. PETERSON. 1977. Disulfiram therapy in alcoholism: Patient compliance studied with a urine-detection procedure. Alcoholism: Clin. Exp. Res. 1: 213–216.
8. ROTH, H. P., H. S. CARON & B. P. HSI. 1969. Measuring intake of a prescribed medication. A bottle count and a tracer technique compared. Clin. Pharmacol. Ther. 11: 228–237.

9. SOUTTER, B. R. & M. C. KENNEDY. 1974. Patient compliance assessment in drug trials: Usage and methods. Aust. New Zeal. J. Med. **4:** 360–364.
10. BOWEN, R. G., R. RICH & R. M. SCHLOTFELDT. 1961. Effects of organized instruction for patients with the diagnosis of diabetes mellitus. Nurs. Res. **10:** 151–159.
11. GORDIS, L., M. MARKOWITZ & A. M. LILIENFELD. 1969. Studies in the epidemiology and preventability of rheumatic fever. IV. A quantitative determination of compliance in children on oral penicillin prophylaxis. Pediatrics **43:** 173–182.
12. RITSON, B. 1969. Involvement in treatment and its relation to outcome amongst alcoholics. Br. J. Addict. **64:** 23–29.
13. ROTH, H. P. & D. G. BERGER. 1960. Studies on patient cooperation in ulcer treatment. I. Observation of actual as compared to prescribed antacid intake on a hospital ward. Gastroenterology **38:** 630–633.
14. JOYCE, C. R. B. 1962. Patient cooperation and the sensitivity of clinical trials. J. Chron. Dis. **15:** 1025–1036.
15. PARK, L. C. & R. S. LIPMAN. 1964. A comparison of patient dosage deviation reports with pill counts. Psychopharmacologia **6:** 299–302.
16. HAYNES, R. B., D. L. SACKETT, E. S. GIBSON, D. W. TAYLOR, B. C. HACKETT, R. S. ROBERTS & A. L. JOHNSON. 1976. Improvement of medication compliance in uncontrolled hypertension. Lancet **1:** 1265–1268.
17. ROTH, H. P. & H. S. CARON. 1978. Accuracy of doctors' estimates and patients' statements on adherence to a drug regimen. Clin. Pharmacol. Ther. **23:** 361–370.
18. RICKELS, K. & E. BRISCOE. 1970. Assessment of dosage deviation in outpatient drug research. J. Clin. Pharmacol. **10:** 153–160.
19. CARON, H. S. & H. P. ROTH. 1968. Patients' cooperation with a medical regimen. JAMA **203:** 120–124.
20. MUSHLIN, A. I. & F. A. APPEL. 1977. Diagnosing potential noncompliance. Physicians' ability in a behavioral dimension of medical care. Arch. Intern. Med. **137:** 318–321.
21. BYINGTON, R. P., J. D. CURB, J. A. GROVER & M. GREENLICK for the BHAT Research Group. May 1983. Assessment of patient blindness at the conclusion of a clinical trial. Presented at the 4th Annual Meeting of the Society of Clinical Trials. Controlled Clinical Trials **4:** 163–164 (abstract).
22. BLACKWELL, B. 1973. Drug therapy? Patient compliance. N. Engl. J. Med. **289:** 249–252.
23. NELSON, E. C., W. B. STASON, R. R. NEUTRA & H. S. SOLOMON. 1980. Identification of the noncompliant hypertensive patient. Prev. Med. **9:** 504–517.
24. ANDERSON, R. J. & C. MATHEWS. 1980. Noncompliance: Failure of the therapeutic partnership. Cardiovasc. Rev. Rep. **2:** 464–470.
25. INUI, T. S., E. L. YOURTEE & J. W. WILLIAMSON. 1976. Improved outcome in hypertension after physician tutorials. A controlled trial. Ann. Intern. Med. **84:** 646–651.
26. LEY, P., P. W. BRADSHAW & D. EAVES. 1973. A method for increasing patients' recall of information presented by doctors. Psychol. Med. **3:** 217–220.
27. LEY, P. 1972. Primary, rate importance, and the recall of medical statements. J. Health Soc. Behav. **13:** 311–317.
28. VINCENT, P. 1971. Factors influencing patient noncompliance: Theoretical approach. Nurs. Res. **20:** 509–516.
29. ZOLA, I. K. 1972. Studying the decision to see a doctor. Review, critique, corrective. Adv. Psychosom. Med. **8:** 216–236.
30. ZOLA, I. K. 1973. Pathways to the doctor from person to patient. Soc. Sci. Med. **8:** 677–689.
31. STIMSON, G. V. 1974. Obeying doctor's orders: View from the other side. Soc. Sci. Med. **8:** 97–104.
32. KASL, S. V. 1975. Issues in patient adherence to health care regimens. Hum. Stress **1:** 5–58.
33. PORTER, A. M. W. 1969. Drug defaulting in a general practice. Br. Med. J. **1:** 218–222.

34. BERKOWITZ, N. H., M. F. MALONE, M. W. KLEIN & A. EATON. 1963. A patient follow-through in the outpatient department. Nurs. Res. **12:** 16–22.
35. DAVIS, M. S. 1967. Predicting non-compliant behavior. J. Health Soc. Behav. **8:** 265–271.
36. JOHANNSEN, W. J., G. A. HELMUTH & T. SORAUF. 1966. On accepting medical recommendations. Arch. Environ. Health **12:** 63–69.

# Role of Higher Nervous Activity in Ventricular Arrhythmia and Sudden Cardiac Death: Implications for Alternative Antiarrhythmic Therapy

PHILIP J. PODRID

*Harvard School of Public Health*
*Brigham and Women's Hospital*
*Boston, Massachusetts 02115*

For thousands of years sudden cardiac death and the fear of dying has been written about extensively. Historians have documented the death of famous persons during times of great emotional stress, while novelists and playwrights have used the association between psychological trauma and death to emphasize the tragedy that can plague human beings. However, a relationship between sudden death and psychological stress factors has not been well studied, although clinical experience would support the supposition that such a relationship exists.

There is increasing evidence that psychological factors and emotional stress can affect health, most evidently with respect to the cardiovascular system. Psychological inputs, which augment neural traffic from the brain, provoke many cardiac manifestations including angina pectoris, congestive heart failure, hypertension, myocardial infarction, a wide array of arrhythmias, and even sudden death. Unfortunately, the relationship between mind and body, the realm of psychosomatic medicine, has no sound scientific foundation and has been relegated to an undistinguished position in medicine with evidential support only from anectodal reports. Nevertheless, a relationship does exist and forms the basis for much of the clinical practice of medicine, especially in cardiology.

During times of emotional stress, patients often complain of "palpitations," "skipped beats," "racing of the heart," or other manifestations of rapid heart action or arrhythmia. Fear, expectation, anger, and even joy and happiness can provoke major alterations in the cardiac rhythm. Moreover, such rhythm disturbances will often abate when stress is relieved and emotional inputs diminished. Often patients learn to avoid those situations likely to produce such disturbances in rhythm. Physicians, lacking scientific data to support a causal relationship, do not generally become involved with these factors, considering them unessential. A major trigger for cardiac arrhythmias, therefore is ignored while the target, the heart, becomes the primary focus of attention.

Psychology and psychiatry remain primitive as regards both understanding and therapy, while the science of neuropharmacology is in its infancy. Nevertheless, there exists a large body of data relating to animals which support the view that psychological triggers play an important role in the genesis of cardiac arrhythmias and sudden death, although human studies are few in number. This paper accordingly will offer a review of important information derived from animal models and clinical experience.

There are several hypotheses that form the framework for investigative endeavors in the field of sudden cardiac death[1] (FIG. 1):

1. The mechanism of sudden cardiac death is ventricular fibrillation.

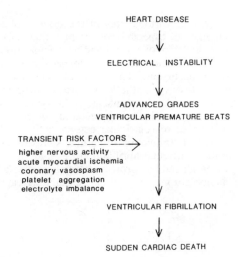

**FIGURE 1.** Hypothesis accounting for sudden death. The presence of heart disease results in myocardial electrical instability, which is manifested by the occurrence of advanced grades of ventricular premature beats. Transient risk factors can alter the electrical properties of the myocardium and trigger ventricular fibrillation, resulting in sudden cardiac death.

2. The myocardium predisposed to the development of ventricular fibrillation is electrically unstable. Such instability long predates the occurrence of sudden death.

3. Certain types of ventricular premature beats, primarily repetitive forms, are the clinical markers of this underlying electrical instability.

4. Transient risk factors, by affecting the electrically unstable heart can trigger ventricular fibrillation.

5. There exist a number of risk factors which include ischemia, platelet aggregation, vasospasm, electrolyte imbalance and metabolic disorders. However, the major factor is that which originates from higher nervous activity.[1] The central nervous system, working through the peripheral autonomic nervous system, has profound effects on myocardial function and electrophysiologic properties (TABLE 1, FIG. 2).

## NEURAL INFLUENCES AND CARDIAC ARRHYTHMIAS

The central nervous system has been shown to have important effects on cardiac function. Ventricular arrhythmia can be provoked when drugs such as nicotine, barium chloride, or epinephrine are injected into certain areas of the brain of anesthetized cats.[2] Electrostimuli delivered through electrodes stereotaxically po-

TABLE 1. Effects of the Sympathetic Nervous System on Cardiac Electrophysiologic Properties

| | |
|---|---|
| Increase the upstroke velocity of action potential | → enhance conductivity |
| Shorten the refractory period of the action potential | → increase excitability |
| Increase the rate of spontaneous depolarization | → enhance automaticity |

sitioned at various sites of the brain profoundly affect cardiac function.[3] Such stimulation, especially of the hypothalamus, can modify heart rate, blood pressure, and provoke atrial and ventricular premature beats. Ventricular fibrillation does not occur, however, unless this structure is stimulated during coronary artery occlusion.[4] The effect of hypothalamic stimulation provides strong evidence that sympathetic pathways are involved in the genesis of arrhythmia.[5] Further evidences implicating the sympathetic nervous system are the observations that cardiac sympathectomy or beta-adrenergic blockade will prevent the occurrence of ventricular ectopic activity when the hypothalamus is stimulated.

Direct stimulation of cardiac sympathetic fibers causes a significant decrease in the ventricular fibrillation threshold,[6] and in the presence of myocardial ischemia produced by coronary artery ligation, such stimulation will provoke ventricular fibrillation.[7] In contrast, circulating catecholamines secreted by the adrenal

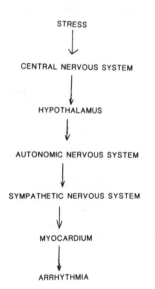

FIGURE 2. Interaction of higher nervous activity and the heart resulting in the provocation of arrhythmia. Any type of stress has profound effects on the central nervous system and can affect hypothalamic function. When the hypothalamus is stimulated, the autonomic nervous system, especially the sympathetic limb, is activated. Neural traffic carried by the sympathetic nervous system can affect myocardial electrophysiologic properties and provoke arrhythmia.

medulla have a much smaller effect on ventricular excitability and cause only a moderate and transient reduction in the ventricular fibrillation threshold.[8]

Equally persuasive evidence supporting the role of the sympathetic nervous system in the genesis of arrhythmia is derived from studies involving sympathetic denervation of the heart. Ventricular fibrillation in the dog can be prevented after acute coronary artery occlusion by prior sympathectomy.[9] Mediastinal neural ablation decreased the incidence of ventricular fibrillation after coronary occlusion from 52% to 0%.[10] Schwartz and coworkers[11] found that ablation or cooling of the left stellate ganglion increases the ventricular fibrillation threshold by 72% when compared with control values, while right stellate ganglion ablation caused a reflex increase in left stellate ganglion activity and a 47% decrease in ventricular fibrillation threshold.

During acute coronary artery occlusion, there is an activation of a sympathetic-cardiac reflex.[12] This reflex occurs within the first minute after coronary arterial obstruction and its time course corresponds closely to that of the change in ventricular fibrillation threshold. Measurements made by direct nerve recording reveal that a close relationship between the enhancement of sympathetic discharges to the heart and the reduction in ventricular fibrillation threshold following coronary artery occlusion.[13] A return of sympathetic neural discharge rate to baseline correlates with the return of the ventricular fibrillation threshold to normal. It is noteworthy that the abrupt and profound decrease of ventricular fibrillation threshold that occurs with coronary artery release is not associated with any change in the degree of sympathetic discharge, a fact which suggests that the decrease in the ventricular fibrillation threshold during this phase has another etiology.

As expected from the studies of vulnerability during acute ischemia, the administration of beta-adrenergic blocking agents protects against the enhanced vulnerability associated with coronary artery occlusion, but not release.[14] This protective effect is exclusively a result of inhibition of beta receptors and is not due to membrane-stabilizing activity. It has been shown that the effect on ventricular fibrillation threshold differs among the various beta-adrenergic blocking agents.[15] Those with intrinsic sympathomimetic activity maintain baseline sympathetic tone and do not cause any change in ventricular fibrillation threshold. Other interventions that decrease sympathetic tone also affect vulnerability. When blood pressure is increased with phenylephrine, a direct alpha-adrenergic agonist, there is a reflex decrease in sympathetic tone, resulting in a decreased propensity toward ventricular fibrillation.[16] Increasing blood pressure during acute myocardial ischemia also has a protective effect.

The sympathetic nervous system also has a significant effect on ventricular refractoriness.[17] Right stellectomy, which causes a reflex in left stellate discharge, shifts the strength interval curve 3–5 msec earlier ($p < 0.005$), indicating a decrease in refractoriness, while left stellectomy shifts the strength interval curve 4–7 msec later ($p < 0.005$), representing an increase in cardiac refractoriness. This is similar to the effect of left stellate ablation or stimulation on the ventricular fibrillation threshold.[11]

## ROLE OF THE PARASYMPATHETIC NERVOUS SYSTEM

Although it had been assumed that vagal innervation of the ventricular myocardium is absent, there is now a large body of evidence that supports the view that the parasympathetic nervous system has an important effect on both the inotropic and chronotropic properties of the ventricle. In the rabbit heart, acetylcholine or direct stimulation of the vagus nerve will decrease the rate of an idioventricular rhythm caused by surgically induced complete AV block.[18] Acetylcholine depresses the slope of phase 4 of the action potential generated by proximal His-Purkinje fibers.[19] Although the sinus and AV node as well as the atria contain a far more extensive amount of vagal innervation, there is histologic as well as histochemical evidence for cholinergic innervation of the ventricular conduction system.[20]

There is also evidence that the parasympathetic nervous system can affect the electrical properties of the ventricular muscle. Kent and coworkers,[21] utilizing an open chest dog preparation, demonstrated that stimulation of the vagus nerve increased the ventricular fibrillation threshold during acute ischemia. In a open chest cat model, Corr and coworkers[22] demonstrated that the presence of intact vagi protected against ventricular fibrillation during coronary artery ligation.

However, when the intact, closed chest animal is studied, stimulation of the vagus nerve has no effect on ventricular fibrillation threshold.[23] Therefore, only in the presence of enhanced sympathetic activity, as produced by stress or direct stimulation of the sympathetic nervous system, is there demonstration of an antifibrillatory effect of the vagus nerve[24] (FIG. 3). When adrenergic blockade is produced with propranolol, direct vagal stimulation has no effect on the ventricular fibrillation threshold.[24] The effect of the vagus nerve on ventricular vulnerability seems to be indirect, opposing the adverse changes resulting from heightened sympathetic tone. Rabinowitz and coworkers[25] demonstrated that an injection of norepinephrine caused a significant decrease in the ventricular fibrillation threshold, which was restored to control levels by stimulation of the vagus nerve. The vagus nerve exerted no protective effect when atropine pretreatment was used. Vagal tone thus modulates the effect on cardiac vulnerability caused by sympathetic discharge. A number of parasympathomimetic agents such as edrophonium, morphine,[26] and especially metacholine[25] will also affect the ventricular fibrillation threshold and decrease susceptibility to ventricular arrhythmias.

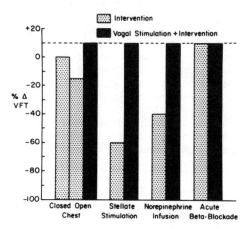

**FIGURE 3.** Effect of the vagus nerve on the ventricular fibrillation threshold (VFT) during enhanced sympathetic tone. When the "closed-chest" animal is used, stimulation of the vagus nerve does not significantly alter the VFT. When an open-chest dog is studied, the VFT is reduced. Vagal stimulation reverses this. The reduction of VFT by stellate stimulation and norepinephrine infusion is also reversed by vagal stimulation. When beta-blockers are given to the animal, vagal stimulation does not change the VFT. (From Lown and Verrier.[69] Reprinted by permission.)

There are a number of studies in man supporting the concept of the role of the vagus nerve in protecting against ventricular arrhythmia. Nathanson[27] provoked multiformed ventricular premature beats after administration of intravenous epinephrine to six patients. When this experiment was repeated after pretreatment with acetyl beta methacholine chloride, ventricular premature beats were no longer observed in four of the six patients. Weiss and coworkers[28] administered phenylephrine to ten patients with ventricular premature beats. In five of them, significant bradycardia developed and ventricular ectopic beats were reduced from 18.2% to 3.2% (p < 0.005). Administration of atropine resulted in reemergence of arrhythmia in two patients. Waxman and coworkers[29] reported that phenylephrine was effective for terminating ventricular tachycardia in six patients. They further demonstrated that pretreatment with edrophonium decreased the dose of phenylephrine necessary to terminate the ventricular tachycardia, while atropine pretreatment increased the dose requirements. Moreover, after edrophonium pretreatment, carotid sinus pressure, which was previously ineffective, now resulted in termination of the ventricular tachycardia. Although the group of patients studied was highly selected and each patient had ventricular tachycardia provoked by exercise, these results lend further support, along with the animal data, to the view that the major effect of vagal action is the negation of changes due to heightened sympathetic tone. Enhanced vagal activity may occur in some patients at the onset of an acute myocardial infarction, but it is unknown whether this protects against ventricular fibrillation in these patients. There are no human studies evaluating the role of the vagus nerve during an acute myocardial infarction.

## PSYCHOLOGICAL FACTORS AND VENTRICULAR ARRHYTHMIA

### Animal Models

The essential question involving the interaction between higher nervous activity and ventricular fibrillation relates to the role of psychological stress factors. It has been observed that a number of psychological stresses will cause myocardial necrosis and infarction in many different species of animals.[30] Interference with the ability of rats to obtain food, aversive avoidance experiments with monkeys, and subjecting pigs to electric shocks while paralyzed with muscle relaxants will result in a significant occurrence of myocardial necrosis and in some cases the development of a cardiomyopathy.[31] These lesions are likely the result of changes induced by high catecholamine levels, since coronary arteries are invariably free of any lesions.

Although there are a number of studies confirming the deleterious effects of psychological stress on the integrity of the myocardial cell, data are lacking correlating psychological stress, higher nervous activity, and the occurrence of ventricular arrhythmia. The absence of an appropriate animal model has been a limiting factor. In order to study the role of psychological inputs and interventions designed in such a way that their effects can be modified, episodes of ventricular fibrillation must be repeatedly induced and terminated. This requires the use of traumatic resuscitation techniques, including defibrillation, which will have profound effects on the measurement of psychological variables and inputs into the heart. Matta and coworkers[32] reported that when test stimuli are added with increasing currents, single repetitive extrasystoles can be induced at a stimulus energy which is 66% of the ventricular fibrillation threshold. Multiple repetitive ventricular responses can be reproducibly provoked when the current energy is 82% of the energy necessary to provoke ventricular fibrillation. Interventions that alter the ventricular fibrillation threshold produce comparable changes in the repetitive extrasystole threshold. This relationship between the ventricular fibrillation threshold and the repetitive extrasystole threshold is maintained in the conscious animal regardless of the intervention, suggesting that the ventricular fibrillation threshold and the threshold for repetitive ventricular responses have a similar electrophysiologic mechanism. The repetitive ventricular response can be used as a marker for vulnerability, allowing for repeated studies of psychological stress factors and their relationship to ventricular fibrillation. Lown and coworkers[33] used transthoracic shocks for conditioning a dog to recognize a Pavlovian sling as an aversive environment. In the cage, a relaxed environment, the animals were left undisturbed, and repetitive extrasystoles (RE) were elicited when a stimulus current of 43 mA was utilized (RE threshold). However, in the sling, at a time when the dogs were stressed and became restless, the RE thresh-

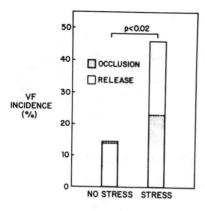

FIGURE 4. Effect of stress on the occurrence of ventricular fibrillation (VF) during coronary artery occlusion and release. The cage-sling model was used to provoke psychological stress in the dog, while in the cage the incidence of VF during occlusion-release was only 15%. However, there was a significant increase in the incidence of VF when the dog was placed in the stressful sling environment.

old was significantly reduced to 14 mA (p < 0.001). This difference could not be ascribed to changes in heart rate, which was held constant by pacing. It can be concluded that psychological stress of whatever type can have profound effects on the threshold for ventricular fibrillation. Beta-adrenergic blocking drugs prevented this stress-induced change in cardiac vulnerability, further supporting the conclusion that such changes are the result of sympathetic neural inputs into the myocardium.[33]

The cage-sling model was also utilized to examine the role of psychological stress during coronary artery occlusion[34] (FIG. 4). A balloon occluder implanted around the left anterior descending artery was inflated, resulting in a myocardial infarction. After recovery from the occlusion, and at a time when there was no spontaneous arrhythmia, the dogs were reexposed to the two environments. While in the cage no arrhythmia occurred; however, upon being placed in the sling, frequent ventricular arrhythmia, including ventricular tachycardia and ventricular fibrillation was provoked. Return to the cage resulted in the restoration of sinus rhythm. Skinner and his coworkers[35] reported similar results when a farm pig was used. When the pigs were adapted to the laboratory environment during a 4–8-day period, ventricular fibrillation after coronary occlusion was prevented. In those animals which had not been adapted to the laboratory, ventricular fibrillation occurred which was not prevented by pretreatment with beta-adrenergic blocking agents. It is unclear whether the failure of the beta blocker was a result of inadequate blockade or the involvement of other factors which may play a role during psychological stress and adaptation.

Others however have found a significant protective role for beta-adrenergic blockade. Rosenfeld and coworkers,[36] using chronically instrumented animals, recorded electrocardiograms and electrograms from ischemic and nonischemic ventricular epicardium during coronary artery occlusion. When dogs were exposed to a variety of behavioral stress, such as an unfamiliar environment or aversive stimuli, there was a significant decrease in the time to onset of arrhythmia, and increased complexity of arrhythmia provoked during occlusion. The emergence of these arrhythmias was prevented by beta-adrenergic blockade. An analog of propranolol (UM 272) devoid of beta-adrenergic blocking properties, but with local anesthetic properties, did not protect against ventricular arrhythmia. It appears that the beneficial effects of the beta-adrenergic blocking agents is not due to their nonspecific local anesthetic effect, but is a result of antiadrenergic activity. The tranquilizing drug diazepam, which reduces sympathetic neural traffic, also had an antiarrhythmic effect.

## Human Studies

Although animal models have clearly shown a relationship between psychological stress factors and vulnerability to ventricular fibrillation, definitive human studies are as yet lacking. This is not unexpected, given the complexity of the problem. Nevertheless, there is a substantial body of evidence suggesting a powerful relationship between the mind and heart. Many years ago Cannon[37] suggested that epinephrine was secreted in response to the occurrence of fear and rage reactions in animals. He considered that epinephrine also played a role in "voodoo death." In a review of psychological stress and its relationship to sudden death, Engel[38] retrospectively examined 170 examples of sudden death felt to be associated with disruptive life events (TABLE 2). These examples were obtained from newspaper reports and only those with a clear association with some precipitating problem were utilized. He established eight categories of stress which provoke sudden death: (1) the collapse or death of a close person, (2) acute grief, (3) the threatened loss of a close person, (4) a period of mourning or an anniversary of a death, (5) loss of status or self-esteem, (6) personal danger or threat of injury, (7) the period after danger is over, and (8) times of triumph, success, or happiness. Engel concluded that the common denominators were overwhelming excitation, loss of control, or giving up. Parkes and his coworkers[39] reported a significant increase in death rate during the first six months after the loss of a spouse. The conclusion was that bereavement increased the susceptibility to sudden death. In a retrospective study, Rahe and coworkers[40] interviewed the families of 226 victims of sudden cardiac death. They observed that there were major life changes such as divorce, grief, and altered work patterns in the six months preceding death as compared with the same time interval one year before. Greene and coworkers[41] interviewed 26 widows who reported that an acute exacerbation of anxiety, anger and changes at work had preceded the deaths of their husbands. It has been shown that in patients who are recovering from an acute myocardial infarction, ward rounds increased the incidence of sudden death fivefold.[42] Interestingly, it was during rounds by the physician-in-chief, which only occurred once per week, that half of the sudden deaths occurred. In a very complete study of a 39-year-old male without heart disease who had experienced ventricular fibrillation, Lown and coworkers[43] observed a clear relationship between emotional stress and the occurrence of ventricular arrhythmia. Complex arrhythmias including ventricular tachycardia were provoked during visits with a

**TABLE 2.** Psychologic Stress Factors Associated with Sudden Death[a]

|  |
|---|
| 1. Death of family member of close friend |
| 2. Grief reaction |
| 3. Threatened loss of family or friend |
| 4. Mourning |
| 5. Loss of status or self-esteem |
| 6. Danger or threat of injury |
| 7. Triumph, achievement, and happiness |
| 8. Significant life changes |

[a] From Engel.[38]

psychiatrist as well as during the REM stages of sleep. Meditation and a beta-adrenergic blocking drug were effective for preventing the ventricular arrhythmia.

Stress in humans is an established provoking factor for ventricular arrhythmia. The stress of public speaking was a sufficient stimulus to provoke ventricular arrhythmia in 6 of 23 healthy young men.[44] The same type of stress provoked more advanced grades of ventricular arrhythmia in those with heart disease. The use of a beta-adrenergic blocking agent prevented the occurrence of ventricular arrhythmia.

Similar observations have been made in patients during an acute myocardial infarction. Certain interactions can provoke arrhythmias in patients in the coronary care unit recovering from an acute myocardial infarction. Lynch and coworkers[45] reported that the touch of a nurse during measurement of radial pulse caused a reduction in ventricular arrhythmia. Donlon et al.[46] reported a clear relationship between the frequency of ventricular premature beats and the state of stress during a psychiatric interview in a 38-year-old man recovering from a myocardial infarction. Arrhythmia had not been provoked by exercise, which produced a much greater acceleration of heart rate and rise in blood pressure.

One of the most interesting relationships between the effect of neural and psychological inputs into the heart is observed in patients who have prolonged Q-T syndromes. These patients have an imbalance between left and right stellate ganglion activity and are at an increased risk for sudden death due to ventricular fibrillation.[47] It has been observed that electric stimulation of the left stellate ganglion can evoke T-wave alternans and ventricular premature beats.[48] Wellens and coworkers[49] reported on a 14-year-old girl who had syncopal episodes when awakened by thunder. In this patient, various stimuli such as an alarm clock, music, or a falling bedpan evoked nonsustained ventricular tachycardia or ventricular fibrillation. There was a reproducible electrocardiographic sequence of sinus tachycardia, prolongation of the Q-T interval, development of T-wave inversion and the emergence of ventricular premature beats, resulting in ventricular tachycardia and fibrillation. The occurrence of these malignant arrhythmias was prevented by the use of beta-adrenergic blocking agents and diphenylhydantoin. The most effective treatment of the prolonged Q-T syndrome involves the sympathetic nervous system and includes stellate ganglionectomy as well as the administration of agents such as propranolol, diphenylhydantoin, and bretylium, which have effects on the central nervous system or the peripheral sympathetic nervous system.[48]

There are very few clinical studies that have addressed the problem of psychological stress factors in ventricular arrhythmia. Lown and DeSilva[50] examined the effect of psychological stress testing in 19 patients who demonstrated complex ventricular arrhythmia on ambulatory monitoring or exercise testing. Fifteen of 19 patients studied had out-of-hospital ventricular fibrillation or ventricular tachycardia. The psychological stress-testing protocol consisted of three parts. The first was mental arithmetic performed under time pressure. The second component was reading from Stroop color cards designed to create color-word confusion. The third was a psychological interview consisting of discussion about illness and emotional aspects of the patient's life, such as job-related stress, marriage, and death. In 11 of 19 patients, ventricular premature beats were increased during the stress test (FIG. 5). In seven of these patients there was a twofold or greater increase. The mean frequency of ventricular premature beats during control was 2.96 per minute compared with 6.62 per minute during the stress period ($p < 0.05$), while heart rates in these patients showed an increase from 71 bpm to 82 bpm during psychological stress ($p < 0.01$). There was a significant concordance between the increase in heart rate and the increase in ventricular premature beat frequency during psychological stress testing. Fourteen of the patients in this group underwent testing of cardiovascular autonomic reflexes. Autonomic profiling included tilting, hyperventilation, right and left carotid sinus massage, Val-

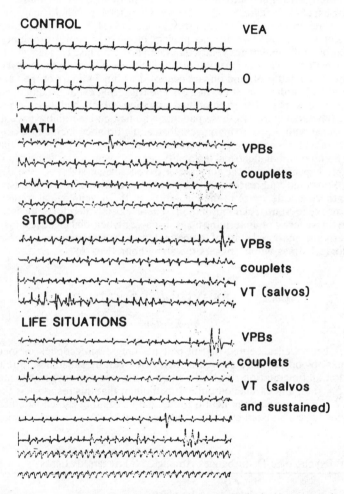

**FIGURE 5.** Electrocardiographic recording during a psychological stress test in a patient receiving antiarrhythmic drugs. During a 30-min control period there is no ventricular ectopic activity (VEA). The patient performed a series of mathematical problems under time pressure, which provoked frequent ventricular premature beats (VPBs) and couplets. More frequent VEA, including salvos of ventricular tachycardia (VT) occurred during testing with Stroop color cards. During a discussion of the fear of dying, a sustained episode of VT occurred.

salva maneuver, and elicitation of the dive reflex. Autonomic testing failed to provoke any significant increase in ventricular arrhythmia. Moreover, comparison of these 14 patients with 10 normal controls failed to reveal any difference in the response to this testing.

In an attempt to identify the psychological factors which provoked arrhythmia, a group of 122 patients who experienced out-of-hospital ventricular tachycardia or fibrillation underwent psychiatric and psychologic evaluation.[51] Patients studied could be stratified into three groups: (1) those who had no unusual psychological or psychiatric features, (2) those who had some psychological stress state present at the onset of the serious arrhythmia, and (3) those with an identifiable "psychological trigger" which was present in close temporal proximity to the precipitation of the malignant ventricular tachyarrhythmias. This last group, numbering 26 patients, was the most interesting. In these patients a major psychological event which had profound impact occurred within 24 hours of the ventricular fibrillation and cardiac arrest (TABLE 3). The triggering event usually occurred in the setting of a preexisting emotional situation which had been present for months. When compared to those patients who had no identifiable psychological trigger, those with a provoking psychological disturbance included a disproportionate number with no structural heart disease. It may be hypothesized that when there is no myocardial electrical instability present, ventricular fibrillation cannot be triggered regardless of the underlying psychological state. As the degree of electrical instability increases, as it does in the presence of more extensive heart disease, there is a decrease in the magnitude of the psychological trigger necessary to provoke ventricular fibrillation. There exists, therefore, an interaction between the severity of underlying heart disease, myocardial electrical instability, the underlying emotional state of the patient, and the superimposition of an acute psychological stress which triggers the arrhythmia (FIG. 6).

## NONANTIARRHYTHMIC DRUG THERAPY

### Meditation

It has been well accepted that in patients taught biofeedback or meditation techniques, blood pressure as well as heart rate can be substantially reduced.[52] Relaxation and meditation result in a marked decrease in oxygen consumption, respiratory rate, and cardiac output.[52] It is thought that this response is the result of a decrease in sympathetic neural traffic and circulating catecholamines. Such techniques have also been effectively applied to patients with arrhythmia. Weiss

TABLE 3. Psychologic Disturbances Among 25 "Trigger" Patients

*Major Disturbances*
Interpersonal conflict
Public humiliation
Threat of or actual marital separation
Bereavement
Business failure

*Affective States*
Acute depression
Fear
Anticipatory excitement
Grief
Agitation and tension

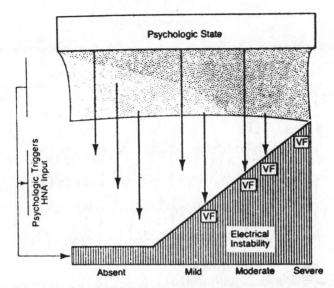

**FIGURE 6.** Interactions between psychological variables and myocardial electrical instability. When myocardial electrical instability is absent, stress does not trigger ventricular fibrillation (VF), regardless of the underlying psychologic state. When electrical instability is marked, and depending upon the underlying psychologic state, little or no stress is necessary to provoke VF. In the intermediate zone there is an interaction between the degree of electrical instability, the underlying emotional state, and the magnitude of the acute stress "trigger." Thus, when myocardial electrical instability is increased or when the underlying psychological state is of a greater degree, the magnitude of the "trigger" to provoke VF is less.

and Engel[53] and Pickering and Miller[54] have reported that learned voluntary control of heart rate with biofeedback techniques can suppress ventricular premature beats. Benson and coworkers[55] observed that in 11 patients with chronic ventricular premature beats, relaxation techniques practiced over a period of several weeks resulted in a substantial decrease in arrhythmia frequency as determined by ambulatory monitoring. Voukydis and Forwand[56] reported similar results in patients with ventricular arrhythmias that did not respond to antiarrhythmic drugs. The theoretical basis for this decrease in ventricular arrhythmia is that mediation and biofeedback decrease central nervous system activity and reduce sympathetic neural inputs to the heart.

In our experience, meditation technique has been useful in some patients with high-density ventricular arrhythmia (FIG. 7). In a group of 20 patients with stable, frequent ventricular arrhythmia during baseline evaluation, a significant decrease in ventricular premature beat frequency occurred during meditation in 13. This reduction in arrhythmia was not associated with a significant alteration of heart rate. We have used meditation as an adjunctive method for arrhythmia control in selected patients with symptomatic ventricular arrhythmias. It has been especially helpful in those in whom there is an established relationship between the occurrence of the arrhythmia and psychologic stress.

## Psychotropic Agents

A number of psychotropic agents including phenothiazines, benzodiazepines and tricyclic antidepressants have been shown to have antiarrhythmic effects. Imipramine has been reported to be an effective agent for suppressing both atrial and ventricular arrhythmias in man. Giardina and coworkers[57] utilized this agent

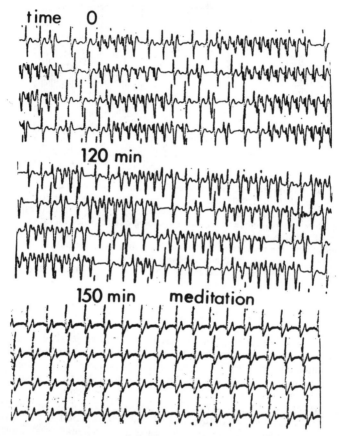

**FIGURE 7.** Example of the effect of meditation on ventricular arrhythmia. During a 2-hour period of observation the patient had a stable level of high-density ventricular arrhythmia, including salvos of ventricular tachycardia. At the end of the 120 minutes he was instructed in meditation. After 30 minutes, ventricular arrhythmia was totally abolished.

in 20 patients with frequent ventricular premature beats, but no psychological depression. They reported that 18 patients responded, with an 80% reduction in frequency of ventricular premature beats as documented by ambulatory monitoring. Intravenous and orally administered diazepam is effective for producing sedation in humans after a myocardial infarction and will significantly reduce the level of circulating catecholamines and the frequency of ventricular arrhythmia.[58]

Van Loon[59] demonstrated that 10–20 mg of intravenous diazepam reproducibly suppressed high grades of ventricular arrhythma and terminated ventricular tachycardia.

The phenothiazines have also been observed to have antiarrhythmic efficacy in animals.[60] It is of interest that a phenothiazine derivative, ethmozine,[61] is an effective antiarrhythmic drug and is currently undergoing investigation.

Morphine sulfate has long been used to treat the pain of myocardial infarction. Administration of morphine sulfate during experimental coronary artery occlusion has a significant protective effect against ventricular fibrillation.[26] Interestingly, morphine sulfate does not change ventricular vulnerability if it is administered after vagotomy or pretreatment with atropine. Moreover, morphine increased the ventricular fibrillation threshold only when it was altered by increased sympathetic tone. Since morphine is a parasympathomimetic agent, these observations support the parasympathetic-sympathetic interaction previously mentioned.

### Neural Transmitters

Since autonomic control of the heart is important, it seems logical to consider the role of neural transmitters.[62] Serotonin has been shown to be one such agent which will inhibit central sympathetic neural traffic. The effect of this drug on ventricular arrhythmia was studied by Rabinowitz and Lown,[63] who observed that an increase in central nervous system serotonin modified ventricular fibrillation thresholds and enhanced electrical stability. Melatonin, a hormone secreted by the pineal gland, causes an increase in brain serotonin. Administration of melatonin will also increase ventricular fibrillation threshold and decreases ventricular vulnerability.[64] An increase in central nervous system levels of norepinephrine has been shown to decrease sympathetic brain neural traffic.[65] This neural transmitter might have significant effects on the ventricular fibrillation threshold. Intravenous administration of L-tyrosine, an amino acid precursor of norepinephrine, increased the central nervous system levels of this substance[66] and resulted in a dose-dependent increase in the ventricular fibrillation threshold.[67] This change in ventricular vulnerability was prevented by bilateral vagotomy and stellectomy,[68] which indicates that the effect of tyrosine was mediated via the autonomic nervous system.

## CONCLUSIONS

Antiarrhythmic drug therapy remains the cornerstone of a treatment program for suppressing ventricular arrhythmia and preventing sudden death. These agents have profound effects on myocardial electrophysiologic properties. Their major role is "stabilization" of the electrical system of the heart by affecting conductivity, excitability, and automaticity. Although there are now a number of antiarrhythmic drugs available, efficacy varies and side effects are frequent, limiting their usefulness. There are many patients at risk for sudden death who would benefit from prophylactic therapy. However, the limitations of the drugs available precludes such widespread use. There is a great need for the development of other approaches for treatment of ventricular arrhythmia and the prevention of sudden death. Evidence is growing that higher nervous activity plays an important role and can trigger serious ventricular arrhythmias. The major effect of such activity on the heart is modulated through the autonomic nervous system. An alternative strategy for arrhythmia suppression involves pharmacologic and nonpharmacologic modification of this neural traffic. A better understanding of the role of psychological stress factors, their central nervous system effects and interaction with neural inputs to the heart and the occurrence of arrhythmia will further aid in the ability to identify patients at risk and substantially improve our capabilities for treating such patients and preventing sudden cardiac death.

## REFERENCES

1. LOWN, B. 1979. Sudden cardiac death—The major challenge confronting contemporary cardiology. Am. J. Cardiol. **43:** 313–328.
2. LEVY, A. G. 1914. The genesis of ventricular extrasystoles under chloroform, with special reference to consecutive ventricular fibrillation. Heart **5:** 299–334.
3. HOFF, E.C., J. R. KELL & M. N. CARROLL. 1963. Effects of cortical stimulation and lesions on cardiovascular function. Physiol. Rev. **43:** 68–114.
4. GARVEY, H. L. & K. I. MELVILLE. 1969. Cardiovascular effects of lateral hypothalamic stimulation in normal and coronary-ligated dogs. J. Cardiovasc. Surg. **10:** 377–385.
5. HOCKMAN, C. H., H. P. MAUCK & E. C. HOFF. 1960. ECG changes resulting from cerebral stimulation. II. A spectrum of ventricular arrhythmia of sympathetic origin. Am. Heart J. **71:** 697–700.
6. KLIKS, B. R., M. J. BURGESS & J. A. ABILDSKOV. 1975. Influence of sympathetic tone on ventricular fibrillation threshold during experimental coronary occlusion. Am. J. Cardiol. **36:** 45–49.
7. HARRIS, A. S., H. OTERO & A. BOCAGE. 1971. The induction of arrhythmias by sympathetic activity before and after occlusion of a coronary artery in the canine heart. J. Electrocardiol. **4:** 34–43.
8. VASSALLE, M., J. H. STUCKEY & M. J. LEVINE. 1969. Sympathetic control of ventricular automaticity: role of the adrenal medulla. Am. J. Physiol. **217:** 930–937.
9. HARRIS, A. S., A. ESTANDIA & R. E. TILLOTSON. 1951. Ventricular ectopic rhythms and ventricular fibrillation following cardiac sympathectomy and coronary occlusion. Am. J. Physiol. **165:** 505–512.
10. EBERT, P. A., R. B. VANDERBEEK & R. J. ALLGOOD. 1970. Effect of chronic cardiac denervation on arrhythmias after coronary artery ligation. Cardiovasc. Res. **4:** 141–147.
11. SCHWARTZ, P. J., N. G. SNEBOLD & A. M. BROWN. 1976. Effects of unilateral cardiac sympathetic denervation on the ventricular fibrillation threshold. Am. J. Cardiol. **37:** 1036–1040.
12. MALLIANI, A., P. J. SCHWARTZ & A. ZANCHETTI. 1969. A sympathetic reflex elicited by experimental coronary occlusion. Am. J. Physiol. **217:** 703–709.
13. LOMBARDI, F., R. L. VERRIER & B. LOWN. 1983. Relationship between sympathetic neural activity and coronary dynamics and vulnerability to ventricular fibrillation during myocardial ischemia and reperfusion. Am. Heart J. **105:** 958–965.
14. CORBALAN, R., R. L. VERRIER & B. LOWN. 1976. Differing mechanisms for ventricular vulnerability during coronary artery occlusion and release. Am. Heart J. **92:** 223–230.
15. RAEDER, E. A., R. L. VERRIER & B. LOWN. 1983. Intrinsic sympathomimetic activity and the effects of beta-adrenergic blocking drugs on vulnerability to ventricular fibrillation. J. Am. Coll. Cardiol. **1:** 1442–1446.
16. VERRIER, R. L., A. CALVERT, B. LOWN & P. AXELROD. 1975. Effect of acute blood pressure elevation on the ventricular fibrillation threshold. Am. J. Physiol. **228:** 923–927.

17. Schwartz, P. J., R. L. Verrier & B. Lown. 1977. Effect of stellectomy and vagotomy on ventricular refractoriness. Circ. Res. **40:** 536–542.
18. Eliakim, M., S. Bellet & E. Tawil. 1961. Effect of vagal stimulation and acetylcholine on the ventricles: Studies in dogs with complete heart block. Circ. Res. **9:** 1372–1379.
19. Bailey, C. J., K. Greenspan & M. V. Elizari. 1972. Effect of acetylcholine on automaticity and conduction in the proximal portion of the His-Purkinje specialized conduction system in the dog. Circ. Res. **30:** 210–216.
20. Jacobowitz, D., T. Cooper & H. Barner. 1967. Histochemical and chemical studies of the localization of adrenergic and cholinergic nerves in the normal and denervated cat heart. Circ. Res. **20:** 289–298.
21. Kent, K. M., E. R. Smith, D. R. Redwood & S. E. Epstein. 1973. Electrical stability of acutely ischemic myocardium: Influences of heart rate and vagal stimulation. Circulation **47:** 291–298.
22. Corr, P. B. & R. A. Gillis. 1974. Role of the vagus in the cardiovascular changes induced by coronary occlusion. Circulation **49:** 86–97.
23. Yoon, M. S., J. Han, W. W. Tse & R. Rogers. 1977. Effects of vagal stimulation, atropine, and propranolol on fibrillation threshold of normal and ischemic ventricles. Am. Heart J. **93:** 60–65.
24. Kolman, B. S., R. L. Verrier & B. Lown. 1975. The effect of vagus nerve stimulation upon vulnerability of the canine ventricle. Role of sympathetic-parasympathetic interactions. Circulation **52:** 572–585.
25. Rabinowitz, S. H., R. L. Verrier & B. Lown. 1976. Muscarinic effects of vagosympathetic trunk stimulation on the repetitive extrasystole threshold. Circulation **53:** 622–627.
26. DeSilva, R. A., R. L. Verrier & B. Lown. 1978. The effects of psychological stress and vagal stimulation with morphine on vulnerability to ventricular fibrillation in the conscious dog. Am. Heart J. **95:** 197–203.
27. Nathanson, M. H. 1935. Action of acetyl beta methylcholin on ventricular rhythms induced by adrenalin. Proc. Soc. Exp. Biol. Med. **32:** 1297–1299.
28. Weiss, T., G. M. Lattin & K. Engelman. 1975. Vagally mediated suppression of premature ventricular contractions in man. Am. Heart J. **89:** 700–707.
29. Waxman, M. B. & R. W. Wald. 1977. Termination of ventricular tachycardia by an increase in cardiac vagal drive. Circulation **56:** 385–391.
30. Raab, W. 1966. Emotional and sensory stress factors in myocardial pathology: Neurogenic and humoral mechanisms in pathogenesis, therapy and prevention. Am. Heart J. **72:** 538–564.
31. Johansson, G., L. Jonsson, N. Lannek, L. Blomgren, P. Lindberg & O. Poupa. 1974. Severe stress-cardiopathy in pigs. Am. Heart J. **87:** 451–457.
32. Matta, R. J., R. L. Verrier & B. Lown. 1976. The repetitive extrasystole as an index of vulnerability to ventricular fibrillation. Am. J. Physiol. **230:** 1469–1473.
33. Lown, B., R. L. Verrier & R. Corbalan. 1973. Psychologic stress and threshold for repetitive ventricular response. Science **182:** 834–836.
34. Corbalan, R., R. L. Verrier & B. Lown. 1974. Psychological stresses and ventricular arrhythmias during infarction in the conscious dog. Am. J. Cardiol. **34:** 692–696.
35. Skinner, J. E., J. T. Lie & H. L. Entman. 1974. Modification of ventricular fibrillation latency following coronary artery occlusion in the conscious pig: The effects of psychological stress and beta-adrenergic blockade. Circulation **34:** 656–667.
36. Rosenfeld, J., M. R. Rosen & B. F. Hoffman. 1978. Pharmacologic and behavioral effects on arrhythmias which immediately follow abrupt coronary occlusion: A canine model of sudden coronary death. Am. J. Cardiol. **41:** 1075–1082.
37. Cannon, W. B. 1942. Voodoo death. Am. Anthropologist **44:** 169.
38. Engel, G. L. 1971. Sudden and rapid death during psychologic stress. Folk lore or folk wisdom? Ann. Intern. Med. **74:** 771–782.
39. Parkes, C. M., B. Benjamin & B. Fitzgerald. 1969. Broken heart: Statistical study of increased mortality among widowers. Br. Med. J. **1:** 740–743.
40. Rahe, R. H., M. Romo & L. Bennett. 1974. Recent life changes, myocardial infarc-

tion and abrupt coronary death. Studies in Helsinki. Arch. Intern. Med. **133:** 221–228.

41. GREENE, W. A., S. GOLDSTEIN & A. S. MOSS. 1972. Psychosocial aspects of sudden death. Arch. Intern. Med. **129:** 725–731.
42. JARVINEN, K. A. S. 1955. Can ward rounds be a danger to patients with myocardial infarction? Br. Med. J. **1:** 318–320.
43. LOWN, B., J. V. TEMTE, P. REICH, C. GAUGH, R. REGESTEIN & H. HAI. 1976. Basis for recurring ventricular fibrillation in the absence of coronary artery disease and its management. N. Engl. J. Med. **294:** 623–629.
44. TAGGART, P., M. CARUTHERS & W. SOMERVILLE. 1973. EKG, plasma catecholamines and lipids and their modifications by oxprenolol when speaking before an audience. Lancet **2:** 341–346.
45. LYNCH, J. J., S. A. THOMAS & D. A. PASKEWITZ. 1977. Human contact and cardiac arrhythmia in a coronary care unit. Psychosom. Med. **39:** 188–194.
46. DONLON, P. T., A. MEADOW & E. AMSTERDAM. 1979. Emotional stress as a factor in ventricular arrhythmias. Psychosomatics **4:** 233–240.
47. JERVELL, A. & F. LANGE-NEILSEN. 1957. Congenital deaf mutism, functional heart disease with prolongations of the QT-interval and sudden death. Am. Heart J. **55:** 59–65.
48. SCHWARTZ, P. J., M. PERITI & A. MALLIANI. 1975. The long QT-syndrome. Am. Heart J. **89:** 378–392.
49. WELLENS, J. H. H., A. VERMEULEN & D. DURRER. 1972. Ventricular fibrillation occurring in arousal from sleep by auditory stimuli. Circulation **46:** 661–665.
50. LOWN, B. & R. A. DESILVA. 1978. Roles of psychologic stress and the autonomic nervous system changes in provocation of ventricular premature complexes. Am. J. Cardiol. **41:** 979–985.
51. REICH, P., R. A. DESILVA, B. LOWN & B.J. MURAWSKI. 1981. Acute psychological disturbances preceding life threatening ventricular arrhythmias. JAMA **246:** 233–235.
52. WALLACE, R. F. & H. BENSON. 1972. The physiology of meditation. Sci. Am. **226:** 84–90.
53. WEISS, T. & B. J. ENGEL. 1971. Operant conditioning of heart rate in patients with premature ventricular contractions. Psychosomat. Med. **33:** 301–309.
54. PICKERING, T. G. & N. E. MILLER. 1977. Learned voluntary control of heart rate and rhythm in two subjects with premature ventricular contractions. Br. Heart J. **39:** 152–156.
55. BENSON, H., S. ALEXANDER & C. L. FELDMAN. 1975. Decreased premature ventricular contractions through the use of the relaxation response in patients with stable ischemic heart disease. Lancet **2:** 380–382.
56. VOUKYDIS, P. C. & S. A. FORWAND. 1977. The effect of elicitation of the relaxation response in patients with intractable ventricular arrhythmias (abstract) Circulation **55**(Suppl III): 157.
57. GIARDINA, E. G. V. & J. T. BIGGER. 1982. Antiarrhythmic effect of imipramine hydrochloride in patients with ventricular premature contractions without psychologic depression. Am. J. Cardiol. **50:** 172–179.
58. MELSOM, M., P. ANDREASSEN, H. MELSOM, T. HANSEN, H. GRENDAHL & L. K. HILLESTAD. 1976. Diazepam in acute myocardial infarction. Clinical effects and effect on catecholamines, free fatty acids and cortisol. Br. Heart J. **38:** 804–809.
59. VAN LOON, G. R. 1968. Ventricular arrhythmias treated by diazepam. Canad. Med. Assoc. J. **98:** 785–789.
60. MADAN, B. R. & V. K. PENDSE. Antiarrhythmic activity of thioridazine (Mellaril). Am. J. Cardiol. **11:** 78–81.
61. PODRID, P. J., H. LYAKISHIV, B. LOWN & N. MAZUR. 1980. Ethmozin. A new antiarrhythmic drug for suppressing ventricular premature complexes. Circulation **61:** 450–457.
62. BAUM, T. & A. T. SHROPSHIRE. 1975. Inhibition of efferent sympathetic nerve activity by 5-hydroxytryptophan and centrally administered 5-hydroxytryptamine. Neuropharmacology **14:** 227–233.

63. RABINOWITZ, S. H. & B. LOWN. 1978. Central neurochemical factors related to serotonin metabolism and cardiac ventricular vulnerability for repetitive electrical activity. Am. J. Cardiol. **41:** 516–522.
64. BLATT, C. M., S. H. RABINOWITZ & B. LOWN. 1979. Central serotonergic agents raise the repetitive extrasystole threshold of the vulnerable period of the canine ventricular myocardium. Circ. Res. **44:** 723–730.
65. SVED, A. F., J. D. FERNSTROM & R. J. WURTMAN. 1971. Tyrosine administration reduces blood pressure and enhances brain norepinephrine release in spontaneously hypertensive rats. Proc. Natl. Acad. Sci. **76:** 3511–3514.
66. GIBSON, C. J. & R. J. WURTMAN. 1977. Physiological control of brain catechol synthesis by brain tyrosine concentration. Biochem. Pharmacol. **26:** 1137–1142.
67. SCOTT, N. A., R. A. DESILVA, B. LOWN & R. J. WURTMAN. 1981. Tyrosine administration decreases vulnerability to ventricular fibrillation on the normal canine heart. Science **211:** 727–729.
68. SCOTT, N. A., R. L. VERRIER, B. LOWN & R. J. WURTMAN. 1981. Mechanisms mediating influence of tyrosine on vulnerability to ventricular fibrillation. Clin. Res. **29:** 240A.
69. LOWN, B. & R. L. VERRIER. 1976. Neural activity and ventricular fibrillation. N. Engl. J. Med. **294:** 1165.

# Future Perspectives in Antiarrhythmic Drugs[a]

DONALD C. HARRISON

*Cardiology Division*
*Stanford University School of Medicine*
*Stanford, California 94305*

## INTRODUCTION

This volume has attempted a concise summary of the existing data on currently available antiarrhythmic drugs, and on selected new agents that are now in clinical study. It further attempts to catalog the data developed for these pharmaceutical products as our understanding of arrhythmias and their treatment has evolved over the past decade. The papers herein clearly demonstrate the need for further studies and for skepticism regarding our present state of knowledge.

My purpose in this article is to emphasize some of the problem areas that have been identified by several of the papers in this volume. In addition, I will attempt to clarify two concepts that have raised controversy but that have been inadequately addressed. Finally, I will present my concept of an ideal antiarrhythmic drug.

## CLARIFICATION OF CONCEPTS

The questions of when it is appropriate to measure therapeutic concentrations of an antiarrhythmic drug as they relate to the therapeutic or toxic window for that drug, and confusion regarding a pharmacologic response versus an individual patient's response to an antiarrhythmic drug, are two recurring problems that I would like to discuss.

### Measurement of Plasma Concentration in Drugs with Carefully Established Therapeutic and Toxic Windows

In order to interpret the plasma levels of an antiarrhythmic drug, carefully established relationships between plasma concentration and drug effect (therapeutic or toxic) must be established. In drugs with long half-lives, active metabolites, or with tissue sequestration, such relationships are difficult to ascertain, and, in general, measurements of plasma concentrations for their use have not been established. With lidocaine, early studies demonstrated effective therapeutic concentrations in plasma at levels below those that were considered toxic.[1] Such plasma concentration ranges have been described as a therapeutic window for the drug.

[a] This work was supported in part by Grants T32-HL 07626 (06) and 1RO-L-HL 29762 (01) from the National Institutes of Health.

The most carefully studied agent in recent years with respect to establishment of a therapeutic window has been tocainide.[2] My colleagues and I performed studies comparing the antiarrhythmic effects of tocainide at low and high doses to values during two placebo periods in 15 patients with frequent and complex ventricular ectopy.[2,3] Thirteen of these patients were unresponsive to available agents or these drugs produced undesirable side effects which prevented their use.[2] The study design is outlined in FIGURE 1. At the end of the administration of the high doses of tocainide, the plasma concentration was measured intermittently along with Holter monitoring determinations of the rate at which ectopic

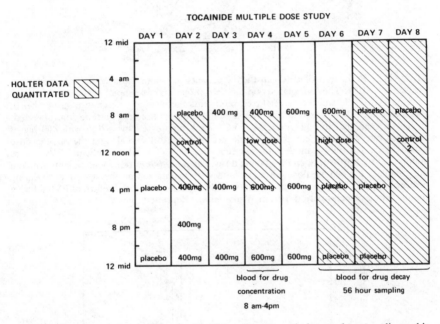

**FIGURE 1.** Study design showing details of drug dosage, ambulatory electrocardiographic (Holter) monitoring of the arrhythmia, and blood-sampling for 15 subjects receiving multiple oral doses of tocainide. Numbers indicate drug dose and time of administration, and the *cross-hatched* areas indicate the periods during which the premature ventricular contractions were quantified. (From Meffen *et al.*[4] Reprinted by permission.)

ventricular activity returned. Eleven of the 15 patients responded with greater than 70% reduction of premature ventricular complexes (PVCs) (FIG. 2), and thus in each patient it was possible to determine quite carefully the relationship between plasma concentration and antiarrhythmic effects of the drug. This permitted the construction of a plasma concentration/effect relationship (FIG. 3). The logarithm of the plasma concentration related to percent reduction in PVC frequency allowed the construction of a sigmoid dose-response curve using modeling techniques.[4,5] This permitted the careful establishment of the therapeutic range necessary to reduce PVCs as being from 4 $\mu$/ml for 60% reduction to 11 $\mu$/ml for greater than 90% reduction. Since tocainide has no active metabolites and is not

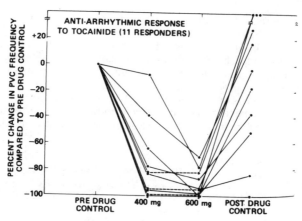

**FIGURE 2.** Reduction of PVCs in the 11 patients in whom these complexes were suppressed by >70%. The four periods on the *horizontal axis* correspond to the cross-hatched areas in FIGURE 1, and the *vertical axis* represents the percent change in total number of PVCs over the 8-hour dose interval compared to the 8-hour pre-drug placebo control period. It can be seen that in eight patients, PVCs were suppressed by >70% with 400 mg of tocainide every 8 hours compared to the pre-drug control period, and the 600-mg dose usually provided only a modest further reduction in PVCs. Three patients' PVCs were suppressed by >70% only on the 600-mg dose. The *dotted lines* represent patients who did not complete the 600-mg dose period or who were maintained on the 400-mg dose during protocol days 4, 5, and 6. The data points on the **right** represent the return of PVCs during the post-drug placebo period. (From Winkle et al.[3] Reprinted by permission.)

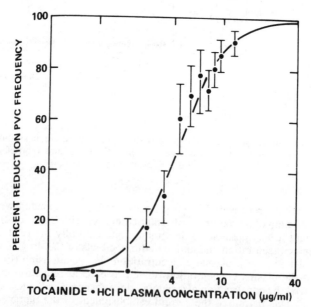

**FIGURE 3.** Plasma concentration–antiarrhythmic response curve for tocainide from studies in 11 patients. Therapeutic range (window) is from 4 to 11 μg/ml. (From Winkle et al.[3] Reprinted by permission.)

sequestered in tissue, this study demonstrates how an effective therapeutic window can be established for an antiarrhythmic drug.

With such a carefully established therapeutic window, measurement of plasma concentration would be very helpful in maintaining a plasma concentration that is effective, yet below the toxic level of the drug. When drugs are to be used prophylactically without available measures for efficacy, plasma concentration measurements are clearly indicated.

### Difference between Pharmacologic Action of a Drug and Individual Patient Response

In their papers in this volume Winkle and Morganroth emphasized the importance of spontaneous variation of ventricular ectopic activity. While individual

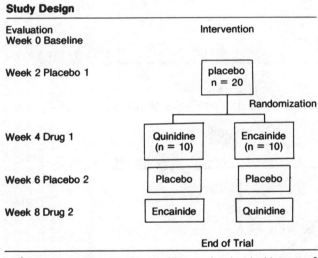

**Study Design**

| Evaluation | Intervention |
|---|---|
| Week 0 Baseline | |
| Week 2 Placebo 1 | placebo n = 20 |
| | Randomization |
| Week 4 Drug 1 | Quinidine (n = 10) — Encainide (n = 10) |
| Week 6 Placebo 2 | Placebo — Placebo |
| Week 8 Drug 2 | Encainide — Quinidine |
| | End of Trial |

Dosage: Encainide, 50 mg every 6 hours; placebo, 1 tablet every 6 hours; quinidine, 300 mg every 6 hours.

**FIGURE 4.** Study design for comparing the antiarrhythmic efficacy of encainide (50 mg every 6 hours), quinidine (300 mg every 6 hours), and placebo (1 tablet every 6 hours). (From Sami et al.[7] Reprinted by permission.)

patient response is difficult to determine, we have recently developed a model for characterizing the variability among individual patients in a group using a linear regression analysis that compares the response to placebo with a baseline recording period on ambulatory monitoring.[6] This permits the establishment of confidence intervals for individual patient response. Such an approach was used to compare the therapeutic effects of encainide and quinidine in 20 postmyocardial infarction patients. The outline of this study[7] is illustrated in FIGURE 4.

In FIGURE 5A, the linear regression analysis comparing baseline and placebo ambulatory monitoring in this group of patients is shown. Ninety-nine and 95% confidence intervals are illustrated. In FIGURE 5B the individual patient's re-

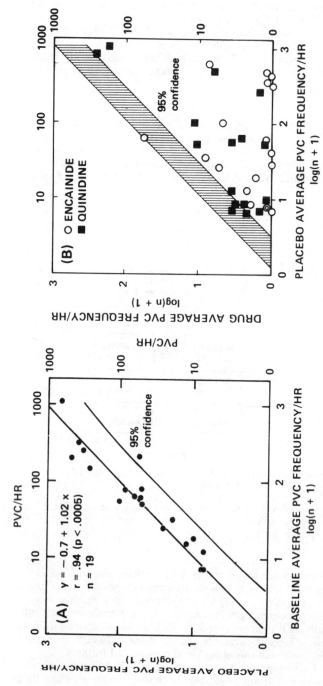

**FIGURE 5. (A)** Linear regression analysis with determination of 95% confidence intervals of variability for baseline versus placebo measurements of average premature ventricular complex (PVC) frequency per hour of ambulatory electrocardiographic recording. Analysis was performed on the log (premature ventricular complex frequency + 1). The corresponding absolute values are shown on the opposing scales. The 95% confidence line represents the one-tailed lower confidence interval for individual data points. The point at which the confidence line crosses the baseline axis determines the "sensitivity threshold," below which even total suppression of premature ventricular complexes cannot be distinguished from spontaneous variability. **(B)** individual responses to encainide (*open circles*) and quinidine (*solid squares*) are plotted. The *hatched area* represents the 95% confidence intervals of variability in premature ventricular complexes. To distinguish true drug response from placebo effect at the 0.05 level of significance, the single point that describes the placebo and post-drug responses must fall below the 95% confidence limit. The higher the average frequency of premature complexes during placebo therapy, the lower the percent reduction required to establish drug efficacy at a given confidence level. (From Sami *et al.*[7] Reprinted by permission.)

sponses to therapeutic doses of encainide and quinidine are illustrated.[7] Clearly, individual patient response can be determined with this approach. However, it should be emphasized that individual patient response to an antiarrhythmic drug does not necessarily mean that the drug has a pharmacologic effect.[8]

In FIGURE 6, the variation of arrhythmia in the same 20 patients during three placebo periods is compared to the average response of the group to quinidine and encainide. The standard deviation around the average baseline and two placebo frequencies is relatively small and there was no statistical difference between the

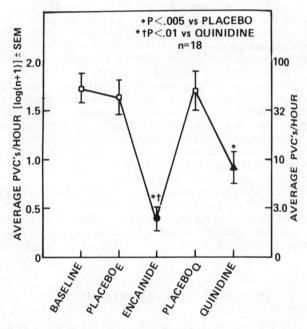

**FIGURE 6.** To demonstrate pharmacologic action rather than individual patient response, the means and SEMs are shown for the average hourly frequency of ventricular ectopic activity on ambulatory monitoring for each of five visits. Paired $t$ tests were used to compare the response of each drug to the preceding placebo response and then to the response of the other drug (encainide versus quinidine). Placebo E period preceded encainide and placebo Q preceded quinidine. There were no statistical differences among baseline average, placebo E, and placebo Q. Clearly, both encainide and quinidine had dramatic pharmacologic effects. (From Sami et al.[7] Reprinted by permission.[7])

mean arrhythmia frequencies in these 18 patients for these three periods. Clearly, the pharmacologic action of the drug is illustrated by the marked reduction in frequency of ectopic activity occurring after the administration of quinidine or encainide.[7] In fact, the pharmacologic response to encainide was statistically greater than that to quinidine. Thus, the considerable statistical manipulation of data that is necessary to determine an individual patient's response to a drug differs markedly from the method used to determine whether an agent has pharmacologic effect in a *group* of patients with arrhythmias. Although the frequency of ectopic activity in an individual patient varies widely, groups of approximately 20 patients studied on several occasions have essentially the same mean frequency of ectopic activity. Thus, pharmacologic agents that change this mean frequency statistically can be assessed as having pharmacologic activity. These two distinctions should be maintained.

### Additional Observations

The subjects of several other presentations in this volume merit additional comment. First, as far as we know, the basis for cardiac arrhythmias is alterations in automaticity and reentry or a combination of the two, little new has been learned about the membrane and cellular mechanisms by which arrhythmias are initiated. Patched clamp techniques allowing study of individual ionic channels in membranes may, in the next decade, permit a mechanism for determining the basis of cardiac arrhythmias in diseased tissues.

Second, the role of the nervous system in the production of arrhythmias and in their response to antiarrhythmic drugs has received only limited interest in recent years. Clearly, central nervous system modifications play a major role in arrhythmia development, as do activities of the parasympathetic and sympathetic nervous system. Many antiarrhythmic drugs have actions on both the nervous system and directly upon the conduction tissues in the heart. Understanding the relationship between the nervous system and the induction of arrhythmias may well lead to a new type of antiarrhythmic drug.

Third, Dr. Vaughn Williams presented exciting new data validating my concept for dividing Class 1 antiarrhythmic drugs into three subgroups: A, B, and C. Although all new agents have not been studied, he presented a mechanism relating to alterations in ionic channels and this mechanism provides a rational basis for this subgroup classification. Further studies will no doubt confirm these hypotheses.

## THE IDEAL ANTIARRHYTHMIC DRUG

Finally, I would like to list the characteristics of what I believe would be the ideal antiarrhythmic drug. Such a drug would (1) be highly effective in arrhythmias of many etiologies; (2) carry only infrequent and minor side-effects; (3) have a high bioavailability; (4) permit both parenteral and oral administration; (5) have a long half-life; (6) allow no accumulation of toxic metabolites; (7) neither promote nor enhance arrhythmias; (8) be shown to favorably alter mortality from arrhythmia; and (9) not reduce ventricular function.

It seems unlikely that a single agent with all of these characteristics will be developed in the next decade. However, agents that meet many of these characteristics are now becoming available for clinical study and as the basic mechanisms for producing arrhythmias are better understood, pharmacologic agents capable of preventing and stopping important cardiac arrhythmias will be developed.

## CONCLUSION

This volume attempts to summarize the basic research and clinical studies on antiarrhythmic drugs that have been carried out in the past decade. In addition, several papers have pointed to the direction that future research must take if we are to discover new therapeutic agents. Careful clinical investigations made on the basis of our past experience will allow us to put such agents in appropriate therapeutic perspective.

## REFERENCES

1. GIANELLY, R., J. O. VON DER GROEBEN, A. P. SPIVACK & D. C. HARRISON. 1967. Effects of lidocaine on ventricular arrhythmias in patients with coronary heart disease. New Engl. J. Med. **277:** 1215–1219.
2. COLTART, D. J., T. B. BERNDT, R. KERNOFF & D. C. HARRISON. 1974. Antiarrhythmic and circulatory effects of Astra W36095, a new lidocaine-like agent. Am. J. Cardiol. **34:** 35–41.
3. WINKLE, R. A., P. J. MEFFIN, J. W. FITZGERALD & D. C. HARRISON. 1976. Clinical efficacy and pharmacokinetics of a new orally effective antiarrhythmic, tocainide. Circulation **54:** 884–889.
4. MEFFIN, P. J., R. A. WINKLE, T. F. BLASCHKE, J. FITZGERALD & D. C. HARRISON. 1977. Response optimization of drug dosage: Antiarrhythmic studies with tocainide. Clin. Pharmacol. Ther. **22:** 42–57.
5. HARRISON, D. C., P. J. MEFFIN & R. A. WINKLE. 1978. Clinical pharmacology and antiarrhythmic actions of tocainide. Br. Heart J. **40:** 83–87.
6. SAMI, M., H. KRAEMER, D. C. HARRISON, N. HOUSTON, C. SHIMASAKI & R. F. DEBUSK. 1980. A new method for evaluating antiarrhythmic drug efficacy. Circulation **62:** 1172–1179.
7. SAMI, M., D. C. HARRISON, H. KRAEMER, N. HOUSTON, C. SHIMASAKI & R. F. DEBUSK. 1981. Antiarrhythmic efficacy of encainide and quinidine: Validation of a model for drug assessment. Am. J. Cardiol. **48:** 147–156.
8. HARRISON, D. C., R. A. WINKLE, M. SAMI & J. W. MASON. 1981. A new and potent antiarrhythmic agent. *in* Cardiac Arrhythmias: A Decade of Progress. D. C. Harrison, Ed.: 315–330. G. K. Hall. Boston, MA.

# Index of Contributors